MORBID CURIOSITIES

Morbid Curiosities

*Medical Museums in
Nineteenth-Century Britain*

SAMUEL J. M. M. ALBERTI

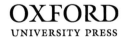
OXFORD
UNIVERSITY PRESS

OXFORD
UNIVERSITY PRESS

Great Clarendon Street, Oxford OX2 6DP

Oxford University Press is a department of the University of Oxford.
It furthers the University's objective of excellence in research, scholarship,
and education by publishing worldwide in

Oxford New York

Auckland   Cape Town Dar es Salaam   Hong Kong   Karachi
Kuala Lumpur Madrid Melbourne Mexico City   Nairobi
New Delhi Shanghai Taipei Toronto
With offices in
Argentina Austria Brazil Chile Czech Republic France Greece
Guatemala Hungary Italy Japan South Korea Poland Portugal
Singapore Switzerland Thailand Turkey Ukraine Vietnam

Oxford is a registered trade mark of Oxford University Press
in the UK and in certain other countries

Published in the United States
by Oxford University Press Inc., New York

ISBN 978-0-19-958458-1

Printed in the United Kingdom by
Lightning Source UK Ltd., Milton Keynes

For Fay, Millie, and Jacob

Acknowledgements

This book has been a long time coming, even in academic terms, and more people have helped than I could mention. *Morbid Curiosities* began its life as a post-doctoral fellowship at the University of Manchester Centre for the History of Science, Technology and Medicine, and colleagues and friends there shaped it from the outset—none more than Duncan Wilson, Mick Worboys, and, especially, John Pickstone. Subsequently, friends in the stimulating and convivial environments of the Manchester Museum and the School of Arts, Histories and Cultures have tolerated and even encouraged the project's incremental progress. My thanks to Kostas Arvanitis, Malcolm Chapman, Mark Crinson, Mel Giles, Asia Haut, Siân Jones, Helen Rees Leahy, Nick Merriman, and Louise Tythacott. Elsewhere I am grateful to Pete Coventry, Nick Hopwood, Anna Maerker, Ruth Richardson, and of course Liz Hallam for their expertise and support. Completing the manuscript was my last act in Manchester before taking up a new post at the Museums and Archives of the Royal College of Surgeons of England—and so the views expressed herein are in no way representative of the College, but are rather the product of a decade at the University of Manchester.

The Wellcome Trust generously funded not only the original fellowship but also a subsequent period of research leave. The Wellcome Library was one of the many wonderful resources I had the pleasure of exploiting—there I would like to thank Anna Smith and Rachael Cross, Wellcome Images, and Simon Chaplin (latterly at the Royal College of Surgeons of England). Elsewhere, I am indebted to staff at the British Library, Glasgow University Special Collections, Edinburgh University Library, and the London Metropolitan Archives; to Sarah Pearson at the Royal College of Surgeons of England; Dawn Kemp, latterly at the Royal College of Surgeons of Edinburgh; James Peters and Dorothy Clayton at the John Rylands University of Manchester; Mary O'Doherty at the Royal College of Surgeons in Ireland Special Collections and Archives; Estelle Gittins at Trinity College Dublin Archives; Samantha Farhall and Katie Ormerod at St Bartholomew's Hospital Archives and Museum; and, especially, Bill Edwards at the Gordon Museum, Kings College London. Seth Cayley and Stephanie Ireland at Oxford University Press made the publication process a pleasure, and their anonymous reviewers improved the book greatly.

Most of all, I would like to thank my family. Hugh, George, and Stephanie advised me on matters medical; Ben and Jo on matters cultural. My wife Fay not only helped me on both fronts, but encouraged, critiqued, and supported me during the entire process. I dedicate this book to her with gratitude, admiration, and affection.

Contents

List of Illustrations

List of Abbreviations

HMSO	Her/His Majesty's Stationery Office
HTA	Human Tissue Authority
LMA	London Metropolitan Archives
MMC	Manchester Medical Collection
RCSI	Royal College of Surgeons in Ireland
TCD	Trinity College Dublin
UCL	University College London
UNESCO	United Nations Educational, Scientific and Cultural Organization

1

Introduction

A Parliament of Monsters

All moveables of wonder, from all parts,
Are here—Albinos, painted Indians, Dwarfs,
The Horse of knowledge, and the learned Pig,
The Stone-eater, the man that swallows fire,
Giants, Ventriloquists, the Invisible Girl,
The Bust that speaks and moves its goggling eyes,
The Wax-work, Clock-work, all the marvellous craft
Of modern Merlins, Wild Beasts, Puppet-shows,
All out-o'-the-way, far-fetched, perverted things,
All freaks of nature, all Promethean thoughts
Of man, his dullness, madness, and their feats
All jumbled up together, to compose
A Parliament of Monsters.[1]

Bartholomew Fair in Smithfield, London, so William Wordsworth told us, presented abnormal humanity at its grotesque extreme (figure 1.1). And yet it was not unique. Deviant bodies, living and dead, were to be found in all corners of the nineteenth-century exhibitionary complex: not

---

[1] William Wordsworth, *The Prelude; or, the Growth of a Poet's Mind. An Autobiographical Poem* (1805; New York: Appleton, 1850), 200–1, written after a visit in 1802. This passage has been cited widely, for example in Richard D. Altick, *The Shows of London: A Panoramic History of Exhibitions, 1600–1862* (Cambridge, Mass.: Belknap, 1978), 36; Tony Bennett, *The Birth of the Museum: History, Theory, Politics* (London: Routledge, 1995), 86; Mark S. Blumberg, *Freaks of Nature: What Anomalies Tell Us About Development and Evolution* (New York: Oxford University Press, 2008), 22; Erin O'Connor, *Raw Material: Producing Pathology in Victorian Culture* (Durham, NC: Duke University Press, 2000), 167; Peter Stallybrass and Allon White, *The Politics and Poetics of Transgression* (London: Methuen, 1986), 120. On the history of Bartholomew Fair, see Jane Goodall, *Performance and Evolution in the Age of Darwin: Out of the Natural Order* (London: Routledge, 2002); Edward Alfred Webb, *The Records of St Bartholomew's Priory and of the Church and Parish of St Bartholomew the Great West Smithfield*, 2 vols. (Oxford: The University Press, 1921); Paul Youngquist, *Monstrosities: Bodies and British Romanticism* (Minneapolis: University of Minnesota Press, 2003).

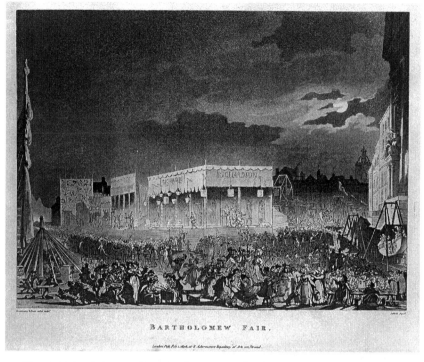

Fig. 1.1. Bartholomew Fair, London: scene of night-time revelry at the fair in Smithfield, outside St Bartholomew's Hospital. Coloured aquatint by J. Bluck after Augustus Charles Pugin and Thomas Rowlandson, 1808. Wellcome Library, London.

only in fairgrounds and freak shows, but also in private cabinets and grand museums, great exhibitions, and shilling anatomy shows. Bartholomew Fair was on one end of a spectrum that stretched to St Bartholomew's Hospital, which a century later would be described as a 'Valhalla of spoils snatched from the dead, the dying, the living, and those who have never been born' (figure 1.2).[2]

This book situates medical museums in these nineteenth-century cultures of display by tracing the passage of dead bodies between them. It is concerned with the afterlives of diseased parts (in particular) in the medical marketplace: how did they come to be in collections? What happened to them there? Students of disease known as 'pathologists'

---

[2] W. R. Bett, 'Sir James Paget and the Hospital Museum', *St Bartholomew's Hospital Journal*, 36 (1929), 140–41 at 140.

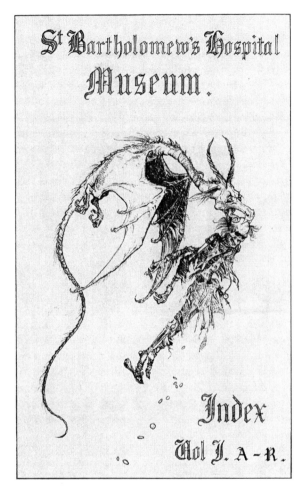

Fig. 1.2. Arthur Rackham, cover for St Bartholomew's Hospital Museum manuscript catalogue, *c.* 1900, reproduced in Harold Burt-White, 'The Museum', *St Bartholomew's Hospital Journal*, 40 (1933), 81–84 at 82. Wellcome Library, London.

dismembered the dead body and preserved the fragments, whether by injection or by storage in fluid, fashioning them into material culture. Such body parts followed complex paths—'harvested' from hospital wards, given to prestigious institutions, or once again fragmented at auction. Human remains acquired new meanings as they were exchanged, the identities of anatomists and collectors obliterating that of the patient. Once in the museum, diseased specimens formed the major proportion of medical collections, re-integrated to form physical maps of disease. Curators juxtaposed organic specimens with paintings, photographs, and models, and rendered them legible with extensive catalogues. Paper, wax and text formed a series of overlapping systems with the morbid body at their centre. They were intended to standardize the educational experience that was the ostensible purpose of most of the museums, and yet visitors refused to be policed, responding powerfully, whether with wonder or disgust. *Morbid Curiosities* is the story of these post-mortem journeys.

Recovering the tales of diseased body parts is a rather esoteric endeavour, and—by definition—a rather morbid one. Why, then, look at the history of pathological collections? By the end of this book I hope to have shown that they can illuminate our understanding of disease and difference; expose the function of museums and the meanings of the objects within them; and illustrate the uses of human remains in nineteenth-century secular culture.

FRAMING MORBIDITY

In a study of diseased fragments, it will be useful to begin by considering an exemplar. A 'typical' pathological specimen, however, is an oxymoron: the normal abnormal. But let us nevertheless contemplate one particular specimen in order to understand just what a morbid curiosity is. If I type 'pathology' and 'specimen' into the catalogue of the Museums and Archives of Royal College of Surgeons of England, among the first items listed is the ulcerated oesophagus shown in figure 1.3. What is it? What is interesting about it?

Perhaps its significant characteristic is that it was once part of a person. In common with anthropology, archaeology, and Egyptology collections, medical museums are storehouses of human remains. As the novelist Hilary Mantel recently reflected,

> In old-fashioned museums you can see the unconscious benefactors of mankind, trapped in glass cases: the freaks and monsters of their day, the anomalies, sometimes skeletonised and entire, sometimes cut into parts and labelled. When we look at them, fascination and repulsion uneasily mixed, we bow our heads to their contribution to knowledge, but it is hard to locate their humanity. The thread of empathy has frayed and snapped. They have become objects, more stone than flesh: petrified, post-human.[3]

---

[3] Hilary Mantel, 'Henrietta's Legacy', *Guardian Review*, 22 May 2010, 7.

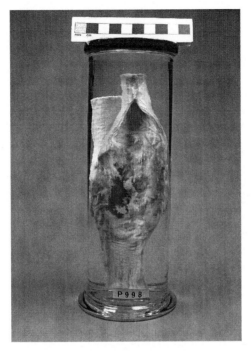

Fig. 1.3. The normal abnormal: an ulcerated oesophagus from a patient of Maxwell Gartshore, prepared by John Hunter in 1783. Copyright the Hunterian Museum at the Royal College of Surgeons of England.

It is likely that the specimen in question was once part of 'Mrs. P—', a fifty-two year-old London woman, patient of the Scottish physician Maxwell Garthshore who practised in the capital. (As we shall see in chapter 3, it is not unusual that we know more about him than her.) Having succumbed to the carcinoma of the oesophagus in 1783, at Garthshore's request this soon-to-be anonymous person's body was the subject of a post-mortem examination by the renowned anatomist John Hunter, who then 'put up' (removed and prepared) the specimen, which became RCSHC/P998.[4]

---

[4] Maxwell Garthshore, 'A Case of Difficult Deglutition Occasioned by an Ulcer in the Oesophagus, with an Account of the Appearances on Dissection', *Medical Communications*, 1 (1784), 242–55; L. W. Proger, *Descriptive Catalogue of the Pathological Series in the Hunterian Museum of the Royal College of Surgeons of England*, 2 vols. (Edinburgh: Livingstone, 1966–72), ii. 113; Simon Chaplin, 'John Hunter and the "Museum Oeconomy", 1750–1800' (Ph.D. thesis, King's College London, 2009).

These acts began to distance the object from any original identity and humanity. 'She' became 'it', representative not of her personality nor story, but rather of gullet cancer; and the patient's identity was subsumed by that of Garthshore and, especially, Hunter. In crafting this once-human object from her corpse, Hunter materialized her illness, rendering an intangible disease concept into a physical thing, to be studied, analysed, displayed, and compared with other objects. This transformation was neither complete nor irreversible, and it is a central tenet of my argument that material culture is more a process than a state. Objects and bodies are constantly in flux—objects made from bodies especially so. It is clear that this process, rendering flesh in material culture, involved considerable work, a complex series of transformative processes. The oesophagus is preserved in fluid, a so-called 'wet specimen', perhaps the mode of preservation most closely associated with medical museums. Other specimens, as we shall see in great detail in chapter 4, were dried, injected with wax, or mounted with wires. Slowing down time (the aim of traditional museum preservation) requires ongoing labour.

The pathological specimen, then, is not only conceptually hybrid (person and thing, subject and object), but also physically hybrid. This specimen is now as much preservative as it is tissue. Others have differing proportions of flesh and fluid, bone and metal, but all are composites. None can substitute for the 'real' (living) thing—the texture, colour, and physicality are merely approximations. Chapter 5 details the ways in which model, picture, and specimen were juxtaposed to give a complete account of a condition, the deficiencies of the small, faded original compensated by the expanded image and colourful wax model. Together they create an impression, an idea of disease; an idea that is interestingly multi-sensory, as discussed in chapter 6.

Given the physical limitations of this specimen, then, why are so many tens of thousands kept in medical museums? The advantages are familiar to any medical student. Specimen RCSHC/P998 illustrates upon demand a condition that might not be encountered in practice; it reveals the inner workings of the body, showing us the physical manifestation of a sickness deep inside the woman's body; it freezes time, rendering the indistinct visible, the ephemeral durable, providing a permanent reference point. Stored alongside the dozens of other oesophagi in the collection, it comprises one page in a three-dimensional encyclopaedia of disease. Western science captures normality in the idealized, singular type specimen—but deviance is limitless. Pathology is the study of the unpredictable diversity of the diseased body.

Perhaps even more significant than its deviance is that the specimen is a fragment. Fragmentation is an important process, and central to this book;

and like other key elements of my study, I am interested in it both as a physical and conceptual act. Fragmentation is both a manual craft and a creative process. Hunter extracted and isolated the woman's disease, preserving only part of her for posterity, in doing so making key decisions about what was important and valued and what was not. (Decisions made by Hunter's successors which would come to light so dramatically in the organ retention scandals discussed in chapter 7.) As such this specimen is barely recognizable as part of a body. It is also rather small: this one 230 by 80 mm, and the great majority of specimens in medical collections are even smaller. It is portable (if delicate), and can be lifted, handled, studied, and, crucially, moved around. Thanks to the anatomist, the dead body has become partible—its parts are divided and separated and are circulated and exchanged within the network of institutions described in the following pages. Parts of the body of one (former) person like this gullet are transferred to other places to join parts of other bodies.

The way I have framed these exchanges and reformulations of the dead body has been informed by anthropological work on the living person. Medical collecting and display may appear to have little in common with Marilyn Strathern's studies of Melanesian society—the classic application of partible personhood—and yet fruitful parallels can be drawn.[5] Strathern and others have shown us that personhood need not necessarily be constrained by the concept of the bounded individual, but rather that some groups frame people in a far more dynamic, relational way, as composite, mutable, multi-authored entities. Clearly I apply the concept in a quite different context, to physical parts of dead bodies rather than elements of living people. This is partibility in a far more literal and physical sense than used by Strathern and other anthropologists—in this sense I have more in common with some archaeologists, as we shall see in chapter 5. Nonetheless it is my contention that to understand human remains in museums it is useful to think about the collection as a dynamic entity, a set of relations (between patients, practitioners, collectors, curators, and audiences) enacted through material (including not only body parts but also models, pictures, and texts). This oesophagus does not share a museum shelf with other parts of the original patient—although parts of the same people are sometimes evident in the same collection—but rather with other examples of the organ or the condition. The extraction of this

---

[5] Marilyn Strathern, *The Gender of the Gift: Problems with Women and Problems with Society in Melanesia* (Berkeley: University of California Press, 1988); Strathern in turn adapted notions of 'dividuality' from McKim Marriott: see for example McKim Marriott and Ronald Inden, 'Toward an Ethnosociology of South Asian Caste Systems', in Kenneth David (ed.), *The New Wind: Changing Identities in South Asia* (The Hague: Mouton, 1977), 227–38.

part of the body during a destructive autopsy was the first step in the construction of a new entity; all the fragments on display together make up a multi-authored, diseased body. It is no longer an individual on display, I argue here (see chapters 3 and 5), but rather a *dividual* body, that is, composed of different separated parts from different sources. The trajectories of the fragments and the identities they carry with them mean that they are more than composites or conglomerates, they are complex sets of relations comprising multiple traces, multi-authored materials that are actively invented and re-invented, the products of considerable work. In constructing the dividual body in the museum (comparable to but distinct from the anthropologists' dividual person), pathologists make something new from the corpses of the patients, generating synthetic knowledge about disease and the body.

RCSHC/P998 is intellectually formative, then; it is also a social object, as revealed in chapter 6, a catalyst for engagement between visitor and curator, student and teacher. Generations of medical students have studied it or other such 'pots' as an essential passage point in their training; countless visitors have gawked at it in a less formal way. The specimen is polysemic—it means very different things to different people as it is part of different kinds of relationships. And different meanings have come to the fore at different times as audiences and their interests wax and wane.

Prevalent among these meanings, as we have already considered, is the significance of the deviance of the specimen. My focus on diseased bodies reflects not only the Victorian fixations with difference, but also recent attention to deviance in historical scholarship. One early and important example is Georges Canguilhem's influential analysis of the biological study of error, in which he demonstrated that 'pathological phenomena' were either considered 'identical to the corresponding normal phenomena save for quantitative variations', or else framed in opposition to health, the morbid *other* (such as germs).[6] Both underlined the co-constitution of normativity and deviance. To understand the normal, the healthy, he showed, we must address the abnormal—which advice holds as true for twenty-first-century historians as it did for nineteenth-century physiologists. Pathology is as much a value judgement as it is a diagnosis. Michel Foucault in particular took this to heart in his studies of 'the large, ill-defined, and confused family of "abnormal individuals," the fear of which

[6] Georges Canguilhem, *The Normal and the Pathological*, trans. Carolyn R. Fawcett (1943; 2nd edn, New York: Zone, 1989), 35; Cristina Chimisso, 'The Tribunal of Philosophy and Its Norms: History and Philosophy in Georges Canguilhem's Historical Epistemology', *Studies in History and Philosophy of Biological and Biomedical Sciences*, 34 (2003), 297–327; Mike Gane, 'Canguilhem and the Problem of Pathology', *Economy and Society*, 27 (1998), 298–312.

haunts the end of the nineteenth century'.[7] He moved beyond Canguilhem's focus on life sciences to root out behavioural (especially criminal), psychological, sexual, and other deviances. The disciplinary institutions of which Foucault was so fond of writing—the hospital, the prison—were designed to enforce the normal by categorizing, controlling, pathologizing, the abnormal. So too, to an extent, the museum.[8]

More recently, the historical study of pathologies has developed in two interesting, but surprisingly unrelated, directions. Social historians and literary scholars have turned their attention to what one might dub 'cultural pathology': that is, the manifestation and representation, whether metaphorical or material, of deviance and transgression—the grotesque— in Western culture.[9] In particular, we have a rich understanding of the (now unpalatable) treatment and exhibition of disability and of living curiosities, those dubbed 'freaks'.[10] By sensitively assessing such attitudes, we are able to unpick how sensibilities concerning corporal and behaviour difference have changed over time and between sites. Historians of medicine, meanwhile, have focussed on disease and difference post-mortem, writing about pathology in clinical and scientific terms, analysing the emergence of a professional community devoted to the study of morbid anatomy.[11] Both of these approaches draw on extensive evidence in art and literature (whether medical or fictional). *Morbid Curiosities* explores

[7] Michel Foucault, *Abnormal: Lectures at the Collège De France 1974–1975*, ed. Valerio Marchetti, Antonella Salomoni, and Arnold I. Davidson, trans. Graham Burchell (1975; London: Verso, 2003), 323; Foucault, *The Birth of the Clinic: An Archaeology of Medical Perception*, trans. Alan M. Sheridan (London: Tavistock, 1976); Foucault, *Discipline and Punish: The Birth of the Prison*, trans. Sheridan (London: Allen Lane, 1977).

[8] Bennett, *The Birth of the Museum*; Eilean Hooper-Greenhill, *Museums and the Shaping of Knowledge* (London: Routledge, 1992).

[9] A range of genres touch on this, including histories of race, queer theory and disability studies; but for broad and reflexive accounts see O'Connor, *Raw Material*; Stallybrass and White, *Politics and Poetics*; Jennifer Terry and Jacqueline Urla (eds.), *Deviant Bodies: Critical Perspectives on Difference in Science and Popular Culture* (Bloomington: Indiana University Press, 1995; Youngquist, *Monstrosities*.

[10] See for example Rachel Adams, *Sideshow U.S.A.: Freaks and the American Cultural Imagination* (Chicago: University of Chicago Press, 2001); Robert Bogdan, *Freak Show: Presenting Human Oddities for Amusement and Profit* (Chicago: University of Chicago Press, 1988); Nadja Durbach, *The Spectacle of Deformity: Freak Shows and Modern British Culture* (Berkeley: University of California Press, 2010); Michael Mitchell, *Monsters: Human Freaks in America's Gilded Age* (2nd edn, Toronto: ECW, 2002); Joe Nickell, *Secrets of the Sideshows* (Lexington: University Press of Kentucky, 2005); Richard Sandell, Jocelyn Dodd, and Rosemarie Garland-Thomson (eds.), *Re-Presenting Disability: Activism and Agency in the Museum* (Abingdon: Routledge, 2010); Rosemarie Garland Thomson (ed.), *Freakery: Cultural Spectacles of the Extraordinary Body* (New York; London: New York University Press, 1996.

[11] Ian A. Burney, *Bodies of Evidence: Medicine and the Politics of the Inquest 1830–1926* (Baltimore: Johns Hopkins University Press, 2000); George J. Cunningham, *The History of British Pathology*, ed. G. Kemp McGowan (Bristol: White Tree, 1992); Russell C. Maulitz,

the ways that abnormality was constructed not only with images and words but also with *objects*. The museum was a crucial site for this material construction, and yet the display of the diseased dead has been overlooked in the study of corporeal deviance (focussed on the circus and the fair) on the one hand, and the history of pathology-as-discipline (in the hospital and the laboratory) on the other.[12]

The collections in museums cannot help but become historical. These things have long back-stories, many layers of experience, meaning and work wrapped around them. After he prepared it in 1783, Hunter retained the oesophagus. It was then transferred to the Company of Surgeons with the rest of his collection at the turn of the century, and so came to occupy the grand premises on Lincoln's Inn Fields that was a key site in the nineteenth-century cultural geography of medical London that is sketched out in chapter 2. This specimen did not move very much

---

Morbid Appearances: The Anatomy of Pathology in the Early Nineteenth Century (Cambridge: Cambridge University Press, 1987).

[12] Which is not to say that medical museums have not attracted scholarly attention. As both exhibition maker and historian, Ken Arnold has assessed the role of the museum in the history of medicine, and vice versa; Ruth Richardson has reflected on historical human remains within them; Elizabeth Hallam's anthropological analyses of anatomy museums have deepened our understanding of the relationship between death, memory and display; and thanks to John Pickstone and Simon Chaplin we know the significance of medical collections for the understanding of health and disease in the eighteenth and nineteenth centuries. See Ken Arnold, 'Time Heals: Making History in Medical Museums', in Gaynor Kavanagh (ed.), *Making Histories in Museums* (London: Leicester University Press, 1996), 15–29; Ken Arnold, 'Museums and the Making of Medical History', in Robert Bud, Bernard Finn, and Helmuth Trischler (eds.), *Manifesting Medicine: Bodies and Machines* (Amsterdam: Harwood Academic, 1999), 145–74; Ken Arnold, *Cabinets for the Curious: Looking Back at Early English Museums*, Perspectives on Collecting (Aldershot: Ashgate, 2006); Ruth Richardson, 'A Potted History of Specimen-Taking', *The Lancet*, 11 March 2000, 935–6; Ruth Richardson, *Death, Dissection and the Destitute* (2nd edn, London: Phoenix, 2001); Ruth Richardson, 'Human Remains', in Ken Arnold and Danielle Olsen (eds.), *Medicine Man: The Forgotten Museum of Henry Wellcome* (London: British Museum Press, 2003), 319–45; Elizabeth Hallam, 'Anatomy Display: Contemporary Debates and Collections in Scotland', in Andrew Patrizio and Dawn Kemp (eds.), *Anatomy Acts: How We Come to Know Ourselves* (Edinburgh: Birlinn, 2006), 119–38; Elizabeth Hallam, 'Anatomical Bodies and Materials of Memory', in Belinda Brooks-Gordon, et al. (eds.), *Death Rites and Rights* (Oxford: Hart Publishing, 2007), 279–98; Elizabeth Hallam, *Anatomy Museum: Death and the Body Displayed* (London: Reaktion, forthcoming); Chaplin, 'John Hunter'; John V. Pickstone, 'Museological Science? The Place of the Analytical/ Comparative in 19th-Century Science, Technology and Medicine', *History of Science*, 32 (1994), 111–38; John V. Pickstone, *Ways of Knowing: A New History of Science, Technology and Medicine* (Manchester: Manchester University Press, 2000). See also two useful theses: Maritha Rene Burmeister, 'Popular Anatomical Museums in Nineteenth-Century England' (Ph.D. thesis, Rutgers University, 2000); Erin Hunter McLeary, 'Science in a Bottle: The Medical Museum in North America, 1860–1940' (Ph.D. thesis, University of Pennsylvania, 2001). The works of these scholars informs this book throughout.

over two centuries, but many others did. *Morbid Curiosities* shows that pathological knowledge was generated and circulated with specimens.

Earlier in this chapter, Hilary Mantel responded to objects similar to specimen RCSHC/P998 partly with horror, part with wonder. This is a common admixture, but it is not universal. As attitudes to death shifted in the modern period, the use, display, and impact of human remains in museums has changed radically over time.[13] Just as the living body has a history, so too the corpse; just as we can better understand the normal by studying the abnormal, so we can glean a great deal about our attitudes to life, self, and personhood from the changing function of dead bodies.[14] This change has been especially marked in the last two decades, but contemporary debates around the repatriation, retention, display, and other uses of bodies in museums have a deep history. We are beginning to understand better the provenances and displays of human remains in other collections, but what of body parts in the medical museum?[15] Chapter 7 addresses recent developments including the legislation leading to the 2004 Human Tissue Act (England and Wales) which licensed and regulated those institutions who could store human remains, and the simultaneous spectacular popularity of Gunther von Hagens's *Body Worlds*. How did such apparently contradictory phenomena come about?

The answers lie in the development and subsequent shifts in the function of museums, and of human remains within them from the late eighteenth-century emergence of pathological anatomy, of which the diseased oesophagus was a part, to the decline in prestige of the medical museum in the inter-war period. This book therefore concentrates on this (very) long nineteenth century. Although informed by important institutional and intellectual development elsewhere—especially France, Italy, and the United States—this is a study of the British Isles.[16] In Britain and

---

[13] On the history of death, see for example Elizabeth Hallam and Jenny Hockey, *Death, Memory, and Material Culture* (Oxford: Berg, 2001); Julie-Marie Strange, *Death, Grief and Poverty in Britain, 1870–1914* (Cambridge: Cambridge University Press, 2005).

[14] Gareth Jones and Maja I. Whitaker, *Speaking for the Dead: Cadavers in Biology and Medicine* (2nd edn, Aldershot: Ashgate, 2009); Christine Quigley, *The Corpse: A History* (Jefferson, NC: MacFarland, 1996); Mary Roach, *Stiff: The Curious Lives of Human Cadavers* (London: Viking, 2003).

[15] Cressida Fforde, *Collecting the Dead: Archaeology and the Reburial Issue* (London: Duckworth, 2004); Jack Lohman and Katherine Goodnow (eds.), *Human Remains and Museum Practice* (Paris and London: UNESCO and the Museum of London, 2006); Laurajane Smith, 'The Repatriation of Human Remains—Problem or Opportunity?' *Antiquity*, 78 (2004), 404–13.

[16] On medical museums in other national contexts, see for example Julie K. Brown, *Health and Medicine on Display: International Expositions in the United States, 1876–1904* (Cambridge, Mass.: MIT Press, 2009); Anna Maerker, *Model Experts: Wax Anatomies and Enlightenment in Florence and Vienna, 1775–1815* (Manchester: Manchester University

Ireland during this period, museums occupied a hegemonic space in the medical marketplace, a key place for the study of disease. *Morbid Curiosities* therefore features the institutions, communities, and, especially, the specimens that comprised and shaped medical collections in order to understand the role of museums in modern medicine, and the role of objects within them. Specifically it will address the meanings adhered to human remains, and how these body parts, these segments of people, became objects. Healthy anatomy features throughout, but is not of principal concern, for as we have seen, to understand normality, we must address the deviant. Abnormality was materially constructed in the nineteenth-century museum with pathological specimens: diseased body parts preserved for posterity.

ANATOMY AND ENLIGHTENMENT

The study of medical museums, then, sits at the historical confluence of some very interesting streams of thought—medicine, collecting, the body—which then flow into contemporary debates about the display and use of human remains. But the source of this macabre river lies much further back.

The preservation and display of human remains was not novel to the modern period. Mediaeval churches housed reliquaries and other collections, including in particular saintly segments—mostly bony, but some dried.[17] 'Humane rarities', including body parts, were then a key element of the Renaissance cabinets of curiosities that have been heralded as the precursors of modern museums.[18] Among the most famous (and macabre)

Press, 2011); Michael Sappol, *A Traffic of Dead Bodies: Anatomy and Embodied Social Identity in Nineteenth-Century America* (Princeton: Princeton University Press, 2002); Thomas Schnalke, *Diseases in Wax: The History of the Medical Moulage*, trans. Kathy Spatschek (Chicago: Quintessence, 1995).

[17] Patrick Geary, 'Sacred Commodities: The Circulation of Medieval Relics', in Arjun Appadurai (ed.), *The Social Life of Things: Commodities in Cultural Perspective* (Cambridge: Cambridge University Press, 1986), 169–91; Arthur MacGregor, *Curiosity and Enlightenment: Collectors and Collections from the Sixteenth to the Nineteenth Century* (New Haven, Conn.: Yale University Press, 2007).

[18] Francis Joseph Cole, 'History of the Anatomical Museum', in Oliver Elton (ed.), *A Miscellany Presented to John Macdonald Mackay* (Liverpool: Liverpool University Press, 1914), 302–17; Harold J. Cook, 'Time's Bodies: Crafting the Preparation and Preservation of *Naturalia*', in Pamela H. Smith and Paula Findlen (eds.), *Merchants and Marvels: Commerce, Science and Art in Early Modern Europe* (New York: Routledge, 2002), 223–47; Lorraine J. Daston and Katharine Park, *Wonders and the Order of Nature, 1150–1750* (New York: Zone, 1998); Paula Findlen, *Possessing Nature: Museums, Collecting, and Scientific Culture in Early Modern Italy* (Berkeley: University of California Press,

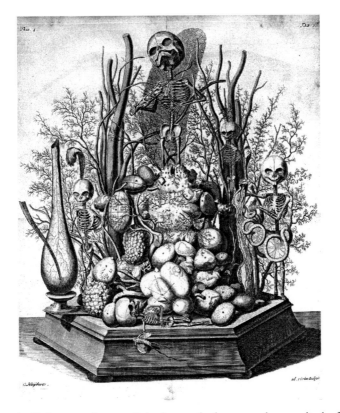

Fig. 1.4. Skeletons and parts of the human body arranged on a plinth, from Frederik Ruysch, *Thesaurus Anatomicus Primus: Cum Figuris Aeneis* (Amsterdam: Wolters, 1703), part iii plate 1. Wellcome Library, London.

were the elaborate tableaux constructed by the Dutch naturalist, surgeon and anatomist Frederik Ruysch, which incorporated multiple infant skeletons (see figure 1.4). Deviance was one of the qualities admired by Ruysch and his peers, so monsters (that is, abnormal births) were prized components of their cabinets, as marvels, portents, prodigies, and spectacles. Collectors understandably preferred durable human remains, especially bones and stones (whether bladder or kidney), but from the mid seventeenth century, new preservation techniques allowed the long-term storage of soft tissues in spirits (as we shall see in chapter 4) and deformed

1994); Julie V. Hansen, 'Resurrecting Death: Anatomical Art in the Cabinet of Dr. Frederik Ruysch', *Art Bulletin*, 78 (1996), 663–79; MacGregor, *Curiosity and Enlightenment*.

foetuses in jars became a regular feature in cabinets of curiosity. Superflui-
ty was popular, from conjoined twins to bicephallic embryos. Juxtaposi-
tions were key to *Wunderkammern*, so that living oddities such as dwarfs
guided visitors around the deformed dead; in death, human monsters sat
alongside deformed animals.

For the most part, cabinets of curiosity were to modern eyes dizzyingly
heterogonous. But some had strengths in particular areas, including the
categories we would now group within medical museums. Apothecaries
were among the most prolific early modern collectors, who used their
cabinets for clinical or research purposes, and teachers at the Dutch and
Italian medical schools displayed their cabinets in anatomical theatres.
From the turn of the seventeenth century, as dissection became more
prevalent in Western Europe, they were joined by an increasing number of
collections dedicated to anatomy gathered by anatomists and surgeons,
and over the course of the eighteenth century anatomy collections proliferated as a distinct museological enterprise. We should not overstate 'the
tension between an Enlightenment, classifying culture, or rational system-
atics, and a waning baroque oral-visual polymathy' that Barbara Maria
Stafford observes, but we can nevertheless discern a shift in collecting and
exhibitionary practices in the eighteenth century, the era of the *Encyclo-
pédie*.[19] Some forty English anatomy museums are evident in the historical
record in the second half of the century; in London alone, forty-nine of
the sixty-nine anatomy teachers in London had access to significant
collections.[20]

The emergence of such collections cannot properly be characterized as
specialization. Anatomists collected many other kinds of objects as well as
human remains, and body parts continued to feature in a range of other
collections throughout the modern era—collectors prized ancient Egyptian mummies in particular.[21] Nevertheless, the proliferation of dedicated
anatomical collections was a qualitative as well as a quantitative development. Anatomy was a broad church, including human and animals (and
plants), diseased and healthy—but at its core was the dissected, preserved,
body. Eighteenth-century anatomists gathered not only prized oddities
but also large numbers of typical specimens, and their collections were not
characterized so much by the kinds of objects therein (human remains and
natural history occurred in other collections), but in the way they were

[19] Barbara Maria Stafford, *Artful Science: Enlightenment, Entertainment, and the Eclipse
of Visual Education* (Cambridge, Mass.: MIT Press, 1994), 220.
[20] Chaplin, 'John Hunter'; Cole, 'History of the Anatomical Museum'. Much of the rest
of this section is informed by the former.
[21] Stephanie Moser, *Wondrous Curiosities: Ancient Egypt at the British Museum* (Chicago:
University of Chicago Press, 2006).

analysed.[22] This abundance of anatomy museums can partly be explained by shifts in the way anatomy was studied in the eighteenth century: with more dissection, with more objects. Surgical anatomy relied on in-depth knowledge of the dead body, which could only be partly provided by fresh dissections, so those who would make a living as instructors needed sizeable collections.

This 'entrepreneurial anatomy' was to be found in a range of settings.[23] Anatomical theatres continued to be a site for the display of medical collections, not only the iconic skeletons but also wet specimens and body parts (see figure 1.5). Many others were to be found in the homes of anatomists, whether displayed there or stored for transport to other teaching sites. London in particular emerged as a key site for medical education in the later eighteenth century, and collections proliferated there (see chapters 2 and 6).[24] Thus emerged what Simon Chaplin has dubbed the 'museum oeconomy'—that is, 'the system of operations by which the collecting and display of preserved body parts allowed the surgeon-anatomist to represent himself as a virtuous and knowledgeable medical practitioner'.[25]

Anatomical collections were at once part of the European Enlightenment and an integral component of the medical marketplace of eighteenth-century consumer society, serving to generate both financial and cultural capital for their collectors.[26] But they were by no means the exclusive concern of medio-surgical collectors and audiences. The distinction between medical educators and anatomical showmen was not clear cut in this period (nor, as we shall see later, would it become so for some time). Organic and wax remains were on display in anatomical shows and fairs from early in the eighteenth century, there to be found alongside living exhibitions of freakery as they had been in earlier eras.[27] *The London Spy*, for example, noted 'abortives put up in pickle' on display in 1703.[28]

---

[22] Pickstone, *Ways of Knowing*.

[23] Anita Guerrini, 'Anatomists and Entrepreneurs in Early Eighteenth-Century London', *Journal of the History of Medicine and Allied Sciences*, 59 (2004), 219–39; Jonathan Simon, 'The Theatre of Anatomy: The Anatomical Preparations of Honoré Fragonard', *Eighteenth-Century Studies*, 36 (2002), 63–79.

[24] Susan C. Lawrence, *Charitable Knowledge: Hospital Pupils and Practitioners in Eighteenth-Century London* (Cambridge: Cambridge University Press, 1996).

[25] Chaplin, 'John Hunter', 11.

[26] For recent studies of the medical marketplace, see Mark S. R. Jenner and Patrick Wallis (eds.), *Medicine and the Market in England and Its Colonies, c. 1450– c. 1850* (New York: Palgrave Macmillan, 2007).

[27] Altick, *Shows of London*; Alan W. Bates, '"Indecent and Demoralising Representations": Public Anatomy Museums in Mid-Victorian England', *Medical History*, 52 (2008), 1–22; Durbach, *Spectacle of Deformity*.

[28] Ned Ward, *The London Spy; the Vanities and Vices of the Town Exposed to View*, ed. Arthur L. Hayward (1703; London: Cassell, 1927), 50.

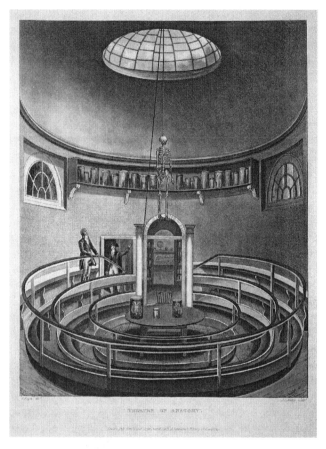

Fig. 1.5. The Anatomical Theatre at Cambridge by J.C. Stadler after Augustus Charles Pugin for William Combe, *A History of the University of Cambridge, Its Colleges, Halls, and Public Buildings,* 2 vols. (London: Ackermann, 1815). Wellcome Library, London.

Notorious showmen included Benjamin Rackstrow, who combined prestigitation, electricity, and morbidity at his 'Museum of Anatomy and Curiosity' on Fleet Street, including alongside organic remains the intricate wax models that we shall meet again in chapter 5.[29]

---

[29] Altick, *Shows of London*; Pamela Pilbeam, *Madame Tussaud and the History of Waxworks* (London: Hambledon and London, 2003); Benjamin Rackstrow, *A Descriptive Catalogue (Giving a Full Explanation) of Rackstrow's Museum* (London: n.p., 1782).

Four aspects of eighteenth-century anatomical objects are of particular importance to the present study: their movement, preservation, exhibition, and reception. Firstly, once within the custody of the anatomist, the body parts were his property, and they were then kept or exchanged by gift or purchase during his lifetime or posthumously. Ruth Richardson has shown that in the decades around 1700 the corpse became a commodity.[30] To endure beyond the immediate study at the point of dissection, and to be sturdy enough to be subject to such exchanges, anatomical objects need to be expertly 'put up', and thus rendered 'preparations'— the very term drawing attention to the work that went into them.[31] They were also stable enough to display. The corpse was fragmented and preserved in order to be experienced—looked at, touched (even smelled) and talked about. Anatomists did not horde them for their own sake, but rather showed them off, as physical evidence of their skills as dissectors, their discernment as collectors, and their ability to acquire rarities. The collection was credibility in material form. Finally, it is important to emphasize the diversity of audiences for these objects, from surgical apprentices to fairground goers to nobility. On the one hand, although Enlightenment anatomy was 'the quintessential impolite science: messy, nasty, and faintly ridiculous', delicate preservation helped to render anatomy virtuous, an acceptable part of fashionable society.[32] On the other, monsters in jars helped to keep it firmly in the cultural gutter, the stuff of nightmares and horror.

Two figures exemplified these aspects of the anatomical collection, looming over the eighteenth-century medical and museological landscapes and casting long shadows over the following century (and therefore this book). The London-based Scottish brothers William and John Hunter independently accumulated the two most important anatomical collections in eighteenth-century Britain.[33] William Hunter arrived in London

---

[30] Richardson, *Death, Dissection and the Destitute*; as corroborated by Guerrini, 'Anatomists and Entrepreneurs'.

[31] See the distinction between 'specimen' and 'preparation' in Chaplin, 'John Hunter', 8.

[32] Guerrini, 'Anatomists and Entrepreneurs', 220; Richard Barnett, *Medical London: City of Diseases, City of Cures*, ed. Mike Jay (London: Strange Attractor, 2008); Bates, '"Indecent and Demoralising Representations"'; Chaplin, 'John Hunter'; Roy Porter, 'William Hunter: A Surgeon and a Gentleman', in William F. Bynum and Roy Porter (eds.), *William Hunter and the Eighteenth-Century Medical World* (Cambridge: Cambridge University Press, 1985), 7–34.

[33] A distinct body of literature has coalesced around each. Recent scholarly work includes Chaplin, 'John Hunter'; C. Helen Brock (ed.), *The Correspondence of Dr William Hunter*, 2 vols. (London: Pickering and Chatto, 2008); Lawrence Keppie, *William Hunter and the Hunterian Museum in Glasgow, 1807–2007* (Edinburgh: Edinburgh University Press, 2007); Helen McCormack, 'A Collector of the Fine Arts in Eighteenth-Century Britain: Dr William Hunter 1718–1783' (Ph.D. thesis, University of Glasgow, 2010).

from Glasgow in 1740 to take up man-midwifery, soon afterwards acquiring the anatomical preparations of James Douglas, to whom he had been apprenticed, which became the nucleus of his extensive collection of anatomy, natural history, books, art, and antiquities. 'I have collected such anatomical apparatus', he later claimed with characteristic immodesty, 'as was never brought together in any age or country.'[34] Establishing himself as a lecturer and anatomist, in 1763 Hunter audaciously proposed to the Government the establishment of a medical school and museum. Unsurprisingly rebuffed, Hunter financed his own school at his home on Great Windmill Street from 1767. By this time, his younger brother John, who had come to London to work for him in 1748, was building up his own collection. Skilled in preparing specimens, the younger Hunter practised as a surgeon and anatomist and eventually set himself up independently of William, with whom he had a turbulent relationship. He also established a thriving school, which from the 1783 operated from premises behind his home in Leicester Square. There he expanded his collection of normal, comparative, and morbid anatomy; by the time he died in 1793, his collection of 14,000 items included over 9,000 preparations of human and animal anatomy, healthy or diseased. These objects, and those of his brother, were at the heart of the nineteenth-century medical museum culture.

A MUSEUM TAXONOMY

The Hunters' museums, like those of most eighteenth-century anatomists, were the private property of the collector.[35] That both brothers' collections constituted the core of institutional museums by the turn of the century (see chapter 2) is illustrative of a shift in governance that renders this study, of nineteenth-century collecting, distinct from those of earlier periods. As one Victorian surgeon reflected of John Hunter and his pupil Astley Cooper:

> This indifference on the part of his associates, as to the preservation of examples of the various diseases which came under their notice, was a circumstance which had offered John Hunter one of his chief opportunities of enlarging his morbid collection, and Mr. Cooper found it equally available

---

[34] William Hunter, *Two Introductory Lectures, Delivered by Dr. William Hunter, to His Last Course of Anatomical Lectures* (London: Johnson, 1784), 93, also cited in Keppie, *William Hunter*, 20.
[35] For the complexities of owning eighteenth-century anatomy collections, see Anita Guerrini, 'Duverney's Skeletons', *Isis*, 94 (2003), 577–603.

in the fulfillment of his object. This was an advantage peculiar to their time, for the scientific value of such collections is too well appreciated now [1843], both by public institutions and individuals, ever to allow any private person to meet with such facilities of accumulating examples of disease or malformation.[36]

Some institutions had collections from early in the eighteenth century, but the large-scale institutionalization of the material culture of anatomy in the second quarter of the nineteenth constituted an unprecedented qualitative and quantitative shift in the form and function of collections. The Enlightenment 'museum oeconomy' gradually merged into the Victorian 'exhibitionary complex', that is, the web of institutions (exhibitions, fairs, museums of art and nature, department stores, arcades, panoramas) connected by disciplinary and power relations, which over the course of the nineteenth century brought objects and bodies—dead and alive—into increasingly public spaces for display.[37]

Which is not say that private collecting declined, or that human remains ceased to feature in personal collections; far from it. Medical practitioners were among the most prolific of collectors of all kinds of objects, and they had privileged access to body parts. Pathological human remains featured in the massive collection of the pharmaceutical baron and obsessive collector Henry Wellcome—the largest medical museum in history and a candidate for the most expansive personal collection of all time.[38] But for many other medical collectors, just what constituted a personal collection was not always clear, and teaching collections blurred the distinction between private and institutional. One of the earliest examples of a genuine institutional medical museum in its current sense, however, was to be found at St Bartholomew's Hospital, probably founded in 1726 (see figure 1.6). Some of the other 'great' London hospitals developed cabinets over the next century, and in the early Victorian period in particular it became clearer that these were the property of the hospital rather than lecturer-clinicians—a process not without pain, as we shall see in chapter 3. The medical departments of the armed forces set up museums in the early nineteenth century; elsewhere infirmaries, lying-in charities, and even asylums

---

[36] Bransby Blake Cooper, *The Life of Sir Astley Cooper, Bart.* 2 vols. (London: Parker, 1843), ii.102.

[37] Tony Bennett, 'The Exhibitionary Complex', *New Formations,* 4 (1988), 73–102. On the quantitative expansion of anatomical museums in the early nineteenth century, see Cole, 'History of the Anatomical Museum'.

[38] Arnold and Olsen, *Medicine Man*; Frances Larson, *An Infinity of Things: How Sir Henry Wellcome Collected the World* (Oxford: Oxford University Press, 2009).

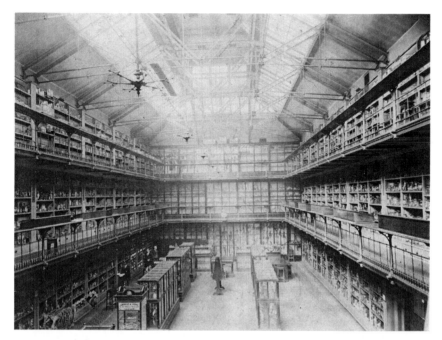

Fig. 1.6. Anatomy and Pathology Museum, St Bartholomew's Hospital, 1899. Copyright St Bartholomew's Hospital Archive, Barts and the London Hospital Trust Archives and Museums.

later followed suit.[39] The museum was a key element of the Victorian hospital.

Few hospital museums survive in the twenty-first century, for reasons explored in chapter 7. Rather, the most prominent collections to be seen today can be found in the royal colleges of surgeons in London, Edinburgh, and Dublin. Although the Edinburgh collection dates back to 1699, these collections were for the most part developed from private collections a century later, most famously in the case of the acquisition of John Hunter's collection for what would become the Royal College of Surgeons of England. The collection in Lincoln's Inn Fields became an

---

[39] On the army medical museum, established in 1816, see Army Medical Museum, *Anatomical Drawings, Selected from the Collection of Morbid Anatomy in the Army Medical Museum, Chatham*, 5 fasciculi vols. (London: Longman, 1824–1850), for which reference I am grateful to Katherine Foxhall; on brain collections in late nineteenth-century asylums, see Cathy Gere, 'A Brief History of Brain Archiving', *Journal of the History of the Neurosciences*, 12 (2003), 396–410.

exemplar for others across the country, and was the measure against which many of the collectors, curators and institutions encountered here measured themselves.[40]

Even in the capitals, however, medical education and practice was not limited to the royal colleges, and certainly this was not the case beyond them. Most of the proprietary anatomy schools that proliferated across the country in the early nineteenth century included collections of healthy, morbid, and comparative anatomy. Rivalling these in the early century and incorporating them towards the end were university museums, whether general faculty collections with anatomical components or specific medical museums. The established universities in London, Oxford, Cambridge, and Scotland were joined by new civic colleges in the English provinces in the second half of the century, which were chartered in the early twentieth century to become the 'Redbrick' universities; most by this time had distinct pathological museums.

Probably the majority of medical museums in the nineteenth century, then, and certainly the institutions that will feature in this study, were sites for formal medical education (as discussed in greater detail in chapter 6). But the exhibitionary complex also consisted of informal and ephemeral collections and displays, intersecting and overlapping with each other and with the established museums already mentioned. Some were gathered by elite groups within the medical establishment, and were thus on the more exclusive end of the spectrum, such as the collections of learned medical associations, especially the pathological societies that were formed in many cities in the middle of the century. Central to their function was the regular discussion of interesting specimens, which sometimes became the core of a society collection (although most were short-lived and few survived).

Other exhibitions, by contrast, were exhibited by those afforded little credibility by these elites, for a far more inclusive audience. Just as the difference between private and institutional collection was unclear, so too the distinction between curator and showman remained hazy. Commercial anatomy shows were evident in the capital in the eighteenth century and in the provinces from the early 1800s, including for example Joseph Woodhead's Museum of Anatomy, allegedly established in Liverpool in 1816. They were especially common in London in the mid nineteenth century, but evidence of their display can be found across the country up

---

[40] The Hunterian collection has a considerable body of historical literature, and it has not been the focus of original research for the present study. See rather Chaplin, 'John Hunter'; Nicolaas A. Rupke, *Richard Owen: Biology without Darwin* (2nd edn, Chicago: University of Chicago Press, 2009).

to the 1870s.[41] Although fewer records and specimens remain for the historian or the curator, and as such they may seem under-represented in *Morbid Curiosities*, the commonalities and contrasts between these and their more orthodox equivalents nevertheless provides a useful balance throughout this book. On the one hand, their different motivation and widely variant audiences provide interesting counterpoints; on the other, we find on closer examination that their exhibitionary strategies and layouts were not as different from other medical museums as their critics suggested.

These, then, are the nodes in the exhibitionary complex with which the account that follows will be most concerned: private anatomy schools, universities, hospital museums, royal colleges, pathological societies, and commercial anatomy exhibitions. The next chapter will account for the emergence of these different kinds of collections in specific locations: London, Edinburgh, and Dublin as British capitals and renowned centres for medical education; and Glasgow and Manchester as other major medical and museological centres. As well as considering other places where relevant, this gives *Morbid Curiosities* significant geographical scope and comparative power.[42] Within these locations we encounter the communities of practice that coalesced around and deployed collections, and through them the role of material culture in the medical marketplace and the construction of pathology as a discipline. Knowledges and practices involve material interactions, and specimens were as much part of the tools of science and medicine as the microscope.[43]

[41] On Liverpool, see [Joseph T. Woodhead], *Descriptive Catalogue of the Liverpool Museum of Anatomy* (Liverpool: Matthews, 1877). Although rarely considered alongside formal medical museums, they have attracted considerable historical attention in their own right: Altick, *Shows of London*; Alan W. Bates, 'Dr Kahn's Museum: Obscene Anatomy in Victorian London', *Journal of the Royal Society of Medicine*, 99 (2006), 618–24; Bates, '"Indecent and Demoralising Representations"'; Burmeister, 'Popular Anatomical Museums'; Hallam, *Anatomy Museum*; Stephen Johnson, 'The Persistence of Tradition in Anatomical Museums', in T. Christine Jespersen, Alicita Rodriguez, and Joseph Starr (eds.), *The Anatomy of Body Worlds: Critical Essays on the Plastinated Cadavers of Gunther Von Hagens* (Jefferson, NC: McFarland, 2009), 68–85.

[42] For studies of medical education in the ancient universities, including the role of human remains, see Elizabeth T. Hurren, 'A Pauper Dead-House: The Expansion of the Cambridge Anatomical Teaching School under the Late-Victorian Poor Law, 1870–1914', *Medical History*, 48 (2004), 69–94; Elizabeth T. Hurren, 'Whose Body Is It Anyway?: Trading the Dead Poor, Coroner's Disputes, and the Business of Anatomy at Oxford University, 1885–1929', *Bulletin of the History of Medicine*, 82 (2008), 775–818; Mark Weatherall, *Gentlemen, Scientists, and Doctors: Medicine at Cambridge, 1800–1940* (Woodbridge; Rochester, NY: Boydell, 2000).

[43] John V. Pickstone, 'Working Knowledges before and after *circa* 1800: Practices and Disciplines in the History of Science, Technology and Medicine', *Isis*, 98 (2007), 489–516; Michael Worboys, *Spreading Germs: Disease Theories and Medical Practice in Britain, 1865–1900* (Cambridge: Cambridge University Press, 2000). On museums and disci-

Having started with the urban locations and then the built environment, then populated them with the professionals (and amateurs), the core chapters of the book focus on specimens—their movement, the practices associated with them, and how they were used in museums. Not so much through details of particular objects (although there will be plenty, beginning with specimen RCSHC/P998 above), but rather the general 'career path' that specimens followed: how they got to collections, what happened to them there, and who viewed them.[44] Chapter 3 begins with the point of origin of the anatomical specimen, that is, the death and dissection of the 'patient'. Thus fragmented, body parts followed complex paths—harvested from hospital wards, given to a prestigious institution or once again fragmented at auction. Human remains acquired new meanings associated with collectors and practitioners as they were exchanged. We find here that the process of objectification, rendering the human body material culture, begins as a conceptual act even before the death of the patient. The accompanying physical processes, namely, the preservative techniques intended to render organic remains stable, are the subject of chapter 4. The messy, contingent business of museum conservation is concealed by the pristine pages of the published catalogues, and this chapter turns to the very materiality of the preparation: the preservative fluids, the jars, and the injected substances. This gives us a rare glimpse into museum practice, the techniques, and the skills involved, and a deeper understanding of the processes of material culture (and material culture as process).

Chapter 5 investigates how specimens were deployed in displays, finding that they were re-integrated to form a physical map of disease—no longer an individual person but a dividual body. Or rather, *bodies*: the healthy body contrasted with the different ways in which parts of it became diseased; the human body compared to the animals (most collections included an element of comparative anatomy); and the corroding, discoloured organic body in the shadow of the ideal perfection of the wax

plines, see Chris Gosden and Frances Larson with Alison Petch, *Knowing Things: Exploring the Collections at the Pitt Rivers Museum 1884–1945* (Oxford: Oxford University Press, 2007); Christopher Whitehead, *Museums and the Construction of Disciplines: Art and Archaeology in Nineteenth-Century Britain* (London: Duckworth, 2009).

[44] For other instances of this tripartite museum historiography, see Samuel J. M. M. Alberti, *Nature and Culture: Objects, Disciplines and the Manchester Museum* (Manchester: Manchester University Press, 2009); Moser, *Wondrous Curiosities*. Most literature on object biographies and the social lives of things stems from Igor Kopytoff, 'The Cultural Biography of Things: Commoditization as Process', in Appadurai, *The Social Life of Things*, 64–91; for a survey, see Samuel J. M. M. Alberti, 'Objects and the Museum', *Isis*, 96 (2005), 559–71.

model or clinical illustration. Paper, wax, and text formed a series of overlapping, intermedial systems that buttressed the organic morbid body.

The narrative pans out again to wider audiences and institutional histories in the closing chapters of the book. Shifting from this production of pathology to its reception, chapter 6 contrasts the intentions of those who constructed these elaborate bodies as far as possible with the responses they elicited. It is concerned with their intended visitor constituencies, from medical students to mechanics. It confirms the suggestion in chapter 2 that the principal intended use of pathological specimens was pedagogic—this book is in a large part a study of medical education, formal and informal. However didactically museums may have been laid out, we find, visitors nevertheless responded with contingent and highly personal mix of enlightenment and wonder, horror, and disgust. The experience of the museum visit was not only visual, as curators intended, but also aural, olfactory, and (especially) tactile. Finally, chapter 7 traces the diminution of these audiences as the medical museum ceased to be such a prestigious site for the construction and reception of pathology.

Overall, then, the central themes of *Morbid Curiosities* are the ways in which human remains became material culture, how parts of people became *things* in medical collections; and, more broadly, the varied associations they accrued during their afterlives—that is, the meaning of specimens in museums. As reflected in the structure of the chapters, I am interested in the mobile, material and contingent character of modern western biomedical knowledge. Human remains are especially potent objects with complex meanings. The collections they constituted were complex, dynamic entities, growing and shrinking, changing over time and place both physically and conceptually. Like other collections, the medical museum was an entangled assemblage, and like all assemblies, it was deeply political: a parliament of monsters indeed.[45]

---

[45] On assemblies, see Bruno Latour and Peter Weibel (eds.), *Making Things Public: Atmospheres of Democracy* (Cambridge, Mass.: MIT Press, 2005); Robert Louis Welsch, 'One Time, One Place, Three Collections: Colonial Processes and the Shaping of Some Museum Collections from German New Guinea', in Michael O'Hanlon and Welsch (eds.), *Hunting the Gatherers: Ethnographic Collectors, Agents and Agency in Melanesia, 1870s–1930s* (New York: Berghahn, 2000), 155–80. On the anatomy museums as an organic entity, especially metaphorically, see Hallam, *Anatomy Museum*.

2

Situating Pathology

A Cultural Cartography

To understand the circulation of diseased body parts, we need first to orient ourselves within the clinical, educational, and exhibitionary sites in which they were moved.[1] This chapter therefore locates the pathological collections introduced above on a number of different scales: civic, architectural, institutional, and finally professional. At each level the perspective on where diseased bodies were displayed is different, as is the role and status of those using them, including not only such medical dynasties as the Hunters, Thomsons, and Monros, but also provincial anatomy teachers including Joseph Jordan and Thomas Turner and showmen such as Joseph Kahn. To understand medical collections we need not only understand the relationships between these practitioners and their audiences, we must also map the borders between disciplines and the boundaries between institutions.

From such a map, we may better understand the fluid and contingent nature of pathology as a discipline, and of disciplinarity more generally. As Ken Arnold writes, museums were 'used to define where one discipline ended and another began, and indeed how they fitted together—which next to which'.[2] The language of territorialism pervades discussions of disciplinarity—we speak of 'fields', of provinces of knowledge, of 'charting' terrain. Where in this cultural landscape were different groups of anatomical specimens (and curators) located? The answers lie on both tangible and intangible factors: not only the location and classification of

---

[1] For helpful surveys of the historical geography of science, see Diarmid Finnegan, 'The Spatial Turn: Geographical Approaches in the History of Science', *Journal of the History of Biology*, 41 (2008), 369–88; David N. Livingstone, *Putting Science in Its Place: Geographies of Scientific Knowledge* (Chicago: University of Chicago Press, 2003).

[2] Ken Arnold, *Cabinets for the Curious: Looking Back at Early English Museums* (Aldershot: Ashgate, 2006), 239; Samuel J. M. M. Alberti, *Nature and Culture: Objects, Disciplines and the Manchester Museum* (Manchester: Manchester University Press, 2009); Christopher Whitehead, *Museums and the Construction of Disciplines: Art and Archaeology in Nineteenth-Century Britain* (London: Duckworth, 2009).

objects within the collection, but also the training and outlook of keepers. The history of collections is a shifting intellectual topography; just as on a political map nations build borders and sign treaties, so on the landscape of the museum curators construct boundaries and ally themselves with different disciplines. 'Cultural cartography is not idle play with Venn diagrams', argues its arch-proponent Thomas Gieryn, 'maps of science give definitions of situations real in their consequences, both for those who rely on them and those who draw them.'[3] The topography of knowledge is messy, contested, and disunified. To exploit the metaphor further: disciplines have jagged borders, contingent cartographies, and internal border disputes. Museums shape disciplines, and disciplines shape museums.

We can only understand the movement and meanings of the material culture followed in later chapters by unpicking the interplay between the institutions, individuals, and spaces that comprised nineteenth-century pathology; and the special peculiarities of British morbid anatomy in particular. We shall see in this chapter the unusually late development of a distinct pathological community in the British Isles, despite the massive growth in size and number of pathological *collections*, first in the early years of the century, then again at its end. To make sense of the development and function of museums we shall need to trace the complex relations between hospitals and universities, clinicians and scientists, and especially the particularities of British medical education (which are addressed again in chapter 6). This gives vital context to the status and duties of pathology collectors and curators, a remarkably small and relatively stable group that of course features prominently throughout *Morbid Curiosities*. Pathological specimens remained vital cultural capital for both individuals and institutions across the century, but their intellectual and clinical contexts changed significantly.

Around 1800, pathological anatomy was one of a number of enterprises to emerge that were fundamentally collection-based, including stratigraphy, phrenology, and comparative anatomy. Its international pedigree in this period is by now familiar to historians of medicine, thanks in particular to Russell Maulitz.[4] In mid-eighteenth-century London, as we

---

[3] Thomas F. Gieryn, *Cultural Boundaries of Science: Credibility on the Line* (Chicago: University of Chicago Press, 1999), 12; see also Thomas F. Gieryn, 'What Buildings Do', *Theory and Society*, 31 (2002), 35–74; Susan Leigh Star and James R. Griesemer, 'Institutional Ecology, "Translations" and Boundary Objects: Amateurs and Professionals in Berkeley's Museum of Vertebrate Zoology, 1907–39', *Social Studies of Science*, 19 (1989), 387–420.

[4] Russell C. Maulitz, *Morbid Appearances: The Anatomy of Pathology in the Early Nineteenth Century* (Cambridge: Cambridge University Press, 1987); George J. Cunningham,

saw in the last chapter, William and John Hunter and other anatomists began to gather morbid examples as well as normal human anatomy. The Hunters' morbid anatomy was largely from a surgical perspective, complemented by the organ-based morbid anatomy elucidated, largely with their collections, by their nephew Matthew Baillie in his *Morbid Anatomy* (1793). But it was in Paris in the work of Xavier Bichat and Théophile Laënnec that pathological anatomy as a distinct and coherent enterprise emerged, generated from a blend of surgical and medical pathology and based on tissues and membranes.[5] Parisian medicine found receptive ears in Edinburgh in the early nineteenth century, especially in the anatomist John Thomson, who dispatched his son William and their friend Robert Carswell to Paris to learn more.[6]

Together with Thomas Hodgkin (of whom much more later), Carswell then carried these ideas back to London to be manifested in print and specimen. Despite the quantity and quality of the collections they developed, however, their bid to institutionalize pathological anatomy was thwarted, and pathology came to occupy a very different place in the British medical establishment than it did elsewhere. Whereas in the German States, for example, Rudolf Virchow lead a thriving community of pathologists who held prestigious and recognized position, in the UK, by contrast, pathology did not reach a professional critical mass until the very late century.[7] The apparent disjuncture between vast collections and a small professional community is at the core of this chapter, and can only

The History of British Pathology, ed. G. Kemp McGowan (Bristol: White Tree, 1992); Toby Gefland, *Professionalising Modern Medicine: Paris Surgeons and Medical Science and Institutions in the Eighteenth Century* (Westport, Conn.: Greenwood, 1980); Elizabeth Haigh, *Xavier Bichat and the Medical Theory of the Eighteenth Century* (*Medical History* Supplement 4; London: Wellcome Institute for the History of Medicine, 1984); Esmond R. Long, *A History of Pathology* (London: Baillére, Tindall and Cox, 1928); Alvin E. Rodin (ed.), *The Influence of Matthew Baillie's Morbid Anatomy: Biography, Evaluation and Reprint* (Springfied, Ill.: Charles C. Thomas, 1973).

[5] Matthew Baillie, *The Morbid Anatomy of the Most Important Parts of the Human Body* (London: Johnson, 1793); Xavier Bichat, *Pathological Anatomy* (Philadelphia: John Grigg, 1827).

[6] Andrew Hull, 'Carswell, Sir Robert (1793–1857)', *Oxford Dictionary of National Biography* (Oxford: Oxford University Press, 2004), www.oxforddnb.com/view/article/4778, accessed 20 June 2008; L. Stephen Jacyna, 'Robert Carswell and William Thomson at the Hôtel-Dieu of Lyons: Scottish Views of French Medicine', in Roger French and Andrew Wear (eds.), *British Medicine in an Age of Reform* (Abingdon: Routledge, 1991), 110–35.

[7] Angela Matyssek, *Rudolf Virchow. Das Pathologische Museum. Geschichte einer Wissenschaftlichen Sammlung um 1900* (Darmstadt: Steinkopff, 2003); Rudolf Virchow, *Die Cellularpathologie in ihrer Begründung auf Physiologische und Pathologische Gewebelehre* (Berlin: Hirschwald, 1858).

be accounted for by understanding the organizational arrangement of material culture and the status of the roles associated with collections: the historical geography of British medical museums.

URBAN CONTEXTS

Nationwide, there were well over 100 pathological collections or museums with considerable morbid components during the nineteenth century, most of them concentrated in the capitals. Even though this chapter will indicate the general shape of the exhibitionary complex rather than account for them all, it pays to be specific to locale, because interesting parallels and contrasts emerge if one raises one's eye from a metropolitan focus. While the configurations of anatomical collections in each city have been touched on by historians, usually as a by-product of the history of medical education, they have not been explicitly juxtaposed and compared, so it will prove useful to devote some pages to introduce the people and places who will feature throughout *Morbid Curiosities*.

The different types of collection presented in the previous chapter—private, proprietary, university, hospital, royal college, learned society, and commercial—are evident in distinct configurations in different cities. In order to build up an image of the urban geography of these museums, I shall sketch out these formations; first in London, then Glasgow, Edinburgh, Dublin, and finally Manchester. The rationale for the selection of these sites was touched on in the last chapter, intended to be a revealing admixture of capitals and major provincial centres, while also providing contrasts between England, Scotland, and Ireland. Only with this comparative institutional framework in place, with the key characters, collections and their connections established, can we go on to explore the spatial, disciplinary and professional characteristics of nineteenth-century medical museums.

London

London was the epicentre of British museum culture, medical or otherwise. As indicated in the previous chapter, in the eighteenth century this was thanks in no small part to the Hunter brothers. The significance of both their collections endured through the nineteenth century and beyond, not only in London but also in Glasgow (see below). After his death in 1793, John Hunter's collection was eventually purchased by the government and given to the Company of Surgeons, having been refused by the Royal Society and the Royal College of Physicians (who would later accept Matthew Baillie's preparations).[8] In 1813, the Hunterian Museum opened on Lincoln's Inn Fields as the material jewel in the Royal College of Surgeons's crown.

By this time, however, the collection had some substantial rivals, especially from the anatomy schools whose museums accounted for many of the proliferating anatomy collections in the period 1810–40 (see figure 2.1). Perhaps the most famous of these was the school on Great Windmill Street, set up by William Hunter but by this time run by the Scottish anatomist Charles Bell (see chapter 3). In 1812 Bell wrote to his brother of the time he took 'putting this *great museum* in order' and that 'It would delight you to see me the proprietor of this museum, which looks great, even now in its great confusion—a noble room nobly filled.'[9] Other significant collections were to be found in schools such as Joshua Brookes's on Blenheim Street, Aston Key's at Maze Pond and Edward Grainger's on Webb Street.[10] The surgeons John Heaviside and George Langstaff displayed their notable collections in their homes, (although of course the distinction between domestic and didactic space was not clear-cut).[11] Just as the Hunterian collection expanded in the Royal

---

[8] Simon Chaplin, 'John Hunter and The "Museum Oeconomy", 1750–1800' (Ph.D. thesis, King's College London, 2009); Jessie Dobson, 'The Place of John Hunter's Museum', *Annals of the Royal College of Surgeons of England*, 33 (1963), 32–40.

[9] Charles Bell (ed.), *Letters of Sir Charles Bell* (London: Murray, 1870), 199, 200, original emphasis; Gordon Gordon-Taylor and E.W. Walls, *Sir Charles Bell: His Life and Times* (Edinburgh: Livingstone, 1958); Great Windmill Street Anatomical Museum, *Description of the Anatomical Museum of the School of Great Windmill Street* (London: Burgess and Hill, 1819); Matthew H. Kaufman, *Medical Teaching in Edinburgh During the 18th and 19th Centuries* (Edinburgh: Royal College of Surgeons of Edinburgh, 2003); Helen McCormack, 'Housing the Collection: The Great Windmill Street Anatomy Theatre and Museum', in Peter Black (ed.), *'My Highest Pleasure': William Hunter's Art Collection* (Glasgow: University of Glasgow in association with Paul Holberton, 2007), 101–16; John H. Teacher, *Catalogue of the Anatomical and Pathological Preparations of Dr. William Hunter in the Hunterian Museum, University of Glasgow*, 2 vols. (Glasgow: MacLehose, 1900); Stewart Craig Thomson, 'The Great Windmill Street School', *Bulletin of the History of Medicine*, 12 (1942), 377–91.

[10] Hector Charles Cameron, *Mr. Guy's Hospital: 1726–1948* (London: Longmans, 1954); Adrian Desmond, *The Politics of Evolution: Morphology, Medicine and Reform in Radical London* (Chicago: University of Chicago Press, 1989); Eilidh Margaret McInnes, *St Thomas' Hospital* (London: Allen and Unwin, 1963).

[11] Alan W. Bates, '"Indecent and Demoralising Representations": Public Anatomy Museums in Mid-Victorian England', *Medical History*, 52 (2008), 1–22; John James Edwards and M. J. Edwards, *Medical Museum Technology* (London: Oxford University Press, 1959); John Heaviside, *Catalogue of the Museum of John Heaviside, Esq.* (London: Woodfall, 1818); George Langstaff, *Catalogue of the Preparations Illustrative of Normal, Abnormal, and Morbid Structure, Human and Comparative, Constituting the Anatomical Museum of George Langstaff* (London: Churchill, 1842); James Paget, *Memoirs and Letters of Sir James Paget*, ed. Stephen Paget (London: Longmans, Green, 1901); George C. Peachey, *John Heaviside Surgeon* (London: St Martin's Press, 1931).

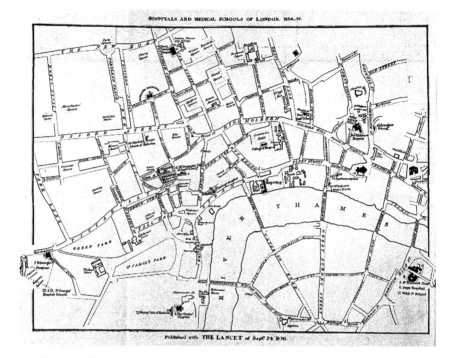

Fig. 2.1. Hospitals and medical schools in London, 1836. *The Lancet* 5 March 1837, facing p. 5. Wellcome Library, London.

College to include more morbid anatomy, so these early nineteenth-century collections included large sections explicitly devoted to pathological specimens.[12]

But morbid collecting on a grand scale was most evident elsewhere, in the site for medical education for which London was most famous: the great teaching hospitals. Their museums emerged alongside and eventually absorbed the private anatomy school collections. The earliest hospital museum in London was probably that at St Bartholomew's, as indicated in the last chapter, which from 1726 boasted a 'repository for anatomical and chirurgical preparations' under the cutting ward, next to the dead room.[13] However, notwithstanding the work on the

[12] See for example Benjamin Wheatley and George Adlard, *Museum Brookesianum. A Descriptive and Historical Catalogue of the Remainder of the Anatomical and Zootomical Museum, of Joshua Brookes, Esq.* (London: Taylor, 1830).
[13] From St Bartholomew's Hospital Minutes of the Governors, 23 June 1726, cited in Frederick S. Eve, 'Our Museum and Its Associations', *St Bartholomew's Hospital Reports*, 17

collection around the turn of the century by the anatomist James Macartney (later so famous in Dublin as we shall see), the Barts collection was to remain rather small until the late 1820s. At this point, the collection would begin to expand considerably, as did that of Guy's Hospital in Southwark under the enthusiastic curatorship of Thomas Hodgkin, the Quaker (would-be) physician. Hodgkin had walked the wards of Guy's for a year before studying in Edinburgh and Paris. He returned to London in 1826 bursting with the pathological anatomy of Bichat and Laënnec, and set about gathering a suitably extensive collection.[14] Gradually, all of the major teaching hospitals followed suit, usually as part of their medical schools. By the mid century, there were twelve hospital medical schools in the capital: Guy's and Barts competed with St Thomas's, King's College, Charing Cross, Middlesex, North London (University College), St George's, Westminster, St Mary's, the London, and St Mark's hospitals, all boasting major collections with significant pathological elements— many of which, as we shall see in the following chapter, stemming from or encompassing the private collections of their staff or of the anatomy schools. Furthermore, staff from the hospitals formed the core of the Pathological Society of London in 1846 whose members met together to display specimens from interesting cases.[15]

As the hospitals built up their collections, a new and significant institution emerged in the intellectual, educational, and material landscape of London.[16] The University of London in Bloomsbury, later University College London (UCL), was modelled on the University of Edinburgh and Scots filled many of the early chairs. The most renowned of the

(1881), 165–84 at 165; see also David Lowe, 'The Pathology Museum', *Bart's Journal* (Autumn 1992), 19.

[14] Thomas Hodgkin, *A Catalogue of the Preparations in the Anatomical Museum of Guy's Hospital* (London: Watts, 1829); Amalie M. Kass and Edward H. Kass, *Perfecting the World: The Life and Times of Dr. Thomas Hodgkin 1798–1866* (Boston: Harcourt Brace Jovanovich, 1988).

[15] There had been an earlier group who met in London in 1840. The first formal group in England was the Reading Pathological Society, founded in 1841. Cunningham, *History of British Pathology*; H. R. Dean, 'The Pathological Society of London', *Proceedings of the Royal Society of Medicine*, 39 (1946), 823–27.

[16] Hugh Hale Bellot, *University College London 1826–1926* (London: University of London Press, 1929); Desmond, *Politics of Evolution*; Negley Harte and John North, *The World of UCL 1828–1990* (2nd edn, London: University College London, 1991); Jacyna, 'Robert Carswell and William Thomson'; Maulitz, *Morbid Appearances*; Pauline M.H. Mazumdar, 'Anatomical Physiology and the Reform of Medical Education: London 1825–1835', *Bulletin of the History of Medicine*, 57 (1983), 230–46; Sarah E. Parker, *Robert Edmond Grant (1793–1974) and His Museum of Zoology and Comparative Anatomy*, ed. Helen Chatterjee and Joe Cain (London: Grant Museum of Zoology, 2006).

founding professors was Charles Bell; Robert Grant, who had also taught anatomy in Edinburgh, was Professor of Comparative Anatomy; and Granville Sharp Pattison, who had trained and taught in Glasgow, briefly and disastrously held the first chair in anatomy. Appointed but absent in the first three sessions was Robert Carswell, holding the first chair of pathological anatomy in Britain, who remained in Paris to continue to gather specimens and 'delineations'. (When he was offered the post Carswell was in Paris at John Thomson's behest, making illustrations of diseases; he proposed to create a museum using these 'delineations', 'together with diseased organs preserved in spirits, and accurate histories of each individual case'.[17]) Bell, who had recently sold the bulk of his collection to the Royal College of Surgeons at Edinburgh, also sold some preparations to the University, but did not build up a collection in Bloomsbury, and in any case neither he nor Pattison remained in post for long. That they and the anatomy demonstrator all used the same preparations in the same space to teach similar courses was not a tenable situation, and the conservative Bell clashed with the radical Grant. But the latter built up a renowned zoology collection during nearly half a century in post and Carswell's pathology collection slowly expanded in the first decade. *The Lancet* reported, 'Twelve years of uninterrupted labour he has devoted to the collection of his museum, and more than two thousand specimens of the common and rare form of disease testify the extent of his talent and industry.'[18]

Less acknowledged yet far more visible were the talent and industry of the many showmen—anatomists who were by this time operating in the capital. Chief among them was Joseph Kahn, a physician of dubious qualifications who arrived from Germany and established an anatomical museum on Oxford Street in 1851. There he rivalled such (equally exotic) shows as those of J. W. Reimers and Signor Sarti.[19] Although the principal attraction for those who paid their shilling to enter were no doubt the models in wax and other media (see chapters 5 and 6), these exhibitions included some morbid specimens, especially when associated with the lurid elements of obstetrics and diseases of the generative organs. Although for the most part they have been studied separately from their more orthodox peers, such commercial ventures were modelled on, exchanged

[17] Robert Carswell to University of London Council, 21 December 1827, University College Archives MS 304; Arthur Hollman, 'The Paintings of Pathological Anatomy by Sir Robert Carswell (1793–1857)', *British Heart Journal*, 74 (1995), 566–70.

[18] *The Lancet*, 23 November 1833, 326.

[19] Bates, '"Indecent and Demoralising Representations"'; Elizabeth Stephens, 'Venus in the Archive: Anatomical Waxworks of the Pregnant Body', *Australian Feminist Studies*, 25 (2010), 133–45.

material with, or otherwise bore striking parallels with the teaching collections, as we shall see in the chapters that follow.

London, then, was undoubtedly the nerve centre of both medical education and display in England, largely due to the concentration of teaching hospitals. But large hospital collections could be found elsewhere, commercial showmen toured their collections and anatomy schools were to be found in the provinces. Even the collection at Lincoln's Inn Fields was not unique, whether as a Royal College collection or even as 'The Hunterian'.

Glasgow

When the government refused to fund his proposed medical school and museum in London, William Hunter, in high dudgeon, bequeathed his massive and varied collection to the faculty of his Alma Mater, the University of Glasgow, having specified that it first be used for thirty years from his death (in 1783) by his nephew Matthew Baillie and Baillie's co-proprietor William Cruikshank at Great Windmill Street. However, Baillie retired from teaching shortly after Cruikshank's death in 1800, so in 1807 the collection—valued at £65,000 in the 1780s—was transported north to Glasgow. With a further bequest of £8,000, the collections were housed in grand neoclassical premises in the gardens behind the College on High Street in central Glasgow.[20]

The Hunterian thereby became the largest and most prestigious anatomy collection in Glasgow; but it was not the first. Although often associated with the university, several prominent practitioners gathered large private cabinets with pathological aspects in the eighteenth century, including Thomas Hamilton, Professor of Anatomy, of whose specimens the *Glasgow Mercury* reported when they were sold at auction in 1791, the 'morbid ones are very valuable, and particularly worthy of attention'.[21] Just as they did in London, the extramural schools of anatomy operating in the town also boasted large collections. In 1797, the brothers John and Allan Burns set up a medical school on College Street, adjacent to the university, and Allan established an extensive collection there. John would later take the chair of anatomy and transfer his collection to the university,

---

[20] James Coutts, *A History of the University of Glasgow* (Glasgow: Maclehose, 1909); Lawrence Keppie, *William Hunter and the Hunterian Museum in Glasgow, 1807–2007* (Edinburgh: Edinburgh University Press, 2007).

[21] *Glasgow Mercury*, 15 March 1791, 81. I am grateful to Anne Cameron for this reference.

where the anatomy department included a collection distinct from that of the Hunterian.[22]

Aside from the university and the College Street School, there were three other medical schools in Glasgow with significant collections. The first was a proprietary anatomy school on Portland Street, not unlike the Burns' establishment and their contemporaries in London. The second was more distinct, however. Anderson's Institution—later 'Anderson's University' and later still 'Anderson's College'—was established on John Street in 1796 thanks to the endowment of John Anderson, professor of natural philosophy at the university.[23] From the turn of the century John Burns taught anatomy there (presumably with his specimens) and Anderson's built a new medical school in 1831 on George Street including a substantial collection of anatomy and pathology. It continued to grow, thanks especially to the anatomist and former teacher at the Portland Street school Robert Hunter (no relation), who added to the museum, then left his own thousand-strong collection upon his retirement in 1860 (the whole collection was later transferred to the University of Glagsow). By this time, however, the third pathological collection had emerged, to rival even the Hunterian. The Glasgow Royal Infirmary opened in 1794 and provided the clinical education for the university.[24] In 1852, presumably because they felt that the morbid anatomy at the Hunterian was insufficiently representative and accessible, its directors ordered a pathological museum to be formed in the hospital, from the seed of a morbid anatomy collection and wax models provided by the Royal College of Physicians and Surgeons of Glasgow.[25] Crucial to its early years was the anatomist Allen Thomson, son of John Thomson of Edinburgh, of whom more below.

---

[22] Allen Thomson, 'Daily Register of Objects Illustrative of Medical Science Added to the Anatomical Museum of the University of Glasgow from October 1848', bound MS, 1848–1877, Glasgow University Special Collections MR 49/4; Coutts, *History of the University of Glasgow*; Alexander Duncan, *Memorials of the Faculty of Physicians and Surgeons of Glasgow 1599–1850* (Glasgow: Maclehose, 1896); Johanna Geyer-Kordesch, Fiona Macdonald, and Andrew Hull, *Physicians and Surgeons in Glasgow: The History of the Royal College of Physicians and Surgeons of Glasgow 1599–1858* (London: Hambledon, 1999); Ronald S. Wade, 'Medical Mummies: The History of the Burns Collection', *The Anatomical Record*, 253 (1998), 158–61.

[23] John Butt, *John Anderson's Legacy: The University of Strathclyde and Its Antecedents 1796–1996* (East Linton: Tuckwell, 1996); John Young, 'Hunterian Treasures', *Glasgow University Magazine*, 5 February 1889, 1–3.

[24] Jacqueline Jenkinson, Michael Moss, and Iain Russell, *The Royal: The History of Glasgow Royal Infirmary, 1794–1994* (Glasgow: Published by the Bicentenary Committee on behalf of Glasgow Royal Infirmary NHS Trust, 1994).

[25] Duncan, *Memorials of the Faculty*; Geyer-Kordesch, Macdonald, and Hull, *Physicians and Surgeons in Glasgow*; David Murray, *Museums: Their History and Their Use*, 3 vols. (Glasgow: MacLehose, 1904); John H. Teacher, 'On the History of Pathology in the

The distance between 'The Royal' and the university was in any case set to increase. Having been engulfed by the factories and slums of the industrial town centre, when the railway companies were enabled by Parliament to purchase the university's land, the faculty welcomed the opportunity to erect new premises in the spacious surrounds of Gilmore-hill, overlooking the city from the west. The Hunterian Museum was removed to the new buildings in 1870. This move broke the geographical and administrative link between the medical parts of the university and the Royal Infirmary. At the hospital the newly appointed pathologist Joseph Coats continued to expand, re-organize, and catalogue the museum until 1875, when he transferred to the new Western Infirmary adjacent to the re-located university.[26] There he oversaw a new, distinct morbid anatomy collection as part of a dedicated department of pathology. His successor, John Teacher, oversaw both the Hunterian and the Royal Infirmary collections. The former began to be broken up in the new century; the anatomical and pathological specimens were first transferred to a new anatomy block and eventually in 1954 to the museum of the Royal Infirmary.[27]

The overall shape of Glasgow's medical museums over the course of the nineteenth century appears to have been similar to that of London, albeit on a smaller scale—alongside a Hunterian collection a number of other museums were developed, among the various anatomy schools, hospitals, and universities. But the different timing is important, with the university dominating earlier and hospital collections only emerging later in the century. Unlike its elders, the Royal Infirmary museum was then a dedicated morbid collection from the outset, which meant that Glasgow punched above its weight as a site for the study of pathology in Britain, perhaps even compared to that of the Scottish capital.

Edinburgh

The roots of nineteenth-century medical museum culture in Edinburgh lie in the Surgeon's Hall on Surgeon's Square, the centre of yet another cluster of proprietary anatomy schools. Chief among these in both repute and collection were the 'extra-academical' schools run by John Bell

Glasgow Royal Infirmary and the Functions of the Pathological Department', *Glasgow Medical Journal* (January 1912), 3–15.

[26] Loudon MacQueen and Archibald B. Kerr, *The Western Infirmary 1874–1974: A Century of Service to Glasgow* (Glasgow: John Horn, 1974).

[27] Keppie, *William Hunter*; Alice J. Marshall and J. A. G. Burton (eds.), *Catalogue of the Preparations of Dr. William Hunter, Sir William MacEwen, Professor John H. Teacher, Professor J. A. G. Burton in the Museum of the Pathology Department, Glasgow Royal Infirmary* (Glasgow: University of Glasgow, 1962).

(where his younger brother Charles learnt his trade before moving south to the Great Windmill Street Museum) and by John Barclay, who amassed a famous anatomy museum. Over the course of the early nineteenth century, these were complemented and absorbed into two major sites: Edinburgh University and the Royal College of Surgeons of Edinburgh. Both ostensibly housed museums in the eighteenth century, but both expanded and diversified their collections in the nineteenth.[28]

The Royal College re-invigorated its eighteenth-century anatomical museum in 1804 with the appointment of John Thomson as the first professor of surgery, and invited members to donate preparations.[29] Thomson had trained at Glasgow, Edinburgh, and with John Hunter in Leicester Square; his son William went to Paris with Robert Carswell, and both William and his brother Allen would go on to hold chairs at the University of Glasgow. Thomson senior presented his own private collection to the Royal College, and he and his assistants supplied many of the specimens acquired in the first years of the museum's existence. But the core of the collection arrived from elsewhere. John Barclay promised his collection, as detailed in the following chapter, provided the college build dedicated accommodation for it. In the mean time the complex web of inter-capital collection exchange became ever more close-knit as the surgeons also purchased Charles Bell's collection from the Great Windmill Street school.[30] Both the Bell and Barclay collections were housed from

---

[28] Violet Tansey and D. E. C. Mekie, *The Museum of the Royal College of Surgeons of Edinburgh* (Edinburgh: The Royal College of Surgeons of Edinburgh, 1982); E. Duval and A. Currie, *The University of Edinburgh Pathology Department. The First 100 Years* (Edinburgh: University of Edinburgh, 1981); Andrew G. Fraser, *The Building of Old College: Adam, Playfair and the University of Edinburgh* (Edinburgh: Edinburgh University Press, 1989); Dugald L. Gardner, 'A Tale of Two Old and Historical Museums', in Robin A. Cooke (ed.), *Scientific Medicine in the Twentieth Century: A Commemoration of 100 Years of the International Association of Medical Museums and the International Academy of Pathology* (Augusta, Ga.: United States and Canadian Academy of Pathology, 2006), 92–98; Matthew H. Kaufman, *The Regius Chair of Military Surgery in the University of Edinburgh, 1806–55*, (Amsterdam: Rodopi, 2003); Kaufman, *Medical Teaching in Edinburgh*; Matthew H. Kaufman, 'John Barclay (1758–1826) Extra-Mural Teacher of Anatomy in Edinburgh: Honorary Fellow of the Royal College of Surgeons of Edinburgh', *The Surgeon: Journal of the Royal College of Surgeons of Edinburgh*, 4/2 (2006), www.thesurgeon.net, accessed 12 January 2009; Dawn Kemp with Sara Barnes, *Surgeon's Hall: A Museum Anthology* (Edinburgh: The Royal College of Surgeons of Edinburgh, 2009).
[29] Jacyna, 'Robert Carswell and William Thomson'; D'Arcy Power, 'Thomson, John (1765–1846)', rev. Anita McConnell, *Oxford Dictionary of National Biography* (Oxford: Oxford University Press, 2004), www.oxforddnb.com/view/article/27316, accessed 19 July 2008.
[30] Elizabeth Hallam, *Anatomy Museum. Death and the Body Displayed* (London: Reaktion, forthcoming); Kaufman, *Medical Teaching in Edinburgh*; Frederick John Knox, *The Anatomist's Instructor, and Museum Companion: Being Practical Directions for the Formation and Subsequent Management of Anatomical Museums* (Edinburgh: Black, 1836); John

1832 in the college's new premises on Nicholson Street, 300 yards to the south.

John Thomson also had a hand in another important collection nearby. In 1806, he had been appointed professor in military surgery at the university, and in 1832 he took up the new chair in general pathology. The medical faculty had been dominated for a century by another Scots medical dynasty, the Monros. Alexander Monro *primus* (who had trained William Hunter) formed the faculty in 1726; his son, Alexander *secundus* donated the extensive anatomical museum he inherited and augmented to the university in 1800. This was further expanded in the opening decades of the nineteenth century by Monro *tertius*, and with pathological specimens from the Royal Infirmary just across South Bridge Street, between the university and Surgeon's Square, further increasing the striking concentration of medical education, practice, and collections in Edinburgh.[31] This density was slightly diluted in 1880, however, when the anatomical museum was removed from the Old College with the rest of the medical school 400 yards west to Teviot Place in the 1880s.

Nevertheless, Edinburgh was striking in the richness of medical collections in a small area. This proximity goes some way to explain which elements of the town's collection configuration it had in common with its fellow capital London, and which with its neighbour Glasgow. Like London, the Royal College collection emerged as the most renowned collection, not necessarily through use or even size, but rather in prestige. Like Glasgow, the university emerged as the major site for the practice and material culture of pathology. Unlike either, there was no significant collection at the hospital, principally because both university and Royal College were so close. But in all three cities we see the form and fate of anatomy museums responding and contributing to shape of medical education: the numerous smaller private and school collections in the early century giving way to fewer, larger, late Victorian museums. One further national context will corroborate this pattern, once again with key local characteristics.

Struthers, *Historical Sketch of the Edinburgh Anatomy School* (Edinburgh: MacLachlan and Stewart, 1867).

[31] Proceedings of the Edinburgh Town Council as to the Anatomical Museum, 25 June 1824, cited in the Royal Commission on the Universities of Scotland, *Minutes of Evidence*, 4 vols. (House of Commons Command Papers 92–95; London: HMSO, 1837), appendix, 174.

Dublin

The roots of the medical museum complex in Ireland's capital closely resembled that of Scotland's, but the development of medical education in Dublin led to a slightly more variegated arrangement, more closely akin to London. Like Edinburgh, Dublin was a renowned centre for medical education, thanks in part to the two oldest institutions (and collections), again at a royal college of surgeons and a university. The size and character of these collections, especially the former, dominated the medical museum complex in the city.

Trinity College Dublin (TCD) was established in 1592, the only university in Ireland until the Queen's colleges in the mid nineteenth century. It housed a medical school from 1711, re-constituted in 1785 in conjunction with what would become the Royal College of Physicians in Ireland as the Dublin School of Physic. Gathered in the anatomy theatre was a small anatomical collection, including waxes crafted by Guillaume Desnoue, and the skeletons of the infamous Irish Giant Magrath and William Clark, the 'ossifed man' (*Myositis ossificans*).[32] The museum of the Royal College of Surgeons in Ireland (RCSI), like many institutional collections, precipitated around a small number of private collections—in this case those of the anatomist John Halahan and the surgeon William Dease.[33] Gathered as a teaching resource in the 1770s, they formed the nucleus of a collection used in the anatomical theatre, later transferred to dedicated space in a building on Mercer Street, behind the main College building.

Both the RCSI and the TCD collections, eighteenth-century cabinets that had fallen into disrepair in the new century, were re-invigorated in the 1820s as part of the minor renaissance in medical collections across the British Isles for which we have already seen evidence. The Trinity collection was refreshed by the new professor of anatomy, James Macartney, who had previously worked on the St Bartholomew's Hospital

[32] Alexander Macalister, *James Macartney: A Memoir* (London: Hodder and Stoughton, 1900); Constantia Maxwell, *A History of Trinity College Dublin 1591–1892* (Dublin: The University Press, 1946); George Newenham Wright, *An Historical Guide to the City of Dublin* (2nd edn, London: Baldwin, Cradock, and Joy, 1825).

[33] Charles Alexander Cameron, *A History of the Royal College of Surgeons in Ireland, and of the Irish Schools of Medicine* (2nd edn, Dublin: Fannin, 1916); John Gilborne, *The Medical Review, a Poëm: Being a Panegyric on the Faculty of Dublin; Physicians, Surgeons, and Apothecaries* (Dublin: Husband, 1775); J. D. H. Widdess, *The Royal College of Surgeons in Ireland and Its Medical School 1784–1984* (3rd edn, Dublin: Royal College of Surgeons in Ireland, 1983).

museum in London.[34] As professor of anatomy at Trinity from 1813, Macartney was prominent among a generation of physicians and surgeons who brought Continental techniques to Dublin and shaped the 'Irish school of medicine'.[35] Immediately upon his appointment he began to gather comparative and pathological anatomy. He oversaw the construction of a new medical school building in 1825 and housed his own considerable collection within it in a huge gallery.

Trinity had a generally uneasy relationship with the Royal College, and this was especially acute when it came to collecting. Unlike the universities in London and Edinburgh, whose relationships with the local royal colleges were aspirational rather than competitive, the RCSI was a teaching as well as an examining institution. From 1820 the college's medical school had its own collection—in a former stable and coach-house—separate from the college's central museum. But in order to emphasize the value of the latter, 'distinct from that used for teaching purposes in the Schools', in 1819 it was resolved 'that it is highly expedient to establish a Museum to contain specimens of Natural History and such other sciences as are subservient to Surgery'.[36] The central museum was awarded extra funding and a dedicated curator, John Shekleton, and invited donations. By 1822, Shekleton had 600 preparations in his care, which doubled the following year. He died in 1824 from an infection contracted while dissecting, however, to be replaced by his apprentice John Houston, a pioneer in the use of the microscope to study morbid growths (after whom Houston's valves in the rectum were named). Houston oversaw the transfer of the collection to new accommodation in 1828, catalogued the collection in detail and continued its expansion.[37]

By this time, however, anatomical collections had proliferated across the city as part of the expansion of medical education. As in other cities, anatomy schools sprang up across town, but in surprising numbers, due in

---

[34] Macalister, *James Macartney*; John Leonard Thornton, 'A Diary of James Macartney (1770–1843) with Notes on His Writings', *Medical History*, 12 (1968), 164–75.

[35] Davis Coakley, *The Irish School of Medicine: Outstanding Practitioners of the 19th Century* (Dublin: Town House, 1988); John Fleetwood, *History of Medicine in Ireland* (2nd edn, Dublin: Skellig, 1983); Elizabeth Malcolm and Greta Jones (eds.), *Medicine, Disease and the State in Ireland, 1650–1940* (Cork: Cork University Press, 1999).

[36] Widdess, *The Royal College of Surgeons in Ireland*, 67.

[37] Anatomy Museum, 'List of Morbid Preps', 10 pp. MS, 1824, Royal College of Surgeons in Ireland Archive RCSI/LO.An/13/4; Abraham Colles, 'Second Communication Relative to the Fatal Consequences Which Result from Slight Wounds Received in Dissection', *Dublin Hospital Report*, 4 (1827), 240–4; Marvin L. Corman, 'Classic Articles in Colonic and Rectal Surgery: John Houston 1802–1845', *Diseases of the Colon and Rectum* 30 (1987), 906–8; John Houston, *Descriptive Catalogue of the Preparations of the Museum of the Royal College of Surgeons in Ireland*, 2 vols. (Dublin: Hodges and Smith, 1834–40).

part to the lack of surgical teaching offered by TCD. Between 1804 and
1880 (later than in London and Scotland, but roughly contemporary with
the English provinces), eighteen anatomy schools appeared, flourished,
and closed again; most, if not all of them, had teaching collections.
Notable among their museums was that of the school set up on Park
Street near Trinity in 1824, large enough to fill a 40-foot gallery and
justify a full-time curator.[38] Its proprietor, the anatomist Hugh Carlile, a
nephew and apprentice of James Macartney, closed the school in 1849
upon his appointment to the Queen's College, Belfast, and took the
museum with him.

As they were elsewhere, the schools were closely connected to the
various hospitals in the city, so that their collections stemmed from the
wards (see chapter 3) and were sometimes housed there: the Ledwich
School, for example, was closely associated with the Coombe Lying-In
Hospital, which has a considerable obstetric collection. There is evidence
of museums at Dr Steevens', St Vincent's, and the Rotunda hospitals
(although none as significant as those of the major London institutions).[39]
Staff in these various sites formed the Dublin Pathological Society in
1838—that is, earlier than in London—and held peripatetic meetings
on Saturday afternoons to exhibit morbid specimens, variously at Park
Street, TCD, and the Richmond Hospital medical school (later re-named
Carmichael College).[40]

The Pathological Society was only one manifestation of the considerable exchange of ideas, specimens, and staff between schools and colleges
in the mid century. John Timothy Kirby had established a school on Peter
Street, the 'Theatre of Anatomy and School of Surgery', in 1809; when he
was appointed Professor of Medicine at the RCSI in 1832, he donated his
collection to the college museum.[41] John Houston went from the Royal
College to the Park Street school, where he catalogued the collection. But
in a pattern that is now familiar in this chapter, towards the end of the

---

[38] Henry Marsh, 'Observations on the Hemorrhages', *Dublin Quarterly Journal of
Medical Science,* 12 (1851), 257–78.
[39] Museum Committee Minutes, 29 June 1886, Royal College of Surgeons in Ireland
Archive RCSI/MUC/2; *Medical Times and Gazette,* 16 September 1854, 297–99; T. Percy
C. Kirkpatrick, *The History of Dr Steevens' Hospital, Dublin 1720–1920* (1924; facsimile
edn, Dublin: University College Dublin Press, 2008); F. O. C. Meenan, *Ceclia Street: The
Catholic University School of Medicine 1855–1931* (Dublin: Gill and Macmillian, 1987);
Douglas Mellon, 'Pathology Services', in Alan Browne (ed.), *Masters, Midwives and Ladies-
in-Waiting: The Rotunda Hospital, 1745–1995* (Dublin: Farmar, 1995), 160–79.
[40] Coakley, *The Irish School of Medicine*; John Fleetwood, 'Dublin's Private Medical
Schools in the Nineteenth Century', *Dublin Historical Journal,* 46 (1993), 31–45.
[41] Museum Committee Minutes, 10 January 1833 [sic—1832], Royal College of
Surgeons in Ireland Archive RCSI/MUC/1.

century the collections were gradually absorbed by a major collection, in Dublin's case that at the RCSI. Philip Bevan gave a large collection to the college in 1875, for example, probably the specimens he had catalogued at the museum of the Dublin School of Medicine, established in 1832. The obstetrical museum of the Coombe Lying-In Hospital was transferred to the Royal College in 1886; three years later Carmichael College and the Ledwich School were absorbed into the RCSI school, bringing to an end the private medical schools in Dublin. Those collections that remained in the schools were perused by the RCSI curator or offered by the proprietor, and the best specimens kept. By this time, the College's museum had expanded into new premises, and was the largest pathological museum in Ireland.[42]

Meanwhile, the TCD collection had suffered a major setback when James Macartney upon his retirement sold his collection to William Clark at the University of Cambridge. By the late 1850s, however, thanks to Macartney's successor Robert Harrison, the museum had recovered, collecting anew over 3,000 specimens, just as the 'main' college museum of natural history had expanded considerably in the mid century. The new anatomy block included a large new museum, ready for use in 1876, but the collection barely filled it.[43] And by this time Trinity was no longer the only university in town. In 1854, the new Catholic University had purchased the Apothercaries' Hall for its faculty of medicine, including the museum of the school of medicine the apothecaries had run there since 1837 (although the Rector John Henry Newman found the museum to be sadly lacking). The faculty worked closely with St Vincent's hospital, and

[42] Museum Committee Minutes, 7 October 1890, 7 February 1893 and Curator's Report for the Year ending 5 April 1889, RCIS/MUC/2, Royal College of Surgeons in Ireland Archive; Philip Bevan, *Descriptive Catalogue of the Anatomical and Pathological Museum of the Dublin School of Medicine, Peter-Street* (Dublin: Goodwin and Nethercott, 1847); Cameron, *History of the Royal College of Surgeons*; Coombe Lying-In Hospital, *The Coombe Lying-in Hospital Dublin 1827–1976* (Dublin: Coombe Lying-In Hospital, 1976); John Houston, *Descriptive Catalogue of the Anatomical and Pathological Museum of the School of Medicine, Park Street, Dublin* (Dublin: Fannin, 1843).

[43] Registry Board Meetings of Trinity College, 12 October 1876, TCD/MUN/V/5/13, Trinity College Dublin Archive; *Returns Relating to Medical Museums in the United Kingdom* (Parliamentary Papers 14; London: House of Commons, 1857); Robert Harrison, *Statement of the Qualifications of Robert Harrison, Candidate for the Professorship of Anatomy and Surgery in the University of Dublin* (Dublin: Hardy, 1837); Robert Harrison, *Catalogue of the Preparations Contained in the Museum of the Medical School of Trinity College, Dublin* (Dublin: The University, 1842); T. Percy C. Kirkpatrick, *History of the Medical Teaching in Trinity College Dublin and of the School of Physic in Ireland* (Dublin: Hanna and Neale, 1912); R. B. McDowell and D. A. Webb, *Trinity College, Dublin, 1592–1952: An Academic History* (Cambridge: Cambridge University Press, 1982); Mark Weatherall, *Gentlemen, Scientists, and Doctors: Medicine at Cambridge, 1800–1940* (Woodbridge; Rochester, NY: Boydell, 2000).

used the museum there before it was absorbed by the Royal College. In the 1890s the Catholic University incorporated fresh museum space in the new anatomical department, just as back at Trinity the new school of pathology included a large museum.[44]

Although it appears more complicated thanks to the sheer number of institutions involved, the general pattern of museum configuration and change in Dublin followed that of other cities in this study. Like London and Edinburgh, the Royal College collection, after an early century kick-start, emerged as the most significant (and enduring) museum, together with the universities, as medical education became more centralized in the later century. But what of the many other British cities without a royal college, and no university for most of the century? Finally, then, our attention turns of the medical museums in Manchester, the largest provincial centre for medical education.

Manchester

Industrialization and urbanization in 'Cottonopolis' brought about not only new health challenges but also a new tier of wealthy middle-classes who were minded to address them. Prominent among them was the surgeon and man-midwife Charles White.[45] In the 1740s White studied at William Hunter's school and became close friends with John Hunter (then a fellow student). After completing his studies in Edinburgh under Monro *secundus*, White brought back Hunterian ideas about classification and collecting to Manchester, building up a collection of over 300 healthy and morbid specimens. White used his collection upon which to base his lectures in anatomy and physiology in conjunction with the Manchester Literary and Philosophical society; his were among the first such lectures delivered in Manchester. Although White withdrew from lecturing at the turn of the century, others used his specimens to teach until 1808 (including P. M. Roget, later of thesaurus fame), when the collection was transferred to the Lying-In Charity (later St Mary's Hospital) that he had established in 1790.[46] Some of them were still used in anatomy and physiology lectures at the Lit and Phil until 1816.

---

[44] Meenan, *Ceclia Street*.

[45] Stella Butler, 'White, Charles (1728–1813)', *Oxford Dictionary of National Biography* (Oxford: Oxford University Press, 2004), www.oxforddnb.com/view/article/29238, accessed 1 June 2007; Jessie Dobson, 'Some Eighteenth Century Experiments in Embalming', *Journal of the History of Medicine*, 8 (1953), 431–41; Charles White, *An Account of the Regular Gradation in Man* (London: Dilly, 1799).

[46] They were destroyed by a fire in 1847. Penny Leach, *St Mary's Hospital Manchester: 1790–1990* (Manchester: St Mary's Bicentenary Appeal for the Care of Patients, 1990);

Other Manchester medical men trained in London, and brought back what they learned to establish Manchester as the pioneer of provincial medical education. After Joseph Jordan studied in London and Edinburgh he set up the first anatomy school in Bridge Street in 1814, incorporating the local lecturing tradition of White and others and giving it a formal, institutional basis. He ensured not only that he had a plentiful supply of bodies for the study of healthy anatomy, but also an extensive morbid anatomy collection.[47] Jordan immediately set about gathering a collection to rival White's, and this was a central part of the custom-built premises he opened on Mount Street in 1826. He explicitly modelled himself and his collection on that at St Thomas's in London, built up by the surgeon Astley Cooper, who had visited Bridge Street. Jordan's nephew and partner, Edward Stephens, trained at Joshua Brooke's anatomy school in London.

Jordan's new building was in part a response to competition from another Manchester native, Thomas Turner.[48] Turner trained in Paris and in London at Guy's and Thomas's, like Jordan under Astley Cooper (very probably listening to some of the earliest lectures on pathology in the capital). Turner had toured Scotland in 1820 and was impressed by Barclay's and Munro's collections in Edinburgh. In Manchester he founded an anatomy school in Pine Street in 1824, which included pathology in its syllabus. Key to the rivalry between the two schools, however, was the lack of collection at Pine Street in contrast to Jordan's expanding museum. Nevertheless, Pine Street had the massive advantage

Peter Mohr and Bill Jackson, 'The University of Manchester Medical School Museum: Collection of Old Instruments or Historical Archive?' *Bulletin of the John Rylands University Library of Manchester*, 87 (2005), 209–23; John V. Pickstone, *Medicine and Industrial Society: A History of Hospital Development in Manchester and Its Region, 1752–1946* (Manchester: Manchester University Press, 1985); Katherine A. Webb, 'Development of the Medical Profession in Manchester 1750–1860' (Ph.D. thesis, University of Manchester, 1988); John Harley Young, *St Mary's Hospital, Manchester* (Edinburgh: Livingstone, 1964).

[47] Leslie Doyle, 'Joseph Jordan (1787–1873): Manchester Anatomist and Surgeon', *Transactions of the Lancashire and Cheshire Antiquarian Society*, 95 (1999), 61–84; F. W. Jordan, *Life of Joseph Jordan, Surgeon, and an Account of the Rise and Progress of Medical Schools in Manchester, with Some Particulars of the Life of Dr Edward Stephens* (London: Sherratt and Hughes, 1904); G.A.G. Mitchell, 'Joseph Jordan 1787–1873 FRCS', in Willis J. Elwood and A. Félicité Tuxford (eds.), *Some Manchester Doctors: A Biographical Collection to Mark the 150th Anniversary of the Manchester Medical Society 1834–1984* (Manchester: Manchester University Press for the Manchester Medical Society, 1984), 65–74.

[48] Jordan, *Life of Joseph Jordan*; E. Bosdin Leech, 'The Pine Street Medical School', *Manchester University Medical School Gazette*, 20/1 (1941), 24–26; 'A Relative', *Memoir of Thomas Turner, Esq.*, intr. David Bell (London: Simpkin, Marshall and Co., 1875); Leslie Turner, 'Thomas Turner, 1793–1873', in Elwood and Tuxford, *Some Manchester Doctors*, 75–82.

of proximity to the Infirmary. A third school emerged in 1829 when John Boutflower and Thomas Fawdington, who had taught pathology for Jordan, broke away from the Mount Street School to set up a new establishment in Marsden Street, which was closer to the Infirmary than Mount Street, but not by much. Fawdington set about building a large collection, a good way of establishing a reputation in Manchester's crowded medical marketplace.[49]

Turner's school on Pine Street grew from strength to strength, however. In the 1830s, he secured the epithet 'Royal' (in a city with no Royal College with which to contend) and absorbed both the Mount Street and Marsden Street schools. He thus eventually secured Jordan's collection, but not Fawdington's, which was purchased by the Infirmary in 1843—as in Glasgow and Birmingham, the hospital needed a morbid collection of its own by the mid century.[50] Turner also purchased the sizeable collection of Gregory Smith, one of the lecturers at the Great Windmill Street School in London. (Windmill Street thereby provided the nucleus of a third collection outside London, after William Hunter's museum went to Glasgow and Charles Bell's to Edinburgh.) As a result, Turner ran the largest provincial medical school in England, and the collection grew to allegedly include 10,000 specimens; *The Manchester Guardian* boasted in 1843, 'except the museum of the Royal College of Surgeons . . . we believe the museum of the Manchester Royal School of Medicine is the largest and richest medical, anatomical and surgical museum in England'.[51] Nevertheless, it is doubtful whether it attracted nearly so many visitors or as much attention as Joseph Kahn's 'Anatomical Museum and Gallery of All Nations', which exhibited at the Royal Exchange in October 1851 as it toured the provinces. He went on to Liverpool, Preston, and Newcastle, allegedly attracting a 'vast influx of visitors'.[52] Whether the local medical profession availed themselves of the offer of a special day for their attendance (*gratis* rather than the usual shilling) is unknown.

[49] Edward Mansfield Brockbank, 'The Early History of the Manchester Medical School', *Manchester Medical Gazette*, 47/3 (1968), 9–17; Thomas Fawdington, *A Catalogue Descriptive Chiefly of the Morbid Preparations Contained in the Museum of the Manchester Theatre of Anatomy and Medicine* (Manchester: Harrison and Crosfield, 1833).

[50] Jonathan Reinarz, 'The Age of Museum Medicine: The Rise and Fall of the Medical Museum of Birmingham's School of Medicine', *Social History of Medicine*,18 (2005), 419–37; Webb, 'Development of the Medical Profession in Manchester'.

[51] Cited in Jordan, *Life of Joseph Jordan*, 110; see also William Stirling, 'The Manchester Medical School', in *Handbook and Guide to Manchester* (Manchester: British Medical Association, 1902), 139–54.

[52] Joseph Kahn, *Atlas of the Formation of the Human Body* (London: Churchill, 1852), back cover—allegedly from the *Sunday Times*, June 1851; 'Dr Kahn's Gallery of All Nations', *Manchester Guardian*, 29 October 1851, 1b; Bates, ' "Indecent and Demoralising Representations" '.

Half a mile south-east, the Royal School, which had operated largely unopposed in the 1840s, found itself in competition with a new school founded on Chatham Street in 1850. The staff there had been at the core of the Manchester Pathological Society, founded in 1846, the same year as its London counterpart, which exhibited specimens at its meetings at the Royal Manchester Institution; plans of 'forming a Pathological Museum' never quite materialized, however, and the Society faded away as its members concentrated on the new school.[53] The facilities at Chatham Street were clearly superior to Pine Street, well-lit and spacious, including 'a brand new museum quite up-to-date', so that when the inevitable amalgamation took place in 1856, the Royal School moved en masse to the Chatham Street premises for five years until the Pine Street premises were suitably adapted.[54] We have seen by now how common such mergers were, and that the bitterest disputes involved concerned the fate of the collections.

In 1860s Manchester, one final amalgamation was in the air. Royal School staff had already spent a decade considering a merger with Owens College, a small teaching outfit founded on Quay Street in 1851.[55] College and medical school finally united in 1872, but at first the new Owens College Faculty of Medicine—mostly Royal School staff— continued to operate in the Pine Street buildings, using the collection there. In 1874 a new medical school building was completed, behind the grand new premises for Owens College a mile south of the city centre on Oxford Road. At its heart was space for a new museum, and the collections at Pine Street gradually moved in over the years that followed. The cabinets of Jordan and Turner, then, formed the basis of the medical museum that would be used in teaching and pathological research at the federal Victoria University, as Owens became in 1880 (obtaining a separate charter in 1903). Owens, the first of the provincial 'university colleges', thereby became the first to absorb the local anatomy school(s)

[53] Cited in Thomas Harris, 'Historical Sketch of the Pathological Society of Manchester', *Transactions of the Pathological Society of Manchester*, 1 (1892), 19–25 at 20; James Davson, 'The Pathological Society of Manchester, 1885–1950', in Elwood and Tuxford, *Some Manchester Doctors*, 20–24; Webb, 'Development of the Medical Profession in Manchester'. The archives are to be found in the Manchester Medical Collection, MMC/ 7/8, John Rylands University Library of Manchester.

[54] A 'former student' cited in Jordan, *Life of Joseph Jordan*, 118.

[55] On the history of Owens and its successor institutions in this period, see Henry Buckley Charlton, *Portrait of a University, 1851–1951: To Commemorate the Centenary of Manchester University* (Manchester: Manchester University Press, 1951); Edward Fiddes, *Chapters in the History of Owens College and of Manchester University, 1851–1914* (Manchester: Manchester University Press, 1937); P. J. Hartog, *The Owens College Manchester: A Brief History of the College and Description of Its Various Departments* (Manchester: Cornish, 1900).

into a medical faculty. Bristol, Sheffield, Leeds, Liverpool, and Birming-ham followed suit in the next two decades, and in most cases a college museum was founded on the basis of the collection at the medical school.[56]

The configuration of collections in Manchester was obviously different from London and the Scottish cities in the lack of a Royal College and late founding of the university. The collections relating to private and propri-etary anatomy teaching, as important as we have seen they were in the capitals, were even more so in the English provinces. The geographical contingencies of medical training were co-constitutive with the location and availability of medical material culture—libraries, dissection facilities, and especially museums. The fate of the specimens was part and parcel of the development of medical practice, research, and education (whether formal or otherwise), so that by the end of the century the magnitude and authority of the museum at the Victoria University ruled out any other collections in the town.

We have seen, then, how closely related different sites for anatomy collections were in training, personnel, and material. By setting out a comparative geographical study of the development of British medical museums for the first time, it is also clear just how close the connections across the country were. Collectors trained elsewhere brought ideas and techniques home with them; collections and parts of collections moved from place to place to augment or catalyse other museums—several times over, as in the case of Great Windmill Street. The parallels and continui-ties of acquisition, technique, and audiences will be discussed in greater detail later in this volume; but in the meantime, having laid out the urban framework for these museums, the second half of this chapter is devoted to their spatial, disciplinary, and professional contexts; each adding a new layer of understanding in this historical geography.

SPACES FOR COLLECTIONS

It has become clear that medical museums were not freestanding entities, and to appreciate their functions one needs to understand their relation-ships with their parent institution. Having located the establishments housing collections within their townscapes, then, we now adjust the

---

[56] Samuel J. M. M. Alberti, 'Civic Cultures and Civic Colleges in Victorian England', in Martin J. Daunton (ed.), *The Organisation of Knowledge in Victorian Britain* (Oxford: Oxford University Press, 2005), 337–56; Edwards and Edwards, *Medical Museum Technol-ogy*; Cunningham, *History of British Pathology*; Reinarz, 'The Age of Museum Medicine'.

scale of analysis to another order of magnification to focus on the physical place of the museums. 'Anatomy had its material territory', as John Pickstone writes: 'the dissecting room and the pathological museum.'[57] By studying the architecture of museums (and of medicine) we better understand the meanings and use of the objects within them.[58]

The (considerable) range of buildings in which pathological specimens were to be found ranged from the grand to the humble. At what we might think would be the latter end of this spectrum, individual collectors stored their specimens wherever they deemed appropriate or could find space within their residences. However, those with sufficient resources set aside (rather large) sections of their homes for the museum. Most famously, both Hunter brothers laid out their collections in the centre of their home-cum-schools. These were large spaces: William's was 50 feet by 27 feet, John's 52 by 28. Each was double height, with galleries and top lighting. These were quasi-public spaces, as discussed in chapter 6 below; collectors such as Charles White allowed visitors into their homes to view their collections, guided either by the host but more often an assistant. But access to these spaces was a complex issue, as Simon Chaplin has shown in his study of John Hunter's house on Leicester Square.[59] In both Hunters' abodes, the collection occupied a liminal space between the polite social world of the home and the seedier environment of the anatomy schools, accessed from the rear of the property—and the museum could be entered from both sides.

In Manchester, Joseph Jordan's collection occupied a similarly interstitial space. His house at 69 Bridge Street connected to his nephew Edward Stephens's next door: 'there was but one yard, and the library formed the connecting link upstairs. The top storey of the two houses being the dissecting room and museum.'[60] The school and collection's growth prompted Jordan to rent part of number 66 as well, until he finally

[57] John V. Pickstone, 'A Profession of Discovery: Physiology in Nineteenth-Century History', *British Journal for the History of Science*, 23 (1990), 207–16, 209; Elizabeth Hallam, 'Anatomy Museum: Anthropological and Historical Perspectives', in Alice Semedo and João Teixeira Lopes (eds.), *Museus, Discursos e Representações* (Porto: Edições Afrantamento, 2005), 111–33.

[58] On the architecture of museums, see for example Suzanne MacLeod (ed.), *Reshaping Museum Space: Architecture, Design, Exhibitions* (London: Routledge, 2005); Thomas A. Markus, *Buildings and Power: Freedom and Control in the Origin of Modern Building Types* (London: Routledge, 1993), 169–244; Carla Yanni, *Nature's Museums: Victorian Science and the Architecture of Display* (London: Athlone, 1999); on the architecture of science and medicine see for example Sophie Forgan, 'Building the Museum: Knowledge, Conflict, and the Power of Place', *Isis*, 96 (2005), 572–85; Peter Galison and Emily Thompson (eds.), *The Architecture of Science* (Cambridge, Mass.: MIT Press, 1999).

[59] Chaplin, 'John Hunter'.

[60] Jordan, *Life of Joseph Jordan*, 127; Mitchell, 'Joseph Jordan'.

moved both the custom-built premises on Mount Street. When the collection was transferred to the Royal School of Medicine on Pine Street, its proprietor Thomas Turner spent £400 on an additional building for the museum, opened in 1842. Although the height of the neighbouring warehouses rendered both dissecting room and museum unsuitably lit for close study, the *Manchester Guardian* nevertheless reported, 'The gallery in which [Jordan and Turners' museum] is now arranged, in most beautiful order, extends the whole length of the building, from Faulkner Street to Pine Street, and is 73 feet in length by 23 feet 5 inches in width.'[61] The museum of the Windmill Street School in London, similarly, was in 'a room admired for its proportions, of great size, with a handsome gallery running round'.[62]

The museum was as essential a space for later, formal medical establishments as the dissecting room and the lecture hall.[63] As proprietary medical schools, hospitals, and royal colleges founded and absorbed collections in the early nineteenth century, they began to erect custom-built premises for their museums. The shape of both Hunterian museums became standard, both in their original contexts and after they were re-housed at the beginning of the century. In 1813 the Royal College in London opened the new premises for John's collection, designed by George Dance and James Lewis: 91 feet by 39, top-lit with a gallery.[64] This was an important exemplar for other museums in London—including dedicated museum spaces incorporated into new anatomy blocks at St Thomas's (1814), Guy's (1825), and Barts (1835)—and other royal colleges.[65] In Dublin, after makeshift accommodation in the early century—described by one contemporary as 'about the size of an ordinary bed-chamber, with one winder to supply it with light',[66]—the RCSI museum (as opposed to the RCSI *school* museum) was housed in a dedicated new wing of the College from 1828, a mock-Grecian construction with a museum room of 84 by 30 feet, with a gallery for morbid anatomy.[67] Later, anatomy and pathology were separated completely, as the former specimens were

[61] Cited in Jordan, *Life of Joseph Jordan*, 110.
[62] Bell, *Letters of Sir Charles Bell*, 200.
[63] Reinarz, 'The Age of Museum Medicine'.
[64] Chaplin, 'John Hunter'; Jessie Dobson, 'The Architectural History of the Hunterian Museum', *Annals of The Royal College of Surgeons of England*, 21 (1961), 113–26.
[65] Cameron, *Mr. Guy's Hospital*; Eve, 'Our Museum'; William Millard, *An Account of the Circumstances Attending the Imprisonment and Death of the Late William Millard* (London: Millard, 1825); F. G.Parsons, *The History of St Thomas's Hospital*, 3 vols. (London: Methuen, 1932–6).
[66] Martin Fallon (ed.), *The Sketches of Erinensis: Selections of Irish Medical Satire 1824–1836* (London: Skilton and Shaw, 1979), 17.
[67] Cameron, *History of the Royal College of Surgeons*.

moved to dedicated space (72 by 36 feet) leaving the morbid specimens in the 'old' museum. In Edinburgh, the dedicated premises that John Barclay demanded for his specimens were designed by William Henry Playfair and completed in 1832. The entire principal floor of the new Royal College was given over to the museum, the first chamber housing Barclay's collection, beyond which a galleried top-lit space, 97 by 40 feet, housed the college's other acquisitions that had been stored in various makeshift accommodation around Surgeon's Square.[68]

In the universities, in contrast to the royal colleges, anatomy collections were not the principal museums. The preparations were only one aspect of the Hunterian Museum in Glasgow, set aside from the rest of the university (and the medical teaching spaces) in the College Gardens to the east of the other buildings, in grand neo-Grecian premises designed by William Stark and opened in 1807 (see figure 2.2). Therein, the 'anatomical room' (38 by 18 feet, around the same dimensions the collection had occupied in Great Windmill Street) was the largest room at the back of the ground floor, behind the minerals and the corals. (A rusticated single-storey extension was added in 1839.) Similarly in Edinburgh, human anatomy occupied only part of the university's museum space. The anatomical collection Monro *secundus* donated had originally been housed in his father's old anatomy block after a new theatre was built in 1764.[69] The anatomy rooms in the new buildings on the 'Old College' quadrangle in the late eighteenth century then included a small museum space adjacent to the double-height anatomy theatre for the museum. But under Monro *tertius* this theatre was truncated at the first floor to create an impressive, octagonal chamber some 60 feet across (the anatomy lecture theatre occupying the same floor space it had, but with half the height). It was nonetheless dwarfed by Robert Jameson's museum of natural history next door.

Monro's new museum space was not ready for use until 1827. By this time, the new University of London was preparing to open its doors, and like its Scottish counterparts, museums were architecturally and conceptually central.[70] Appropriately for an institution inspired by the

---

[68] 'The Deeds of Settlement and Catalogue of the Barcleian Museum', bound MS, 1824–8, Royal College of Surgeons of Edinburgh Museum Archive; Charles W. Cathcart, 'Some of the Older Schools of Anatomy Connected with the Royal College of Surgeons, Edinburgh', *Edinburgh Medical Journal*, 27 (1882), 769–81; Kemp with Barnes, *Surgeon's Hall*; Tansey and Mekie, *The Museum of the Royal College of Surgeons of Edinburgh*.

[69] Fraser, *Building of Old College*.

[70] Bellot, *University College London*; William Filmer-Sankey and Lucy Markham, *University College London Library DDA Works PPG15 Justification* (London: Alan Baxter and Associates, 2004); Harte and North, *World of UCL*.

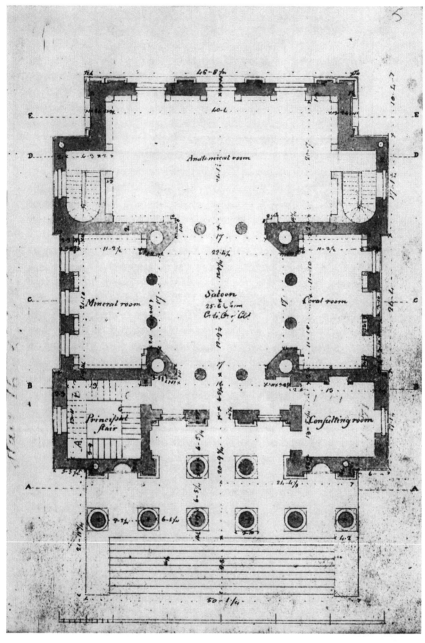

Fig. 2.2. Plan of the principal floor of the Hunterian Museum, University of Glasgow, designed by William Stark and completed in 1807. The 'anatomical room' can be seen at the top of the image. Glasgow University Library, Department of Special Collections.

philosophy of Jeremy Bentham, its collections presented an anatomical panopticon. Passing through the pillared portico, built at once to mimic and to dwarf the University of Edinburgh Old College building erected in the 1790s and which echoed the Hunterian in Glasgow, students turned left away from the grand library, and passed first through the massive natural history museum before entering the smaller museum of anatomy. As at Edinburgh, the space of Robert Grant's natural history collection dwarfed that provided for the medical collections used by Bell, Pattison, and Carswell. Only in 1859 did the collections switch places, so that the 'Museum of Anatomy and Pathology' occupied one of the largest and most privileged halls in the university, and occupied probably the largest footprint of any medical museum in the country—118 by 50 feet (beating by just 3 feet in length that of Trinity College School of Physic in Dublin).[71]

Whatever their relative sizes, the human anatomical collections in the universities tended to be located within or near the natural history collections. For other institutions, museums were carefully arranged near post-mortem and dissecting rooms, which functioned as important sources for anatomical and pathological 'raw material', as discussed in the next chapter. The Hunters' collections were housed adjacent to their teaching and dissecting spaces, and their successors over the century followed suit. Joseph Jordan's dissecting room in Manchester was next to his museum; access was a problem, however, especially for the grim cargo of the Resurrectionists: bodies had to come up via ladder from the back yard (the Alexanders Monro had originally used a tunnel from the back of Edinburgh University). In London, both the anatomy blocks built in 1814 at St Thomas's and in 1826 at Guy's situated the museum alongside the dissecting and post-mortem spaces (for the production of preparations) and the anatomical lecture hall (for their use).

If such facilities were not in the same building, the institutions were best served by being as close together as possible—medical schools such as the Royal School in Manchester and the University of Edinburgh were situated close to the infirmaries. The former was considered at a great disadvantage when absorbed into Owens College, a mile from the hospital. Here it was housed at the heart of the building Alfred Waterhouse designed for the College, around 50 by 30 feet, triple height with two galleries (see figure 2.3); its upper floors were adjacent to the well-lit dissecting room and the 'bone room'.[72] As one of the Professors who

[71] Wright, *Historical Guide to the City of Dublin*.
[72] Owens College *Calendar* (1874–5), 64 and (1883–4), John Rylands University Library of Manchester University Archives; Hartog, *Owens College Manchester*.

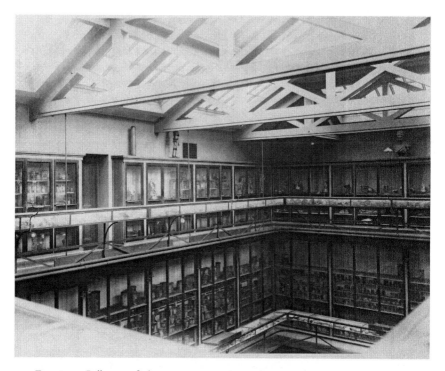

Fig. 2.3. Galleries of the Victoria University of Manchester Medical School Anatomy Museum, *c.* 1894. Manchester Medical Collection, reproduced by courtesy of the University Librarian and Director, The John Rylands University Library, The University of Manchester.

used it insisted, 'The Lecture room should be near the *museum.*'[73] Eventually the Manchester Royal Infirmary itself was moved from its original city centre location to be closer to the University of Manchester (which also received specimens regularly from three other hospitals), just as Glasgow's Western Infirmary, with a separate building for the pathological institute including a single-storey museum, had been erected next to the University after its removal from the city centre to Gilmorehill. Proximity to the dissecting room was a major driver in the fragmentation

[73] Victoria University, Report of the Medical Section of the Senate, 1889, 2, handwritten marginalia, original emphasis, John Rylands University Library of Manchester University Archives; Victoria University of Manchester, *Victoria University of Manchester Medical School* (Manchester: Manchester University Press, 1908).

of the Hunterian collection in Glasgow, which was debated from the 1880s.[74]

Over the course of the century, then, medical museums across the country had expanded considerably in both quantity and space. This growth was one significant driver for the disaggregation of the morbid anatomy sections from the wider collections. At Guy's, for example, the pathological preparations had expanded to fill much of the original anatomy block in the wake of the comparative and healthy anatomy, which were removed to the ground floor of another building, 'Hunt's House'. For those collections without new space, it became common practice to have pathology arranged on the gallery and healthy anatomy on the ground floor, or vice versa. In Edward I'Anson's grand 1881 neo-Florentine Portland stone museum and library block at St Bartholomew's, for instance, the anatomy museum was displayed in the gallery, separate from the pathology collection.[75] By the turn of the century, many collections were broken up entirely. At UCL the pathology collection was transferred to the Rockefeller building adjacent to University College Hospital in 1907.[76] Furthermore, the pathological institutes set up at this time included sizeable museums (see figure 2.4). We shall meet the professional communities who developed these institutes in the final part of this chapter, but better to understand how they emerged, we must first explore the other disciplines from which they distinguished themselves.

THE DISCIPLINARY LANDSCAPE

We may understand the place of collections not only through their physical location but also their conceptual situation. Spatial and disciplinary territories were co-constitutive in complex and interesting ways, as Frances Larson notes in her study of the intellectual landscape of the Oxford University Museum:

> the material substance and the intellectual character of . . . disciplines were less distinct then than might now be assumed. Negotiations concerning

---

[74] Keppie, *William Hunter*; A. E. Maylard, 'A Visit to the Human Anatomy Section of the Hunterian Museum, Glasgow University', *Glasgow Medical Journal*, 22 (1884), 9–18.

[75] Geoffrey Yeo, *Images of Bart's: An Illustrated History of St Bartholomew's Hospital in the City of London* (London: Historical Publications Ltd, in association with the Archives Department, St Bartholomew's Hospital, 1992).

[76] Bellot, *University College London*; Rickman John Godlee, *The Past, Present and Future of the School for Advanced Medical Studies of University College, London* (London: Bale and Danielsson, 1907); see also H. Campbell Thomson, *The Story of the Middlesex Hospital Medical School* (London: Murray, 1935).

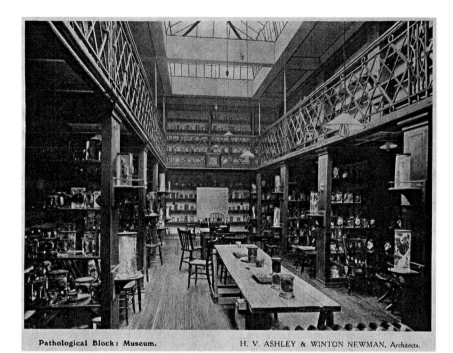

Pathological Block: Museum.　　　H. V. ASHLEY & WINTON NEWMAN, Architects.

Fig. 2.4. The interior of the museum in the pathological block, Royal Free Hospital, London, 1913. Process print, Henry Victor Ashley and Francis Winton Newman, Architects. Wellcome Library, London.

physical resources—in this case, collections and the buildings and facilities they required—were, in effect, negotiations regarding intellectual demarcations. These tangible entities not only shaped the geographies of academic identity but also provided, in a very unambiguous sense, the raw material for knowledge.[77]

Within and beyond medical museums, intellectual territory was carved out with specimens and other material, and this disciplinary landscape is the third scale of analysis deployed in this chapter in an effort to situate pathology in relation to cognate endeavours, especially (normal) anatomy, comparative anatomy, and anthropology.

Early medical collections were rarely formally demarcated, but their catalogues reveal that morbid anatomy dominated. Bichat's conception of

[77] Frances Larson, 'Anthropological Landscaping: General Pitt Rivers, the Ashmolean, the University Museum and the Shaping of an Oxford Discipline', *Journal of the History of Collections*, 20 (2008), 85–100 at 87.

the morbidity as a qualitative variation rather than the opposite of normal encouraged the juxtaposition of healthy and diseased parts in the museum, and, further, ensured the latter outnumbered the former. Hodgkin's museum at Guy's had examples of many morbid conditions to match each healthy specimen, by an average of two to one in his first catalogue.[78] The Mount Street School's museum in Manchester was 'rich in morbid specimens illustrating pathology', as was its counterpart on Marsden Street.[79] Pathological anatomy was nonetheless part of a physically and conceptually combined collection—when absorbed into the Manchester Royal School of Medicine they comprised 'both healthy and morbid conditions of the various bones, organs and processes ... illustrative, both of the pathology of disease, and of the healthy functions of the human frame'.[80] The Edinburgh University collection was not uncommon in being referred to as the 'Anatomical and Pathological Museum'.[81]

Over the course of the century, however, the sheer volume of diseased parts overwhelmed the healthy specimens. At the Middlesex in the 1890s, for example, normal anatomy and physiology occupied only the tables in the museum and pathology was arranged on manifold shelves from floor to ceiling. By the end of the century the major catalogues listed only the pathological specimens, indicating the conceptual independence of pathology.[82] Although they continued to be stored in the same space, at both Manchester and Edinburgh universities the morbid collection was by this time referred to as the 'Pathological Museum'.[83] The emergence of a pathological enterprise distinct from anatomy in the 1880s was thereby not only marked by the distinct spaces discussed above but also by a separation of the healthy and morbid anatomy within medical museums. Furthermore morbid specimens began to be used at a different stage in medical education—normal anatomy studied at foundation level, pathology included in advanced instruction.

Collections varied not only according to anatomical and pathological emphases, but also in their application to medicine or surgery, which

[78] Hodgkin, *Catalogue of the Preparations*.
[79] Edward Stephens, cited in Jordan, *Life of Joseph Jordan*, 41; Fawdington, *Catalogue Descriptive Chiefly of the Morbid Preparations*.
[80] 'A Relative', *Memoir of Thomas Turner*, 153.
[81] Royal Commission, *Minutes of Evidence*, appendix.
[82] See for example James Lorrain Smith, *A Catalogue of the Pathological Museum of the University of Manchester* (Manchester: Manchester University Press, 1906); Teacher, *Catalogue of the Anatomical and Pathological Preparations*.
[83] Owens College, *Catalogue of the Instruments Contained in the Obstetric Portion of the Medical Museum of the Owens College, Manchester* (Manchester: Sowler, 1884); Owens College, *Catalogue of the Preparations Contained in the Anatomical Portion of the Medical Museum of the Owens College, Manchester* (Manchester: Sowler, 1884).

varied from institution to institution and over time. Guy's curators were physicians, whereas the St Thomas's collection, so shaped by Astley Cooper, was more a surgeon's museum. The latter's interest, as his nephew wrote, 'led him to frame the plan for a museum to be composed principally of specimens connected with the study of the several diseases which came under the notice of the surgeon'.[84] Some museums had distinct medical and surgical parts, as St George's had in the middle of the century and University College towards the end.[85] Other more distinct areas such as obstetrics are gradually evident within the collections.[86] Such material fiefdoms within museums are nicely encapsulated in the University of Glasgow's daily register of accessions:

> October 1st 1850. On Dr Laurie succeeding to the Chair of Surgery the casts found in Dr Burns classroom + museum together with other preparations were divided between the professors of Midwifery + Dr Laurie the former taking those preparations illustrative of obstetrics, the latter taking those illustrative of surgery. A number of preparations were left by both, wh. being strictly Anatomical were taken care of by Dr A. Thomson.[87]

In the mid century, collections were clearly demarcated by staff and space.

Many museums also included dentistry, whether within the main medical museum or as a distinct area, which 'odontological' collections were especially strong in comparative anatomy because of the interest in the jaws and teeth of animals.[88] These were by no means the only point of overlap between human and other fauna, however. John Hunter was as much a naturalist as he was an anatomist, and William's collection was

---

[84] Bransby Blake Cooper, *The Life of Sir Astley Cooper, Bart.*, 2 vols. (London: Parker, 1843), ii. 99.

[85] John W. Ogle and Timothy Holmes (eds.), *Catalogue of the Pathological Museum of St George's Hospital* (London: Wertheimer, 1866); Charles Stonham, *Descriptive Catalogue of the Specimens Illustrating Medical Pathology in the Museum of University College, London* (London: University College, 1890).

[86] See for example Owens College, *Catalogue of the Instruments*; John Williams and Charles Stonham, *Descriptive Catalogue of the Specimens Illustrating the Pathology of Gynaecology and Obstetric Medicine Contained in the Museum of University College, London* (London: University College, 1891).

[87] Thomson, 'Daily Register of Objects', 14. On fiefdoms within museums, see Alberti, *Nature and Culture*.

[88] On the Guy's dentistry collection see P. H. Pye-Smith, *Catalogue of the Preparations of Comparative Anatomy in the Museum of Guy's Hospital* (London: Ash, 1874); on the Birmingham Dental School Museum, see John Humphreys, *Catalogue of the Collection of Skulls and Teeth in the Odontological Museum of the University of Birmingham* (Birmingham: Cornish, 1916); Reinarz, 'The Age of Museum Medicine'.

very strong in natural history.[89] As a result, the Royal College of Surgeons collection had a strong zoological element: visitors were met with a veritable stampede of quadrupeds as they entered the main gallery. Thanks to John Barclay, so did its counterpart in Edinburgh. The boundaries between anatomist and naturalist, surgeon and veterinarian were permeable—as in the case of Joshua Brookes, with his renowned comparative osteological collection; among the students he trained there was Edward Stephens of Manchester, who not only taught at Mount Street and Pine Street but also acted as surgeon to the zoological gardens in Higher Broughton.[90] Zoological specimens were common features of medical museums throughout the nineteenth century, whether as complete mounts in the centre of the galleries (see figure 2.5) or partial preparations juxtaposed with the human fragments in the cases. The first specimen acquired by the Birmingham Medical School Museum was the head of a hippopotamus, and at many other hospital and medical school museums, comparative specimens were distributed liberally among the human anatomy.[91] Those medical collections without animal specimens were often nevertheless adjacent to natural history collections, as we saw earlier. The comparative anatomy at Guy's originally occupied the left wing of the 1825 museum block; in the 1830s it expanded into the old dissecting room before moving to its own space in Hunt's House in the mid century.[92] In Manchester, the human anatomy collection was the first functioning museum at the new premises of Owens College in

---

[89] On the Hunters as naturalists, see C. Helen Brock, 'Dr William Hunter's Museum, Glasgow University', *Journal of the Society for the Bibliography of Natural History*, 9 (1980), 403–12; Simon Chaplin, 'Nature Dissected, or Dissection Naturalized? The Case of John Hunter's Museum', *Museum and Society*, 6 (2008), 135–51; Stephen J. Cross, 'John Hunter, the Animal Oeconomy, and Late Eighteenth-Century Physiological Discourse', *Studies in History of Biology*, 5 (1981), 1–110; Keppie, *William Hunter*; W.D. Ian Rolfe, 'William and John Hunter: Breaking the Great Chain of Being', in William F. Bynum and Roy Porter (eds.), *William Hunter and the Eighteenth-Century Medical World* (Cambridge: Cambridge University Press, 1985), 297–319.

[90] Jordan, *Life of Joseph Jordan*; on Astley Cooper as zoologist, see Druin Burch, *Digging up the Dead: Uncovering the Life and Times of an Extraordinary Surgeon* (London: Chatto and Windus, 2007).

[91] Joseph Jordan, 'Catalogue of the Preparations of the Mount Street School Belonging to Joseph Jordan', MS ledger, 1824–37, Manchester Medical Collection, 23.1.58, John Rylands University Library of Manchester; Reinarz, 'The Age of Museum Medicine'; Anthony A. Bowlby, *A Descriptive Catalogue of the Anatomical and Pathological Museum of St Bartholomew's Hospital* (London: Churchill, 1884); J. Jackson Clarke, *Descriptive Catalogue of the Pathological Museum of St Mary's Hospital* (London: Morton and Burt, 1891); Fawdington, *Catalogue Descriptive Chiefly of the Morbid Preparations*; James Paget, *A Descriptive Catalogue of the Anatomical Museum of St Bartholomew's Hospital* (London: Churchill, 1846); 'A Relative', *Memoir of Thomas Turner*.

[92] See for example Pye-Smith, *Catalogue of the Preparations of Comparative Anatomy*.

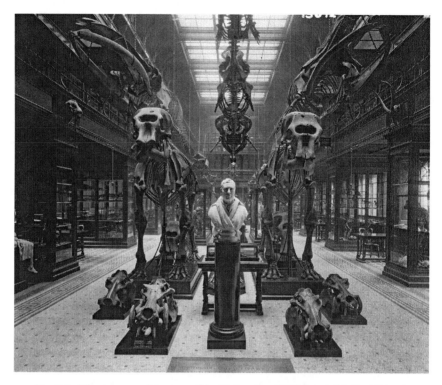

Fig. 2.5. The Anatomy Museum of the University of Edinburgh Medical School, Teviot Place, Edinburgh, 1898. Copyright the Royal Commission on the Ancient and Historical Monuments of Scotland; B/64386. Licensor www.scran.ac.uk.

Manchester, but in the 1880s the college also erected a large natural history museum, and there was considerable traffic between the two.[93]

Disciplinary divisions were not only evident between human and animal specimens but also between different kinds of human remains. The relationship between anatomy and the emerging field of ethnology was complex, but medical museums were commonly sites for the comparison of different races as well as different diseases.[94] Eighteenth-century

[93] Alberti, *Nature and Culture*.

[94] Cressida Fforde, *Collecting the Dead: Archaeology and the Reburial Issue* (London: Duckworth, 2004); Elizabeth Hallam, 'La Fabrication du Savoir sur le Corps en Écosse, de 1880 à 1930 [Anthropometric Laboratory: Making Knowledge of the Body in Scotland *c.* 1880–1930]', *Ethnologie Française*, 37/275–284 (2007); Hallam, *Anatomy Museum*; Helen MacDonald, *Human Remains: Dissection and Its Histories* (London: Yale University Press, 2006).

medical collectors often included extra-European human remains in their collections, especially ancient Egyptian mummies. Human remains from elsewhere in the world found their way into medical museums in great numbers as part of the various ethnological endeavours in the nineteenth century. Skulls were of particular interest. Charles White in Manchester is alleged to have measured heads of different peoples passing through the port of Liverpool; no doubt he also constructed his notions of racial hierarchy from the specimens in his collection.[95] Craniologists and phreno- nologists found a secure disciplinary home within medical museums, often the obvious site for storing the hundreds of skulls they used for comparison. In 1873 Allen Thomson in Glasgow for example accepted a 'Skull of a Female Bosjesman from the Cape of Good Hope. . . . the body had been buried the skeleton was exhumed by Mr J. B. Knobel student and the skull presented to me in exchange for one macerated in the rooms'; by the turn of the century, the University of Glasgow sported nearly 300 crania.[96] In 1886, the University of Edinburgh incorporated the huge collection of the Edinburgh Phrenological Society into the anatomy museum.[97] As pathology collections emerged as distinct material encyclopaedias of difference in the later century, other non-European specimens were often classified within them, as deviations from the European anatomical norm.[98] Rudolf Virchow, the doyen of Euro- pean pathologists, included what we would now term anthropology firmly within his remit, and his renowned Pathological Institute in Berlin included a vast collection of human remains from across the globe. Anthropology overlapped significantly with pathology as the sciences of deviance.[99]

Nevertheless, by 1900 diseased body parts were at the core of pathology as a discrete disciplinary endeavour. There were undoubted similarities with other neighbouring fields and objects: natural history also involved organic specimens; anthropology, archaeology, and Egyptology also involved fragmented human remains, many of them deviant; and there is an extent to which all collections comprise scattered parts of people.[100]

[95] White, *Account of the Regular Gradation in Man*.

[96] Thomson, 'Daily Register of Objects', 10; John Cleland, *Catalogue of the Crania in the Museum of the Anatomical Department of the University of Glasgow* (Glasgow: MacLe- hose, 1909).

[97] Kaufman, *Medical Teaching in Edinburgh*.

[98] See for example Jordan, 'Catalogue of the preparations'; Thomson, 'Daily Register of Objects'.

[99] Matyssek, *Rudolf Virchow*; Roslyn Poignant, *Professional Savages: Captive Lives and Western Spectacle* (New Haven, Conn.; London: Yale University Press, 2004).

[100] Janet Hoskins, 'On Losing and Getting a Head: Warfare, Exchange, and Alliance in a Changing Sumba, 1888–1988', *American Ethnologist*, 16 (1989), 419–40;

But the emergence of pathology as a discrete enterprise depended on distinguishing the diseased body part from these other potentially similar objects. The following chapters will reveal more details of such disciplinary territories as they were materially manifested in collections. But such territories are established with museum things by museum people, and the final element of the groundwork necessary to understand the role of morbid specimens in this cultural cartography is to assess the function and apparently anomalous status of those who had custody of them in Britain.

THE STATUS OF PATHOLOGY

Morbid anatomy, then, had a considerable material presence in the British medical marketplace by the 1820s. Tens of thousands of diseased body parts accumulated in medical schools, universities and royal colleges. And yet as historians of pathology tell us, unlike France, pathological anatomy failed as a professional enterprise in Britain; and unlike Germany, there was no distinct profession of pathology at all until the late century.[101] If, as I have argued, disciplines are writ large in material culture, why this disparity between collections, ideas, and personnel? Why did pathology 'fail' in Britain in the early century? The answer lies in the location of pathology and its objects within the particularities of the British medical profession.

Robert Carswell was appointed *in absentia* to the first chair in pathology in Britain and the University of London in 1828; he actually took up his post as his friend and mentor John Thomson was appointed to the second in Edinburgh in 1831; in the mean time, Herbert Mayo, who would later establish the Middlesex Hospital Medical School, had been appointed to a chair of anatomy, physiology, and pathology at King's.[102] This did not, however, usher in a fully fledged profession as they might have hoped: like many medical teaching appointments in Britain, these posts were part-time; none remained in post for more than a decade; and Carswell and Thomson were reliant on anatomical collections under others' jurisdiction

Susan M. Pearce, *On Collecting: An Investigation into Collecting in the European Tradition* (London and New York: Routledge, 1995).

[101] Maulitz, *Morbid Appearances*; Cay-Rüdiger Prüll, 'Pathology and Politics in the Metropolis, 1900–1945: London, Berlin and the Third Reich', in Margit Szöllösi-Janze (ed.), *Science in the Third Reich* (Oxford: Berg, 2001), 139–83.

[102] Cunningham, *History of British Pathology*; W.D. Foster, *Pathology as a Profession in Great Britain and the Early History of the Royal College of Pathologists* (London: Royal College of Pathologists, 1983); H. Willoughby Lyle, *King's and Some King's Men* (Oxford: Oxford University Press, 1935).

(respectively Richard Quain at UCL and Monro *tertius* in Edinburgh). For the next fifty years, the few pathology positions there were in Britain were low-prestige, poorly paid, early career posts, taken by would-be physicians or surgeons as a step to a medical or surgical appointment. At the Manchester proprietary schools, for example, pathology was taught by one of the junior lecturers—in both Jordan's and Turner's schools, by their nephews (Edward Stephens and William Smith respectively).

Although these teaching posts depended on the collections (see chapter 6), such staff did not always have responsibility for the museums. Curating a hospital collection was usually the duty of the inspector of the dead, usually taken for a short period *en route* to a full hospital appointment.[103] Their principal duty was the autopsy, viewed as a service for the clinician on the case. Even such a committed pathological anatomist as Thomas Hodgkin at Guy's was so keen to take the next step on the career ladder that he resigned the curatorship while lobbying for the assistant physicianship at Guy's.[104] (He failed, thanks largely to his stark political differences with the treasurer Benjamin Harrison.) Among the more prominent of his successors—all of whom went on to a full position at Guy's after the mid century—was Samuel Wilks (who coined 'Hodgkin's Lymphoma' in honour of his predecessor), who held the curatorship while assistant physician, but resigned when appointed full physician.[105] Elsewhere, luminaries such as James Paget held museum appointments (in his case at Bartholomew's) early in their careers.[106] Those few who wanted to follow a museum career tended to be zoologists. Richard Owen and William Henry Flower both curated a hospital collection and the Royal College of Surgeons on their way to becoming first and second directors of the British Museum (Natural History).[107] Positions connected to morbid anatomy collections, and pathology more generally, remained ancillary to practice until the 1880s in Britain, whereas in the German states, by contrast, from the mid century, pathological institutes provided secure

[103] Zachary Cope, *The History of St Mary's Hospital Medical School or a Century of Medical Education* (London: Heinemann, 1954); Foster, *Pathology as a Profession*; L. Stephen Jacyna, 'The Laboratory and the Clinic: The Impact of Pathology on Surgical Diagnosis in the Glasgow Western Infirmary 1875–1910', *Bulletin of the History of Medicine*, 62 (1988), 384–406; Prüll, 'Pathology and Politics'; Reinarz, 'The Age of Museum Medicine'.

[104] Hodgkin Manuscript Material, Wellcome Library WMS/PP/HO/D/B75–100; Kass and Kass, *Perfecting the World*.

[105] Guy's Hospital Museum, Minute Book, 1904, Gordon Museum Archive, King's College London; William Hale-White, 'In Memoriam. Samuel Wilks', *Guy's Hospital Reports*, 67 (1913), 1–39.

[106] Foster, *Pathology as a Profession*; Paget, *Memoirs and Letters*.

[107] Charles J. Cornish, *Sir William Henry Flower* (London: MacMillan, 1904); Rupke, *Richard Owen*.

institutional bases for full-time pathologists.[108] Only in the 1880s did developments elsewhere in the medical firmament render pathology a more prestigious career route, and shift the character of the personnel associated with medical museums.

As germ theories of disease began to proliferate in Britain, pathologists were in high demand to understand disease at a cellular level. Michael Worboys encapsulates this change:

> Pathologists were the medical specialists best placed by expertise and opportunity to pursue bacteriological work, because of their skills in microscopy, the handling of morbid specimens and prior studies of inflammation. Many pathologists had used their extended repertoire and the demands for teaching to convert their hospital and museum appointments from part-time to full-time, and there was an optimism in the late 1880s that pathology was at a new dawn as the 'science of disease'.[109]

By the 1890s, the demand for clinical diagnostic pathology was sufficient to support service laboratories in hospitals and universities, such as those at King's College and St Thomas's in London. The first full-time professional pathologists in Britain, therefore, were clinical bacteriologists. This 'bacteriological revolution' depended as much on the existing material resources of morbid anatomy as it did on clinical and intellectual developments. Worboys astutely views the emergence of germ theories of diseases as the production of social and material practices; in establishing pathology as the science of disease, medical museums were a key part of these materials. The new pathologists found they already had at their disposal vast encyclopaedias of disease in gross and microscopic form.

When academic positions associated with pathology became more prestigious in the 1880s, then, they tended to be in institutions already associated with large pathological anatomy collections.[110] The University of Cambridge appointed its first chair in pathology in the 1880s. Edinburgh's was the only professor of pathology in Scotland until 1882, when a new chair was established in Aberdeen, which had a sizeable collection. Joseph Coats, pathologist at the Glasgow Royal and Western infirmaries in Glasgow (and curator at both) had been teaching pathology for a quarter of a century before he was finally appointed to the independent

---

[108] Prüll, 'Pathology and Politics'.

[109] Michael Worboys, *Spreading Germs: Disease Theories and Medical Practice in Britain, 1865–1900* (Cambridge: Cambridge University Press, 2000), 215–16; John Waller, *The Discovery of the Germ: Twenty Years That Transformed the Way We Think About Disease* (Cambridge: Icon, 2002).

[110] Cunningham, History of British Pathology; Hallam, *Anatomy Museum*; Jacyna, 'Laboratory and the Clinic'; Teacher, 'On the History of Pathology'.

pathology chair at the University in 1894. In Dublin, the Catholic University Medical School established a chair in 1891, while Trinity College only had a separate lectureship from 1895.

In Manchester, the accomplished morbid anatomist Julius Dreschfeld's responsibilities as lecturer in pathology at Owens College from 1875 included caring for the morbid preparations at the medical museum. In 1881 he was appointed to the first chair.[111] Dreschfeld was always part-time, however, and followed the earlier established route to the chair of medicine in 1891. His successor, Sheridan Delépine, who had been pathologist and curator at St George's Hospital in London, was the first full-time professor of pathology.[112] In contrast to Dreschfeld's older clinical approach, Delépine did not practice but was a pioneering bacteriologist, and he set up a thriving public health laboratory. In 1903 the chair was split to reflect this, and James Lorrain Smith was appointed to the chair of pathology and pathological anatomy. Dreschfeld and Delépine had been closely involved with the museum and Smith spent his first years in post compiling a massive catalogue of the now-distinct pathology collection.[113] They were also at the heart of the re-launched Pathological Society of Manchester. Emerging from the Microscopical Section of the Manchester Medical Society in 1885, the society was far larger than its mid-century predecessor (see above). 'The cultivation and promotion of Pathology,' were its aims, 'by the Exhibition of Specimens, Microscopic Preparations, Casts, Models etc., illustrative of Morbid Conditions; by the investigation of Morbid Products'.[114] Clearly morbid preparations remain vital to late nineteenth-century pathology.

[111] Owens College *Calendar* (1974–5), John Rylands University Library of Manchester University Archives; Peter D. Mohr, 'Dreschfeld, Julius (1845–1907)', *Oxford Dictionary of National Biography* (Oxford: Oxford University Press, 2004), www.oxforddnb.com/view/article/32891, accessed 14 July 2008; Samuel Oleesky, 'Julius Dreschfeld', *Manchester Medical Gazette*, 51 (1971), 14–17, 58–60, 96–99; Pickstone, *Medicine and Industrial Society*; Helen K. Valiér, 'Between Science and Clinical Practice: A History of Pathology in Manchester, c.1870–1905' (M.Sc. thesis, University of Manchester, 1997).

[112] R.M. Stirland, 'Auguste Sheridan Delépine, 1855–1921', in Elwood and Tuxford, *Some Manchester Doctors*, 107–12, Valiér, 'Between Science and Clinical Practice'.

[113] Smith, *Catalogue of the Pathological Museum*; R. M., 'James Lorrain Smith 1862–1931', *Journal of Pathology and Bacteriology*, 34 (1931), 683–96.

[114] Pathological Society of Manchester, *Laws of the Pathological Society of Manchester* (Manchester: Meredith, 1898), 1; Archive of the Pathological Society of Manchester, PSM/4/1/1, John Rylands University Library of Manchester University Archive; Davson, 'The Pathological Society of Manchester'; Harris, 'Historical Sketch'; T. N. Kelynack (ed.), *The Transactions of the Pathological Society of Manchester for the Session 1891–2* (Manchester: Heywood, 1892); James Peters and Elizabeth Gow, *The John Rylands University Library MMC Manchester Medical Collection Sections 3–8*, Archive Description (Manchester: John Rylands University Library, 2005); Valiér, 'Between Science and Clinical Practice'.

By this time, however, specimen-based morbid anatomy was only one of a range of pathologies. In the museum, as we have seen, pathology bordered other museum disciplines: zoology, anatomy, anthropology. Likewise in British medicine, these collections operated alongside other sites and media. Ian Burney has demonstrated the relationship between forensic pathology and the inquest.[115] Clinical pathology was practised on the living as other pathologies were on the dead: the ward was a vital site for the British tradition that emerged in the late nineteenth century, especially in London where the hospitals remained all-powerful.[116] But the laboratory is the site that has been afforded the most historical attention for this period. Bacteriology was first and foremost a laboratory activity, and every hospital and university mentioned here had a laboratory by the turn of the century.[117] Nevertheless, bacteriologists continued to rely on large banks of slide specimens that were often stored in museums, and early twentieth-century pathological institutes, like their German forebears, commonly included laboratory and museum spaces in juxtaposition.[118] At Charing Cross for example, 'The Hospital and the School have for many years been in possession of an exceptionally good and well-arranged Pathological Museum containing over 3,000 to 4,000 prepared specimens. The additional Laboratory provision now made for Pathology gives the Hospital one of the most commodious and well-adapted Pathological Institutes attached to any Hospital or School of Medicine.'[119]

Throughout the century, especially in the 1830s and again with renewed vigour in the 1880s and 90s, the medical museum lent physicians, surgeons, and (later) pathologists raw material, positions, and credibility.[120] Those who would build disciplines did so with collections.

---

[115] Ian A. Burney, *Bodies of Evidence: Medicine and the Politics of the Inquest 1830–1926* (Baltimore: Johns Hopkins University Press, 2000).

[116] Prüll, 'Pathology and Politics'; Cay- Rüdiger Prüll (ed.), *Traditions of Pathology in Western Europe: Theories, Institutions and Their Cultural Setting* (Herbolzheim: Centaurus, 2003).

[117] Cooke, *Scientific Medicine*; Cunningham, *History of British Pathology*; Foster, *Pathology as a Profession*; Prüll, 'Pathology and Politics'.

[118] On the development of microscopic techniques in mid-century pathology, see L. Stephen Jacyna, '"A Host of Experienced Microscopists": The Establishment of Histology in Nineteenth-Century Edinburgh', *Bulletin of the History of Medicine*, 75 (2001), 225–53; Worboys, *Spreading Germs*.

[119] William Hunter, *Historical Account of Charing Cross Hospital and Medical School* (London: Murray, 1914), 247.

[120] Samuel J. M. M. Alberti, 'The Status of Museums: Authority, Identity and Material Culture', in David N. Livingstone and Charles W. J. Withers (eds.), *Geographies of Nineteenth-Century Science* (Chicago: University of Chicago Press, 2011).

MATERIALITY AND DISCIPLINARITY

'At an early period diseased parts were preserved in private collections, and afterwards in museums', observed *The Lancet* in 1833. 'These have rapidly multiplied. Every medical school and hospital has its museum.'[121] Formally or otherwise, a collection was a requisite for any anatomy teaching. The Edinburgh anatomist Frederick Knox argued that 'he who attempts to teach anatomy without a museum *bona fide* his own, and, if possible, made by himself, as strictly deserves the name of impostor... every museum takes its character, as it were, from the person who may have formed that collection'.[122] Similarly, staff of the Glasgow Royal Infirmary insisted in 1852,

> a museum seems to be really necessary in order that the institution may keep pace as a school of medicine with the facilities and advantages of a like description which are afforded by most recognized hospitals in the kingdom; and certainly a collection of illustrative specimens would greatly enhance the value of clinical instruction carried on in the infirmary.[123]

The layered map of medical museums presented in this chapter has revealed how closely they related to the institutional configuration of medical education, practice, and research in nineteenth-century Britain, and hinted at their use for entertainment (see chapter 6).

Despite the strangely late birth of the pathology profession, morbid specimens were always significant in medical training (if nothing else). As the status of pathology ebbed and flowed over the century, taken up in different sites for different reasons, collections were a constant presence. The relationship between communities of practice and a collection was complex and contingent; the precipitation of specialisms did not necessarily map directly onto the shape of collections. Before 1880, there were massive pathological anatomy collections, but few pathologists; yet these collections played a key (and overlooked) role in the construction of a professional community of pathologists around the turn of the century.

Pathology, like many other late-Victorian disciplines that condensed around and gave rise to massive collections, was fundamentally material.

[121] 'Pathological Anatomy', *The Lancet*, 23 November 1833, 326–31 at 326–7. On collections and credibility, see Alberti, 'The Status of Museums'; Bates, '"Indecent and Demoralising Representations"'; Desmond, *Politics of Evolution*; Reinarz, 'The Age of Museum Medicine'.
[122] Knox, *The Anatomist's Instructor*, 5.
[123] Minutes of the Pathological Museum Committee of the Glasgow Royal Infirmary 1852, cited in Teacher, 'On the History of Pathology', 12.

The intellectual and organizational basis of a whole set of endeavours in Britain, not yet disciplines, had been laid down in collections in the first half of the century; they then expanded and differentiated in the period 1880–1930. This chapter has charted only one of these, pathological anatomy, which was bordered in the museum by other anatomies (comparative, normal) and operated in conflict and concert outside the museum with other pathologies (clinical, forensic). Museum things were not just boundary objects, however, but were at the heart of pathology, and of medicine. Disciplinary foundation, development, and even 'failure' can be traced through the historical geography of museums, when assessed on a range of levels as we have here. In short, if we want to understand the natural and medical sciences, we need to know about the museums on which they were built. We need to understand the particular configuration of practitioner, built environment, and object in and around nineteenth-century museums. And yet, although pathological facts are locally situated and materially embedded, charting them is not enough. We need to understand how they were collected and the meanings they accrued; the practices enacted upon them; and how they were arranged, used, and experienced.

3

Collecting Pathology

Fragmentation and the Traffic in Morbid Flesh

The famous caricature of William Hunter's museum at Great Windmill Street (figure 3.1) illustrates well the somatic fragmentation brought about by medical collecting, and the anxiety generated by such violations of the integrity of the body. In 'The Resurrection' two of the unfortunate corpses argue over a dismembered limb: 'What this! . . . Devil burn me if it be not my own I know it by the lump on my skin here', to which his neighbour rebuts, 'Damn me Sir that's—my Legg'. The corpulent gentleman on the right has lost his stomach, and another is in even worse straights: 'Where's my Head'? The elderly lady is aghast at the transgression of her inviolability, demanding that Hunter 'Restore to me my Virgin-boner[,] did I keep it inviolated 75 years to have it given up at last'? Hunter, meanwhile, is more concerned for the integrity of his collection: 'O what a smash among my Bottles & Preparations! never did I suppose that such a day would come'. Nevertheless, two centuries later, his museum endures at the University of Glasgow, material evidence of how much he valued these fragments.

So far this book has been concerned with the institutions and individuals that comprised the medical marketplace and the exhibitionary complex in nineteenth-century Britain. This chapter now sets these webs in motion, following the paths of diseased bodies through them as they were broken up and exchanged, analysing the relationships they engendered, and the accompanying shifts in their meaning and value. It assesses how pathological specimens came to be in collections by tracing the trajectories of such objects from their source to the museum shelf: the social (after)life of morbid body parts. Before arriving at the museum, specimens followed complex paths involving different kinds of exchanges, and tracking their passage gives us glimpses of key moments and practices. Just as bodies experience transformative processes during life, so after death, body parts are subject to significant physical and symbolic alterations. What happened to them during their conceptual journey from person to the museum? What layers of meaning

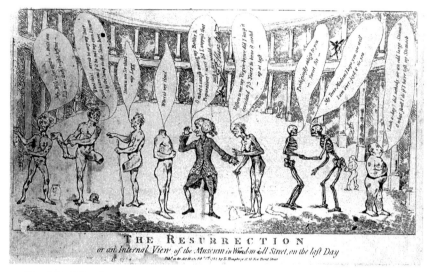

Fig. 3.1. 'The Resurrection or an internal view of the Museum [of William Hunter] in Windmill Street, on the last Day', attributed to Thomas Rowlandson, 1782. Wellcome Library, London.

adhered to these fragments during autopsy, donation, and purchase? What social and intellectual function did these exchanges serve?

As well as explaining the mechanics of nineteenth-century medical museum acquisition, answering these questions deepens our understanding of the movement of human remains for other purposes at other times. Organ transplants and tissue trafficking in the twenty-first century, for example, have long histories, and setting them in this rich context benefits their cultural analysis. Recent legislation regulating the transport and storage of human remains for anatomical study is only the latest chapter in a story that stretches for centuries.

DISMEMBERMENT

Our journey begins with bodily dismemberment—whether in a domestic setting or in an operating theatre, on the dissecting table or the autopsy slab. We then follow the general passage of these partible somatic fragments, especially how they were exchanged as gifts and at auction sales, and then conclude by reflecting on the impact of these processes on the meaning and value of the body parts, their transformation from *subject* to *object* (a process, we shall see, that began even before death). Anthropologists, historians, and philosophers have addressed the psychological and ethical issues thrown up by the traffic in bodies: here we are concerned with the material and museological implications of the circulation of human remains in the nineteenth century. This will provide much-needed historical context to contemporary debates around the market in tissue cultures and organs, emphasizing that the commodification and exchange of body parts was not novel to the late twentieth century. But while drawing parallels between contemporary and Victorian movements of fragmented bodies, we should also be sensitive to differences in meaning and consequences of this traffic over time. We can find evidence of mobilized corpses in many different times and places—from saintly relics to the reburial of political heroes in post-socialist Europe—but the uses and values of dead bodies are not universal.[1]

Figure 3.1 vividly demonstrates the polysemy of human remains, the tensions between person and thing, between the collector seeking to categorize and the stubborn resistance of the object-people in medical museums. These tensions arise especially around the removal and (mis-) use of parts. One later visitor to William Hunter's museum considered what he observed to be 'disgusting, lacerated fragments'.[2] In many ways fragmentation is and was the most significant and problematic aspect of the use of dead bodies for medical purposes. And yet in the expansive

---

[1] On the similarities, see Linda F. Hogle, *Recovering the Nation's Body: Cultural Memory, Medicine, and the Politics of Redemption* (New Brunswick, NJ: Rutgers University Press, 1999); Nancy Scheper-Hughes, 'Bodies for Sale—Whole or in Parts', in Nancy Scheper-Hughes and Loïc J.D. Wacquant (eds.), *Commodifying Bodies* (London: Sage, 2002), 1–8. On the differences, see Bronwyn Parry and Cathy Gere, 'Contested Bodies: Property Models and the Commodification of Human Biological Artefacts', *Science as Culture*, 15 (2006), 139–58; Michael Sappol, *A Traffic of Dead Bodies: Anatomy and Embodied Social Identity in Nineteenth-Century America* (Princeton; Oxford: Princeton University Press, 2002); Duncan Wilson, 'Whose Body (of Opinion) Is It Anyway? Historicising Tissue Ownership and Problematising Public Opinion in Bioethics', in Barbara Katz Rothman, Elizabeth M. Armstrong, and Rebecca Tiger (eds.), *Bioethical Issues, Sociological Perspectives*, Advances in Medical Sociology 9 (Amsterdam: Elsevier, 2008), 9–32. See also Lori Andrews and Dorothy Nelkin, *Body Bazaar: The Market for Human Tissue in the Biotechnology Age* (New York: Crown, 2001); Donna Dickenson, *Body Shopping: The Economy Fuelled by Flesh and Blood* (Oxford: Oneworld, 2008); Renée C. Fox and Judith P. Swazey, *Spare Parts: Organ Replacement in American Society* (Oxford: Oxford University Press, 1992); Erin O'Connor, *Raw Material: Producing Pathology in Victorian Culture* (Durham, NC: Duke University Press, 2000); Lesley A. Sharp, *Strange Harvest: Organ Transplants, Denatured Bodies, and the Transformed Self* (Berkeley: University of California Press, 2006); Lesley A. Sharp, *Bodies, Commodities, and Biotechnologies: Death, Mourning, and Scientific Desire in the Realm of Human Organ Transfer* (New York: Columbia University Press, 2007); Katherine Verdery, *The Political Lives of Dead Bodies: Reburial and Postsocialist Change* (New York: Columbia University Press, 1999).

[2] Benjamin Silliman, *A Journal of Travels in England, Holland and Scotland*, 2 vols. (2nd edn, New Haven, Conn.: Converse, 1812), ii. 293.

literature on the traffic of corpses for dissection (especially concerning the sordid activities of the grave-robbing 'Resurrection Men' and scandals such as the murdering activities of William Hare and William Burke) there is little on the results of the dismemberment of the cadavers.[3] For although most corpses travelled no further than the incinerator, for those organs, tissues and bones that were selected for preservation and further study, the dissecting table was only the beginning. This study addresses the fate of these body parts after dismemberment and the physical and symbolic effects of their fragmentation. Anthony Shelton observes that all museum objects are fragments: 'masks without costumes; figures without shrines; shrines without sacrifices; architectural pieces removed from their buildings... The meaning of objects is hybrid, [exposing the] tension between their previous lives and the stories of their removal and reincorporation'.[4] But different objects bear these meanings in distinct ways, and the movement of separate body parts is especially characteristic of the acquisition routes that led to pathological anatomy collections.

In modern Europe, the revulsion at the prospect of dismemberment stemmed from early Christian attitudes to complete bodily resurrection.[5]

---

[3] Michael J. Durey, 'Bodysnatchers and Benthamites: The Implications of the Dead Body Bill for the London Schools of Anatomy, 1820–42', *The London Journal*, 2 (1976), 200–25; Cressida Fforde, *Collecting the Dead: Archaeology and the Reburial Issue* (London: Duckworth, 2004); John Fleetwood, *The Irish Body Snatchers: A History of Body Snatching in Ireland* (Dublin: Tomar, 1988); Elizabeth T. Hurren, *Dying for Victorian Medicine: English Anatomy and Its Trade in the Dead Poor, 1870 to 1929* (London: Palgrave Macmillan, forthcoming); Fiona Hutton, 'The Working of the 1832 Anatomy Act in Oxford and Manchester', *Family and Community History*, 9 (2006), 125–39; Matthew H. Kaufman, 'Transfer of Bodies to the University of Edinburgh after the 1832 Anatomy Act', *Journal of the Royal College of Physicians of Edinburgh*, 34 (2004), 228–36; Helen MacDonald, *Human Remains: Dissection and Its Histories* (London: Yale University Press, 2006); Helen MacDonald, 'Procuring Corpses: The English Anatomy Inspectorate, 1842 to 1858', *Medical History*, 53 (2009), 379–96; Helen MacDonald, *Possessing the Dead: The Artful Science of Anatomy* (Melbourne: Melbourne University Publishing, 2010); Ruth Richardson, *Death, Dissection and the Destitute* (2nd edn, London: Phoenix, 2001). Studies that *do* address fragmentation in the medical museum context include Simon Chaplin, 'Nature Dissected, or Dissection Naturalized? The Case of John Hunter's Museum', *Museum and Society*, 6 (2008), 135–51; Elizabeth Hallam, *Anatomy Museum. Death and the Body Displayed* (London: Reaktion, 2011); Anna Maerker, '19th-Century Anatomical Models: Fragmentation and Normativity in French Papier-Mâché Anatomies' (M.Phil. thesis, Cambridge University, 1998).

[4] Anthony A. Shelton, 'Curating *African Worlds*', in Laura Peers and Alison Brown (eds.), *Museums and Source Communities* (London: Routledge, 2003), 181–93 at 187. On the metaphorical fragmentation of illness, see Jessica Hughes, 'Fragmentation as Metaphor in the Classical Healing Sanctuary', *Social History of Medicine*, 21 (2008), 217–36.

[5] Caroline Walker Bynum, *Fragmentation and Redemption: Essays on Gender and the Human Body in Medieval Religion* (New York: Zone, 1991); Caroline Walker Bynum, *The Resurrection of the Body in Western Christianity, 200–1336* (New York: Columbia University Press, 1995); Lucia Dacome, 'Resurrecting by Numbers in Eighteenth-Century England', *Past and Present*, 193 (2006), 73–110.

Images such as the Windmill Street caricature demonstrate the enduring popular importance of total bodily integrity for the afterlife: on the day of judgement, one needed one's whole body—that murderers were dissected was the final ignominy, the ultimate punishment for their crimes.[6] Not only that, but this indignity was then compounded if the fragments were sold (and often cheaply, as we shall see). Changing notions of individuality were closely bound up with the inviolability of the body, and the shifting attitudes to medical dismemberment assessed here and in chapters 6 and 7 may help us to appreciate the historical contingency of the individual and even what constitutes the self in the modern West.[7] The diseased dead were rendered partible; separated, re-distributed and circulated, their fragmented bodies carrying relations between them through different kinds of exchange. Anthropologists have long understood gifts as exchanging parts of people—here we see this in a far more literal sense. This is not persons transferring parts of themselves, but rather different people transferring parts of others on the way to the medical museum. By the time they were re-constituted, as I shall argue in chapter 5, they were no longer individual, but *dividual*. Curators re-composed these partible bodies as encyclopaedias of disease—not the partible living persons anthropologists observe, but like them multi-authored dividuals composed of relations, with different parts from different places.[8]

Given the troubling associations of dismemberment, how did anatomists establish their fragmentary accumulations on the grand scale outlined in the previous chapter? How did the small number of eighteenth-century collections of the Hunters and their colleagues give rise to so many museums of thousands upon thousands of body parts? To understand this phenomenon is to acknowledge that the social disadvantages of dismemberment were far outweighed (for collectors at least) by the cultural authority of the fragment

---

[6] Douglas Hay, et al., *Albion's Fatal Tree: Crime and Society in Eighteenth-Century England* (London: Allen Lane, 1975); Paul Rabinow, 'Severing the Ties: Fragmentation and Dignity in Late Modernity', in David J. Hess and Linda L. Layne (eds.), *Knowledge and Society: The Anthropology of Science and Technology* (Greenwich, Conn.: JAI, 1992), 169–87 Richardson, *Death, Dissection and the Destitute*.

[7] On the history of the concept of the self, see Jerrold Seigel, *The Idea of the Self: Thought and Experience in Western Europe since the Seventeenth Century* (New York: Cambridge University Press, 2005); Charles Taylor, *Sources of the Self: The Making of the Modern Identity* (Cambridge, Mass.: Harvard University Press, 1989).

[8] On partibility and personhood, see Cecilia Busby, 'Permeable and Partible Persons: A Comparative Analysis of Gender and Body in South India and Melanesia', *The Journal of the Royal Anthropological Institute*, 3 (1997), 261–78; Chris Fowler, *The Archaeology of Personhood: An Anthropological Approach* (London: Routledge, 2004); Marilyn Strathern, *The Gender of the Gift: Problems with Women and Problems with Society in Melanesia* (Berkeley: University of California Press, 1988).

in other contexts. Morbid anatomy was only one of a raft of new analytical ways of knowing around 1800 that objectified nature by breaking it down into pieces.[9] Men of science dismembered natural entities to understand them; collectors wrested fragments of nature from their contexts and brought them to museums. More generally, literary and architectural fragments—ancient and recent, planned or accidental—were key elements of romanticism. Ruins were alluring, and human remains in anatomy museums mirrored architectural and statuary remains elsewhere.[10] Whole body écorché and waxes were imbued with classical traditions—Hunter's 'Smugglerius', for example, was cast in the pose of the Roman *Dying Gaul*—so too dismembered body parts had classical equivalents in the fragments of statuary and classical ruins that flooded Northern European galleries from Italy and Greece.[11] These and other fragments implicitly legitimated the collecting practices of anatomists. Physicians and surgeons were part of the social class who demonstrated their gentility by collecting fragments of antiquity—the marble arm and the pickled hand moved in the same cultural milieu. After it was incorporated into the College of Surgeons, John Hunter's collection looked out over Lincoln's Inn Fields at that most archetypal collection of architectural and sculptural fragments, Sir John Soane's Museum, each in its own way 'a Pandora's box of cultural fragments'.[12] In the formative decades of the medical museum, fragments were key.

Fragmentation had both conceptual and pragmatic implications. Although collectors liked the massive and the spectacular, when selecting run-of-the-mill museum pieces, whether classical, pathological, or ethnographic, collectors tended to favour remnants of a particular size and shape—to fit in their gallery, shelf, or in the hand for the pathology viva voce (see

[9] John V. Pickstone, *Ways of Knowing: A New History of Science, Technology and Medicine* (Manchester: Manchester University Press, 2000).

[10] Elizabeth Wanning Harries, The *Unfinished Manner: Essays on the Fragment in the Later Eighteenth Century* (Charlottesville, VA: University of Virginia Press, 1994); David A. Hillman and Carla Mazzio (eds.), *The Body in Parts: Fantasies of Corporeality in Early Modern Europe* (New York: Routledge, 1997); Linda Nochlin, *The Body in Pieces: The Fragment as a Metaphor of Modernity* (London: Thames and Hudson, 1994); Michael S. Roth, Claire Lyons, and Charles Merewether (eds.), *Irresistible Decay: Ruins Reclaimed* (Los Angeles: Getty Research Institute, 1997); Sophie Thomas, 'Assembling History: Fragments and Ruins', *European Romantic Review*, 14 (2003), 177–86; Christopher Woodward, *In Ruins: A Journey through History, Art, and Literature* (London: Chatto and Windus, 2001).

[11] Hallam, *Anatomy Museum*; Martin Kemp and Marina Wallace, *Spectacular Bodies: The Art and Science of the Human Body from Leonardo to Now* (London; Berkeley: Hayward Gallery; University of California Press, 2000).

[12] Didier Maleuvre, *Museum Memories: History, Technology, Art* (Stanford, Calif.: Stanford University Press, 1999), 276; Margaret Richardson and MaryAnne Stevens (eds.), *John Soane, Architect: Master of Space and Light* (London: Royal Academy of Arts, 1999); Tim Knox, *Sir John Soane's Museum, London* (London: Merrell, 2009).

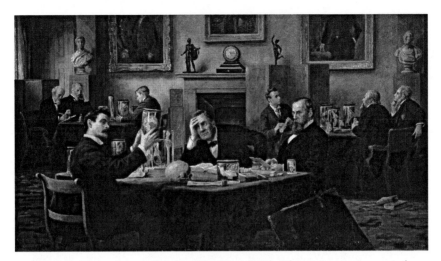

Fig. 3.2. Henry Jamyn Brooks, *The Viva*, 1894. The viva voce in surgical pathology set in the council room of the Royal College of Surgeons. Copyright the Royal College of Surgeons of England.

figure 3.2 and chapter 6).[13] Museums framed and contained specimens, both literally and metaphorically. Certain objects were selected rather than others for their size, shape, and durability—to fit the cabinet as well as the classification. Later in the century, frame and specimen alike shrank as pathologists took smaller and smaller samples: the development of histopathology relied on huge collections of tiny slides.[14] In the late twentieth century, commodified body fragments reduced further to the cellular and even genetic scale. In both contexts, to anatomize was to atomize.[15]

But for the most part nineteenth-century morbid anatomy collections were stocked with gross specimens in jars. Concentrating largely on the early decades of the nineteenth century as the formative years of British medical museums, the rest of this chapter is concerned with the routes that brought these fragments to the collections, whether taken from hospital

[13] On selection in these other contexts, see Shelly Errington, 'What Became Authentic Primitive Art?' *Cultural Anthropology*, 9 (1994), 201–26; Susan Stewart, *On Longing: Narratives of the Miniature, the Gigantic, the Souvenir, the Collection* (Durham, NC: Duke University Press, 1993).

[14] Stephen Baycroft, et al., *Histopathology Collections in London* (London: London Museums Service, c. 1990).

[15] Russell C. Maulitz, *Morbid Appearances: The Anatomy of Pathology in the Early Nineteenth Century* (Cambridge: Cambridge University Press, 1987); Bronwyn Parry, *Trading the Genome: Investigating the Commodification of Bio-Information* (New York: Columbia University Press, 2004).

wards, donated or purchased, tracing them through a dynamic collecting network.[16] These exchanges shifted the status of such specimens, and ultimately objectified and de-humanized human remains. They shared some characteristics and values with bodily fragments in other times and places, and yet were distinct, given particular meanings by the processes outlined below.

MANUFACTURING SPECIMENS

We have seen that the circulation of body parts is not only a recent phenomenon. Medieval churches and reliquaries housed and exchanged pieces of saints; renowned individuals such as René Descartes had the dubious posthumous honour of their body parts entering circulation; and Renaissance cabinets of curiosity sported anatomical preparations, especially 'monsters' that travelled between collectors.[17] But surgeons and anatomists began to accumulate body parts in greater numbers from the late eighteenth century. The healthy specimens in their collections were derived largely from dissections of corpses procured illicitly from graves or later under the auspices of the 1832 Anatomy Act. The unclaimed bodies of those who died in public institutions—principally poorhouses and hospitals—could be used for anatomical education. But although it actually specified that all remains should be buried decently after eight weeks, the Act did not directly address the supply of specimens for anatomical museums.

In any case, only rarely did a dissection reveal a diseased body part of interest to the pathologist.[18] Unclaimed bodies could only supply morbid specimens coincidentally, if the person in question happened to have suffered from a particular condition. Pathological anatomy was more commonly found during an autopsy—meaning 'to see for oneself'—which

---

[16] Chris Gosden and Frances Larson with Alison Petch, *Knowing Things: Exploring the Collections at the Pitt Rivers Museum 1884–1945* (Oxford: Oxford University Press, 2007); Hallam, *Anatomy Museum*.

[17] Patrick Geary, 'Sacred Commodities: The Circulation of Medieval Relics', in Arjun Appadurai (ed.), *The Social Life of Things: Commodities in Cultural Perspective* (Cambridge: Cambridge University Press, 1986), 169–91; Susan C. Lawrence, 'Beyond the Grave—the Use and Meaning of Human Body Parts: A Historical Introduction', in Robert F. Weir (ed.), *Stored Tissue Samples: Ethical, Legal and Public Policy Implications* (Iowa City: University of Iowa Press, 1998), 111–42; Arthur MacGregor, *Curiosity and Enlightenment: Collectors and Collections from the Sixteenth to the Nineteenth Century* (New Haven, Conn.: Yale University Press, 2007); Christine Quigley, *The Corpse: A History* (Jefferson, NC: MacFarland, 1996).

[18] See for example *Guy's Hospital Report* 31 (1871).

provided far richer pickings for morbid specimens. Most preparations in the pathology museum thereby came from patients, whether of the surgeon-collector who gathered the cabinet, or from the wards of a hospital. These distinctions in acquisition routes between healthy and diseased anatomies are too rarely acknowledged, and yet they had significant ramifications for the value and use of specimens.

Although the Hunter brothers and their nephew Matthew Baillie under-took post-mortem examinations, they were otherwise rare in the eighteenth century. As preservation methods began to improve in the early nineteenth century (see chapter 4), more practitioners began to remove interesting parts from their patients. Surgeons kept and preserved the results of interesting operations—the 'off-cuts' of the diseased or damaged body—for their own collections. In one Irish collection, for example, the catalogue entry for a cyst of the Bartonlini gland has a scrawled but encouraging pencilled note—'cured'—but otherwise, rare was the patient fortunate enough to survive.[19] Physicians and surgeons alike kept an interested eye on patients with unusual conditions and removed them post-mortem. Sir William Lawrence, President of the Royal College of Surgeons, sergeant-surgeon to the Queen and surgeon at St Bartholomew's, was not too busy to play a long game in acquisition for the hospital museum. Treating a patient for a head injury, the Baronet subsequently 'watched this man of years, until, on the patient's death, he obtained the skull for the Museum'.[20] Similarly at St Thomas's, 'the old fellow...was kept in the Hospital on purpose that a preparation might be made of him'.[21]

Lawrence was not alone in objectifying his patients even before death. Helen MacDonald has shown how the craniologist Joseph Barnard Davis viewed his patients as 'potential skulls'—but no-one was so brash as the prominent surgeon-Baronet, Astley Cooper.[22] As he informed the anatomy Select Committee in 1828, 'there is no person, let his situation in life

[19] St Ronan's Catalogue of Museum specimens, n.d., Royal College of Surgeons in Ireland Archive RCSI/LO An/8/4.

[20] Frederick S. Eve, 'Our Museum and Its Associations', *St Bartholomew's Hospital Reports*, 17 (1881), 165–84 at 171.

[21] Hampton Weekes to Richard Weekes, 24 September 1801, in John M. T. Ford, *A Medical Student at St Thomas's Hospital, 1801–1802: The Weekes Family Letters (Medical History* Supplement 7; London: Wellcome Institute for the History of Medicine, 1987), 43.

[22] On Davis, see Helen MacDonald, *Human Remains*, 102; on Cooper, see Samuel J. M. M. Alberti, 'Owning and Collecting Natural Objects in Nineteenth-Century Britain', in Marco Berretta (ed.), *From Private to Public: Natural Collections and Museums* (New York: Science History Publications, 2005), 141–54 (in which Bransby Blake Cooper is erroneously referred to as Astley's son, rather than his nephew); Druin Burch, *Digging up the Dead: Uncovering the Life and Times of an Extraordinary Surgeon* (London: Chatto and Windus, 2007).

be what it may, whom, if I were disposed to dissect, I could not obtain'.[23] As well as his own practice, Cooper utilized a large network of colleagues to alert him of interesting cases, and at his home on Broad Street he amassed possibly the most significant private collection of anatomical, pathological, and zoological specimens in London after that of his teacher John Hunter. His initial motivation was to gather specimens to illustrate his lectures, which 'led him to frame the plan for a museum to be composed principally of specimens connected with the study of the several diseases which came under the notice of the surgeon'. Cooper's pupil (and later successor at Tom's) Benjamin Travers had been articled for all of two days when they set off for Newington Green at night to examine a recently deceased woman: he returned with 'a precious, though not over fragrant, relic of the old lady's interior upon [his] person'.[24]

Such body parts were considered to be the property of the practitioner—and we shall return below to the thorny issue of ownership—and given the choice, many patients were not happy to have their organs removed and displayed in this way. Although he 'had very little difficulty in obtaining any specimen he might require from the Hospital, whether they had been removed from his own patients, or from those of the other surgeons', Cooper complained when anyone objected to the practice of post-mortem examination at the behest of the surgeon:

> There was more difficulty in obtaining the examples of the various diseases which occurred to him in the course of his private practice. The repugnance which is felt to submit the bodies of deceased persons to the examination of surgeons, or, among many, even to permit the diseased parts which have been removed by operation, to be subjected to scientific critical examination, sometimes proved of great annoyance.

Cooper's powers of persuasion, however, were formidable: he argued that it would be a shame to lose this rare disease to medical science, and presented the possible life-saving benefits of such a donation. 'If they still persisted in refusing his request, after such an appeal, he would argue with them that they had no right, from merely selfish feeling, to deprive those who professed the practice of surgery of such a source of information.'[25]

---

[23] Select Committee on Anatomy, *Report, Minutes of Evidence, Appendix* (London: House of Commons, 1828), 18.

[24] Bransby Blake Cooper, *The Life of Sir Astley Cooper, Bart.*, 2 vols. (London: Parker, 1843), ii. 99; i. 317. For more examples of Cooper's audacity in obtaining cadavers, see Charles Symonds, *The Hunterian Oration* (London: Ash, 1921).

[25] Cooper, *Life of Sir Astley Cooper*, ii. 101–3. On sacrifice in science, see Michael Lynch, 'Sacrifice and the Transformation of the Natural Body into a Scientific Object: Laboratory Culture and Ritual Practice in the Neurosciences', *Social Studies of Science*, 18 (1988), 265–89.

Even if the patient afflicted with an interesting condition had met their demise in a hospital, their remains might still be obtained for Cooper's or other surgeons' private collections. George Langstaff was Surgeon to the Cripplegate Dispensary, but nonetheless received specimens from his Alma Mater, St Bartholomew's.[26] But as the century progressed, such specimens were more likely to be retained for the hospital's own museum, as the practice of routine post-mortem examinations in London hospitals was gradually imported from Paris.[27] Whereas the anatomist James Macartney was unusual in instituting a system of autopsies at St Bartholomew's in the 1790s (which was discontinued upon his departure to Trinity College Dublin), the practice slowly began to take hold in Britain in the early 1900s.[28] In 1816 army medical officers were ordered to carry out post-mortems, and that 'in all cases if a nature calculated to furnish contributions to Pathological knowledge, preparations should be carefully made'.[29] Likewise at Guy's Hospital, noted Thomas Hodgkin, who was both 'inspector of the dead' and curator of the museum:

> it was expressly understood, that all specimens of morbid structure, met with in subjects either dissected by the Pupils or inspected at the request of the Medical Officers, should be preserved, as the property of the Hospital. Nevertheless [until Hodgkin's appointment in 1826], the accessions to the Museum were far from being numerous; probably from the circumstance, that no one was specifically charged with the preservation of the preserved parts.[30]

Upon his arrival at Guy's, Hodgkin, keen both to make an impression and to implement his Paris training, had thrown himself into the museum and post-mortem work. He arranged a regular and frequent autopsy system, rearranged the museum and expanded it sixfold. Aston Key, who as assistant surgeon had been responsible for post-mortems in the years

[26] George Langstaff, *Catalogue of the Preparations Illustrative of Normal, Abnormal, and Morbid Structure, Human and Comparative, Constituting the Anatomical Museum of George Langstaff* (London: Churchill, 1842).

[27] George J. Cunningham, *The History of British Pathology*, ed. G. Kemp McGowan (Bristol: White Tree, 1992); Maulitz, *Morbid Appearances*; Lawrence, 'Beyond the Grave'.

[28] Alexander Macalister, *James Macartney: A Memoir* (London: Hodder and Stoughton, 1900); John Leonard Thornton, 'A Diary of James Macartney (1770–1843) with Notes on His Writings', *Medical History*, 12 (1968), 164–75.

[29] Army Medical Museum, *Anatomical Drawings, Selected from the Collection of Morbid Anatomy in the Army Medical Museum, Chatham*, 5 fasciculi vols. (London: Longman, 1824–50), preface.

[30] Thomas Hodgkin, *A Catalogue of the Preparations in the Anatomical Museum of Guy's Hospital* (London: Watts, 1829), v.

previous to Hodgkin's appointment, carried out around fifteen per year; the new curator performed nearly fifty. He ensured that interesting specimens from the inspection were kept for the museum on a regular basis, rather than haphazardly as before. And unlike the surgeons who previously carried out post-mortems and controlled supply to the museum, Hodgkin was interested in general morbid specimens, rather than only preparations that displayed the results of particular surgical procedures.

Another early and important site for this practice was University College London, where in 1834 it was decreed that post-mortems should be carried out, and in the following year that all specimens of disease removed from patients in the hospital be sent to the museum. There they were examined by Robert Carswell, occupant (as we saw in the previous chapter) of the first chair of morbid anatomy in the country. Other medical schools in the capital and elsewhere gradually followed suit.[31] Similar formal appointments to other hospital museums were made from the 1830s—curator and pathologist were often the same person or worked very closely together—and autopsies became regular practice. Where possible, as at Guy's, hospital museums were situated adjacent to the post-mortem room. Even so, the Steward's permission had to be secured in order to inspect the body, using a pro forma: '—, late a patient in—Ward, being now dead, I request permission for the Body to be inspected, considering it to be an important Case, from which the Profession may derive much satisfactory information.'[32]

Unlike Astley Cooper's wealthy clients, there is little evidence of the extent to which hospital patients or their next of kin sanctioned or condemned this practice: one of the prized specimens in the early Guy's collection, an enlarged head, was taken to the museum after a mock burial carried out for the benefit of the patient's family.[33] At the Glasgow Royal Infirmary the Pathological Museum Committee was even firmer, claiming 'full powers to render available for the purposes of clinical instruction,

---

[31] W. D. Foster, *Pathology as a Profession in Great Britain and the Early History of the Royal College of Pathologists* (London: Royal College of Pathologists, 1983); W. R. Merrington, *University College Hospital and Its Medical School: A History* (London: Heinemann, 1976); Isambard Owen, *A Supplementary Catalogue of the Pathological Museum of St George's Hospital: A Description of the Specimens Added During the Years 1866–1881* (London: Churchill, 1882); H. Campbell Thomson, *The Story of the Middlesex Hospital Medical School* (London: Murray, 1935).

[32] Printed on every page of Guy's Hospital, Post-Mortem Book, 1821–3, Gordon Museum Archive, King's College London. See also Letters and memoranda accompanying specimens sent to the Museum, 1894–5, MU9/2/9, St Bartholomew's Hospital Archive.

[33] William Millard, *An Account of the Circumstances Attending the Imprisonment and Death of the Late William Millard* (London: Millard, 1825); Richardson, *Death, Dissection and the Destitute*.

and the advancement of medical science, the many rare and valuable specimens of diseased structure which are constantly occurring in the wards of the infirmary'.[34] Negotiations were also complex between medical staff, as for example in Manchester, where

> Pathology was taught at Owens College and specimens were sent there as well as to the Pathological Registrar at the Manchester Royal Infirmary. The specimens belonged to the Infirmary staff unless the Consultant failed to claim them in two weeks. Then they were owned by the Professor at Owens College, but could be used by the Infirmary staff by borrowing them after filling a form.[35]

Collections expanded correspondingly. From Hodgkin's very first autopsy, of Eliza Swindon, a patient of Richard Bright's, he preserved three specimens for the museum.[36] In the late 1820s, there were 250–300 deaths per year in the 421 Guy's beds, providing ample material. The pathological collection increased by a factor of four when Hodgkin first arrived, then threefold again between 1829 and 1857.[37] By 1892 there were around 500 post-mortems each year at Guy's, and his successor the physician Samuel Wilks estimated that he had personally examined nearly 3,000 bodies in his fifteen years as inspector of the dead.[38] Autopsy books and other records were commonly kept with the collections, forming a key element of the textual body discussed in chapter 5 below.

Under Hodgkin and like-minded inspectors of the dead, the post-mortem room became a factory, where pathological assistants transformed bodies into objects for museological consumption. Anthony Carlisle, surgeon to the Westminster Hospital, spoke of anatomists 'manufacturing their own raw material'; Joseph Coats in Glasgow considered incoming body parts 'morbid products'.[39] And so although Erin O'Connor has

[34] Glasgow Royal Pathological Museum Committee Minute, 1852, cited in John H. Teacher, 'On the History of Pathology in the Glasgow Royal Infirmary and the Functions of the Pathological Department', *Glasgow Medical Journal* (January 1912), 3–15 at 13.

[35] Samuel Oleesky, 'Julius Dreschfeld', *Manchester Medical Gazette*, 51 (1971), 14–17, 58–60, 96–9 at 59.

[36] Joseph J. Daws, 'Thomas Hodgkin and the Museum at Guy's Hospital', *Cancer Treatment Reviews*, 25 (1999), 145–9; Guy's Hospital, Green Inspection Book 1 (1826); Guy's Hospital, Post-Mortem Book, 1821–3, Gordon Museum Archive, King's College London.

[37] Hodgkin, *Catalogue of the Preparations*; Samuel O. Habershon, *Pathological Catalogue of the Museum of Guy's Hospital*, 2 vols. (2nd edn London: MacKenzie, 1857).

[38] Samuel Wilks, *Lectures on Pathological Anatomy* (London: Longman, Brown, Green, Longmans, and Roberts, 1859); Samuel Wilks and George Thomas Bettany, *A Biographical History of Guy's Hospital* (London: Ward, Lock, Bowden, 1892).

[39] Charles Bell to Joseph George Bell, 30 November 1804, in Charles Bell (ed.), *Letters of Sir Charles Bell* (London: Murray, 1870), 22; L. Stephen Jacyna, 'The Laboratory and the

argued 'that what the factory system really mass-produces is pathology itself', in a more literal sense the medical museum was embedded within industrialized Britain as a manufactory of pathology.[40] Hospital wards produced morbid specimens for the museum as technical factories manufactured goods for consumption in the shop fronts, and the abattoir fragmented and processed animal meat for distribution and consumption.[41]

Among the specimens garnered from the wards were the least valued items in the museum, the stock-in-trade of the medical museum. These 'tank specimens' were used for regular teaching, often used to destruction: St Bartholomew's, for example, had a 'stock-pot' of such specimens in the work-room.[42] Curators thereby kept the inundation of new acquisitions in check by discarding those specimens that were damaged or deteriorated, reducing what would have been an exponential expansion either to a manageable growth or to an even size. Common afflictions could soon be replaced from the wards. A steady-state system was established, with the collection in a regular system of acquisition, disposal, and refreshing. 'The external appearance of our collection may at any time be completely changed,' explained one Barts curator, 'even to the extent of completely replacing a large number of preparations'.[43] Even more so than other forms of museum, the anatomical collection was a dynamic organism, growing and shrinking, changing over space and time.

GIFTING BODIES

Stock-in-trade specimens harvested from the wards, then, were rarely afforded particular value beyond their rarity. Specimens *given* to the museum, however, came with an added layer of worth and meaning. There is an expansive literature devoted to donation of bodies and body

Clinic: The Impact of Pathology on Surgical Diagnosis in the Glasgow Western Infirmary 1875–1910', *Bulletin for the History of Medicine*, 62 (1988), 384–406 at 389.

[40] O'Connor, *Raw Material*, 7. See also Simon Chaplin, 'John Hunter and The "Museum Oeconomy", 1750–1800' (Ph.D. thesis, King's College London, 2009).

[41] Jonah Siegel, *Desire and Excess: The Nineteenth-Century Culture of Art* (Princeton: Princeton University Press, 2000); Noélie Vialles, *Animal to Edible*, trans. J. A. Underwood (Cambridge: Cambridge University Press, 1994). See chapter 6 below for the parallels drawn by visitors between flesh and meat.

[42] Ernest H. Shaw, 'Pathology at Bart's in the Nineteenth Century', *St Bartholomew's Hospital Journal*, 5 (1949), 75–78 at 77; Guy's Hospital Museum, Minute Book, 15 February 1889, Gordon Museum Archive, King's College London; Erin Hunter McLeary, 'Science in a Bottle: The Medical Museum in North America, 1860–1940' (Ph.D. thesis, University of Pennsylvania, 2001).

[43] Eve, 'Our Museum', 184.

parts, which applies anthropological understandings of exchange to good effect; but such work tends to focus on the gift of one's own blood, remains, or organs; and it tends accordingly to concentrate on the later twentieth century.[44] Just as the recent traffic in body parts has a historical precursor, however, so such 'gifts of life' have interesting antecedents in and around nineteenth-century museums. The selfless card-carrying twentieth-century donors were not the first to give body parts: those same medical practitioners who plundered their patients for medical preparations gifted human remains to each other and to anatomical museums (and even left their own remains to their colleagues). This sense of giving reveals very different meanings and power relations enacted around and through human remains.

'I am sorry Dr. [George] Fordyce is so near his end', lamented a medical student in 1802. 'I wonder what he will do with his Museum[? I] think he will give it to some person.'[45] Many institutional museums in hospitals, anatomy schools, and royal colleges were established with the gift of an entire collection, whether during the lifetime of the donor or posthumously, as in the case of the Hunterian Museum in Glasgow (see chapter 2). But transfer from private to institutional hands did not always run smoothly. Many collections suffered from proprietary ambiguity, as in the case of the Guy's Hospital Museum, the roots of which lie in the 'Great Quarrel' between Guy's and Thomas's. The dispute, which resulted in the separation of the medical teaching at the Borough hospitals (as they were together known), precipitated around the disputed ownership of specimens.[46] Late eighteenth- and early nineteenth-century lectureships belonged to the teachers rather than their hospital, as did the income and material culture associated with them. When Sir Astley Cooper resigned his position at St Thomas's in favour of Bransby Cooper, his nephew and anointed successor, to his surprise this routine nepotism was challenged by the hospital board, and John Flint South was appointed instead. The belligerent Baronet sought to remove his part of the Tom's museum to give

---

[44] Fox and Swazey, *Spare Parts*; Susan E. Lederer, *Flesh and Blood: Organ Transplantation and Blood Transfusion in Twentieth-Century America* (Oxford: Oxford University Press, 2008); Margaret Lock, *Twice Dead: Organ Transplants and the Reinvention of Death* (Berkeley: University of California Press, 2002); Sharp, *Strange Harvest*; Sharp, *Bodies, Commodities, and Biotechnologies*.

[45] Richard Weekes to Hampton Weekes 17 April 1802, in Ford, *A Medical Student*, 160.

[46] Hector Charles Cameron, *Mr. Guy's Hospital: 1726–1948* (London: Longmans, 1954); Cooper, *Life of Sir Astley Cooper*; P. K. B. Davis, *The Work and Teaching of Sir Astley Paston Cooper, Bart.*, ed. J. B. Kinmonth (London: privately printed, 1964); John Flint South, *Descriptive Catalogue of the Preparations in the Museum of St Thomas's Hospital* (London: Renshaw, 1847).

to the fledgling Guy's Medical School. Alleging that Cooper's original agreement with his fellow surgeon Henry Cline stipulated the collections remain intact, St Thomas's Governors refused to split the collection. After a long and bitter dispute that ran over the pages of the newly founded *Lancet*, Cooper accepted £1,000 for his share and built up a new collection at Guy's instead. References to museum ownership were subsequently ordered expunged from the St Thomas's Governors' Court documents (but fortunately the text remains legible under heavy scoring).[47]

The Royal College of Surgeons of Edinburgh narrowly avoided a similar fiasco. John Barclay, identified in the last chapter as one of several anatomy teachers operating in Surgeon's Square, responded to the college's call for specimens in 1821 by offering his thousand-strong collection, largely of comparative anatomy, on condition the college build a hall to house it—for gifts rarely came without strings attached.[48] Furthermore, he insisted in the 1824 deed of settlement:

> the said John Barclay did thereby further recommend to the said Trustees to continue and appoint the said Robert Knox Keeper and Conservator of the aforesaid Museum while the same should remain under their charge . . . Doctor Robert Knox should be in like manner continued and appointed by them Keeper and Conservator thereof for life when the same should be delivered over to the said Royal College.[49]

Grudgingly, the College gave Knox the care of the pathological portion of their museum. At the time he was a rising naturalist and anatomy teacher, working as Barclay's assistant; they became partners in the anatomy school the following year. The year after that, 1826, Barclay's death meant that Knox took possession of the anatomy school, its classes, and the museum. The Royal College, displaying remarkable prescience, had appointed Knox conservator of the entire museum three months before Barclay's death, and he was apparently more than happy to have the collection transferred to the College. Barclay in effect gifted the College

[47] F. G. Parsons, *The History of St Thomas's Hospital*, 3 vols. (London: Methuen, 1932–6).
[48] Matthew H. Kaufman, 'John Barclay (1758–1826) Extra-Mural Teacher of Anatomy in Edinburgh: Honorary Fellow of the Royal College of Surgeons of Edinburgh', *The Surgeon: Journal of the Royal College of Surgeons of Edinburgh*, 4/2 (2006), www.thesurgeon.net, accessed 12 January 2009; Henry Lonsdale, *A Sketch of the Life and Writings of Robert Knox the Anatomist* (London: Macmillan, 1870); Violet Tansey and D. E. C. Mekie, *The Museum of the Royal College of Surgeons of Edinburgh* (Edinburgh: The Royal College of Surgeons of Edinburgh, 1982).
[49] The Deeds of Settlement and Catalogue of the Barcleian Museum Bequeathed to the Royal College of Surgeons of Edinburgh by John Barclay, Fellow of the Royal College of Physicians and Honorary Fellow of the College of Surgeons of Edinburgh, 1828, 12–13, Royal College of Surgeons of Edinburgh Museum Archive. The original deed was dated 16 July 1824.

a conservator—about which the Council was none too pleased, especially after the gruesome events surrounding Knox in 1828. Although he was never officially indicted in the trial of Burke and Hare, increasingly bad relations with the College authorities prompted his resignation in 1831. Barclay's collection, however, remained in their museum.

Nearby, the University of Edinburgh was also the site of proprietary controversy. For although Alexander Monro *primus* had given his anatomical preparations to the University outright, his son and successor argued that since he had paid for their upkeep and expansion, he retained a claim on them. The Monros' collection was only the core of the university's holdings, however, and tension arose between *secundus* and his colleagues in the nearby infirmary, who wanted to retain some control over the morbid specimens deposited at the university from the hospital; *tertius* later bickered with the town council over responsibility for the family cabinet.[50]

Once their title had been successfully transferred, founding collections attracted further donations: a large museum became a centre of gravity for later acquisitions. These often came from practitioners associated with the institution through their professional life or training. At Dublin, for example, after John Timothy Kirby deposited a large collection from his medical school in the nascent Royal College of Surgeons in Ireland museum, others quickly followed suit. The curator acknowledged 'donations from the members and licentiates of the college, and from several other professional gentlemen, who have politely contributed to its advancement'.[51] Such additions *augmented* the collection as a whole, not only by making 'an honourable addition' but also by raising it 'in estimation or dignity'.[52] Glasgow University's Professor of Anatomy Thomas Bryce remarked of the Hunterian over a century after the collections arrived: 'Additions have been made to the collections in greater number than any previous period. . . . we must commemorate to-day, along with William Hunter, a long list of donors too numerous to mention individually.'[53] Hunter himself had benefited from the donations of many former

[50] Proceedings of the Edinburgh Town Council 25 June 1824, cited in Royal Commission on the Universities of Scotland, *Minutes of Evidence*, 4 vols. (House of Commons Command Papers 92–5; London: HMSO, 1837), appendix 1; Andrew G. Fraser, *The Building of Old College: Adam, Playfair and the University of Edinburgh* (Edinburgh: Edinburgh University Press, 1989).

[51] John Houston, *Descriptive Catalogue of the Preparations of the Museum of the Royal College of Surgeons in Ireland*, 2 vols. (Dublin: Hodges and Smith, 1834–40), i. 7–8; Museum Committee Minutes 20 December 1833 [sic—1832], and MS ledger catalogue, 1840s, Royal College of Surgeons in Ireland Archive RCSI/MUC/1 and MUC/3.

[52] *Oxford English Dictionary*, s.v. 'Augment'.

[53] Thomas H. Bryce, *William Hunter and His Museum: An Oration* (Glasgow: MacLehose, 1922), 4.

pupils and medical friends, eager to contribute to one of the largest collections, public or private, in the country. Indeed, the collection became so renowned that he maintained its very status as a private museum was in doubt. 'I look upon every thing of this kind which is given to me, as a present to the public;' Hunter wrote, 'and consider myself as thereby called upon to serve the public with more diligence.'[54]

Countless specimens arrived as single or small groups of items associated collectors, surgeons, and alumni. Curators entreated these good men to send them interesting specimens, soliciting gifts with circulars, as for example from Dublin, where the Royal College curator implored colleagues publishing in medical journals 'that the value of their communications would be enormously enhanced by having the specimens illustrating them permanently displayed on the shelves of the largest Pathological Museum in Ireland' and furthermore:

> individual members of the College Council might themselves use their influence in the various Hospitals to which they are attached, so that not only gynæcological material, but material of every description, which is not made use of in the Hospitals, should be sent to the College Museum. There must be an enormous amount of operative and post-mortem specimens annually thrown away which would be of great value if sent *while fresh* to the museum. Such material would give the Curator the opportunity of selecting, and adding to the Museum, representative diseased conditions prepared by modern methods.[55]

Catalogues identified gaps in collections that were desiderata for further donations, and a major justification for the expense of printing and distributing these hefty tomes was their potential for attracting further donations.[56] They revealed an acquisition network stretching the length of the country and the width of the empire. In the pathological section of the 1829 Guy's Catalogue, those British donors whose geographical location was noted were from Birmingham, Borough, Bournemouth, Brighton, Chichester, Clifton, Deptford, Derby, Ealing, Feversham, Fleet Street, Gravesend, Guernsey, Hull, Hythe, Kingston, Newcastle-upon-Tyne, Plaistow, Rotherhithe, Royston, Rye, Sheffield, Spital Square, Tottenham,

---

[54] Samuel Foart Simmons and John Hunter, *William Hunter, 1718–1783: A Memoir*, ed. C. Helen Brock (1783; East Kilbride: University of Glasgow Press, 1983), 25.

[55] Curator's Report for the Year ending 5 April 1889; Report of the Curator 4 November 1908, Royal College of Surgeons in Ireland Archive, original emphasis RCSI/MUC/2. See also [William Clift], *Invitation to Surgeons, and Naturalists, for Donations to the Museum of the Royal College of Surgeons in London* (London: Carpenter, 1826).

[56] See for example John H. Teacher, *Catalogue of the Anatomical and Pathological Preparations of Dr. William Hunter in the Hunterian Museum, University of Glasgow*, 2 vols. (Glasgow: MacLehose, 1900), i. 144.

Walworth, Woolwich, and Wrexham.[57] Later in the century, Imperial routes became more pronounced, bringing to the collection for example 'the hand of a leper, showing the characteristic ulceration and deformity of the fingers ... presented by Dr. Beavan Neave Rake, of the Leper Asylum at Trinidad' and 'a rare calcareous mass which Surgeon-Major Bovill crushed and removed from the nostril of a Hindu'.[58] Specimens followed a complex path, from patient (be they unborn or ancient, living or dead) sometimes via their family, sent by a doctor or surgeon to the hospital, often by way of a renowned metropolitan practitioner. Although museums were qualitatively shaped most significantly by gifts in their early decades, the volume of gifts peaked in the decades around 1900, matching acquisition patterns in natural history museums.[59]

Whether as part of a founding collection or a subsequent augmentation, gifted body parts brought with them to collections different meanings and value than those that arrived straight from the ward. For giving is rarely altruistic. As with any process of gift exchange, donation constituted a reciprocal relationship between benefactor and museum. As Susan Pearce writes, 'to give material freely to museums is a meritorious act which conveys famous immortality'.[60] Collecting was civilizing, and subsequently to donate to a worthy museum ensured that such an act remained visible in perpetuity. Although Astley Cooper's nephew insisted that the Baronet 'was not instigated to make the collection by the mere desire of possession, which too often influences those who engage in such undertakings: with him it arose from the true love of science which the preparations contributed to illustrate', Cooper knew that by collecting and especially by depositing it in a pubic institution, he gained considerable *regard*, a key

[57] Hodgkin, *Catalogue of the Preparations*; see also Hallam, *Anatomy Museum*; Jonathan Reinarz, 'The Age of Museum Medicine: The Rise and Fall of the Medical Museum of Birmingham's School of Medicine', *Social History of Medicine*, 18 (2005), 419–37.

[58] James F. Goodhart, 'List of Specimens Added to the Pathological Museum During the Year 1884–5', *Guy's Hospital Reports*, 43 (1886), 309–320 at 310, specimen 1620[61]; G. Newton Pitt, 'List of Specimens Added to the Pathological Museum During the Years 1886–88', *Guy's Hospital Reports*, 45 (1888), 437–65 at 438, specimen 1682[100].

[59] See for example Teacher, *Catalogue of the Anatomical and Pathological Preparations*; see also Samuel J. M. M. Alberti, 'The Status of Museums: Authority, Identity and Material Culture', in David N. Livingstone and Charles W. J. Withers (eds.), *Geographies of Nineteenth-Century Science* (Chicago: University of Chicago Press, 2011); Robert E. Kohler, *All Creatures: Naturalists, Collectors, and Biodiversity, 1850–1950* (Princeton: Princeton University Press, 2006).

[60] Susan M. Pearce, *On Collecting: An Investigation into Collecting in the European Tradition* (London: Routledge, 1995), 407; Roy Porter, 'William Hunter: A Surgeon and a Gentleman', in William F. Bynum and Roy Porter (eds.), *William Hunter and the Eighteenth-Century Medical World* (Cambridge: Cambridge University Press, 1985), 7–34.

element of the gift economy in maturing capitalism.[61] The Hunters had likewise known (or at least hoped) that their names would live on in their collections. On a smaller scale, an isolated rural practitioner with appropriate metropolitan contacts sent a specimen from his practice to the hospital with the hope of securing potentially useful patronage, or even better, minor fame in a label, report, or catalogue.

Donated items retained their connection to their collector(s). As Marcel Mauss established, in gift exchange 'objects are never completely separated from the men who exchange them'.[62] Anthropological writing abounds with analyses of the inalienability of gifts, which, as opposed to commodities, are in principle singular, part of a continued relationship between giver and recipient, and they cannot be transferred. Even if they *are* nevertheless circulated, the bond between object and original owner endures, in the medical museum as in other contexts. On the large scale, eponymous museums are enduringly associated with the 'founder' long after the number of original specimens was swamped by later additions, as in both Hunterian collections, and these founding specimens were especially prized. In 1839, William Thomson of Edinburgh inspected the Hunterian on behalf of the Royal Commission visiting the University of Glasgow and reported that the specimens were not kept in a state worthy of the memory of their donor, spurring the university to action regarding the collection.[63] The faculty had, after all, 'in accepting custody of that collection . . . undertaken the guardianship of his scientific reputation'.[64] The university had only 'custody' of the collection— Hunter in effect retained posthumous ownership.

But even those specimens donated piecemeal were not generally as disposable as 'manufactured' remains were, thanks to the reciprocity integral to even such minor gift exchange. 'Great indeed would have been the courage of a Curator', remembered Arthur Voelcker of the Middlesex Hospital, 'to destroy these [donations] for the most useless objects were held in such esteem by the donors [especially] if he were aspiring to a future post on the staff.'[65] One St Bartholomew's curator wrote of donors,

---

[61] Cooper, *Life of Sir Astley Cooper*, ii. 117; Avner Offer, 'Between the Gift and the Market: The Economy of Regard', *Economic History Review*, 50 (1997), 450–76.

[62] Marcel Mauss, *The Gift* (1925; New York: Norton, 1976), 31; Annette B. Weiner, *Inalienable Possessions: The Paradox of Keeping-While-Giving* (Berkeley: University of California Press, 1992).

[63] Commissioners for visiting the University of Glasgow, *Report* (London: HMSO, 1839), 86.

[64] William Thomson (ed.), *Deeds Instituting Bursaries, Scholarships, and Other Foundations, in the College and University of Glasgow* (Glasgow: Maitland Club, 1850), 242.

[65] Cited in Thomson, *Story of the Middlesex Hospital*, 84.

The memory of these Olympians is very tenacious, especially for distant events, and since with us the supply of material is so abundant that it cannot all be housed, even temporarily, the possibility has to be faced that the treasured object has long since reached the furnace. In such cases the quantity of tact necessary to support the occasion with success is almost immeasurable.[66]

In Glasgow, in his capacity as Hunterian curator, the American geologist Henry Darwin Rogers endured an earful from a donor because a specimen he had donated 15 years previously was not on display, and a donor to the Royal College in Dublin was likewise concerned that its collection was 'unclassified and uncared for' and pointedly asked about a specimen he had presented some years previously.[67] Rogers and other curators were thereby victims of the paradox of 'keeping-while-giving', the tyranny of the gift.[68] Clearly, whatever the law stated, such objects were treated as the property of the donor and subsequently the recipient museum; but not the original patient. This chapter returns to the traces of identities that inhere to donated human remains after exploring the final and possibly most troubling of the three principal acquisition routes that brought items to medical museums: the purchase of the human body.

COSTLY REMAINS

Human remains that had been procured from wards or given to collectors might also be exchanged for money on their way to (and from) museums. The human body, so often assumed to be sacred and inalienable, was bought and sold in large quantities in the nineteenth-century medical marketplace. Although this exchange network bore similarities to earlier practices and to twentieth-century body markets, it nonetheless demonstrated particular characteristics. Furthermore, the contrasts between modes of acquisition were not as stark as one might assume, for gift and commodity are not discrete states: objects may acquire characteristics of both.

Purchasing body parts was common practice in the thriving 'museum œconomy' of Georgian London. William Hunter, for example, established his teaching collection by buying the cabinets of other collectors including

---

[66] William P. S. Branson, 'Of the Museum, and Some of Its Recent Additions', *St Bartholomew's Hospital Journal*, 17 (1910), 23–27 at 24.

[67] James Banks to Henry Darwin Rogers, 9 September 1859, MR 50/33, Glasgow University Special Collection; Patsy Gerstner, *Henry Darwin Rogers, 1808–1866: American Geologist* (Tuscaloosa: University of Alabama Press, 1995); Museum Committee Minutes 26 June 1890, Royal College of Surgeons in Ireland Archive RCSI/MUC/2.

[68] Lock, *Twice Dead*; Weiner, *Inalienable Possessions*.

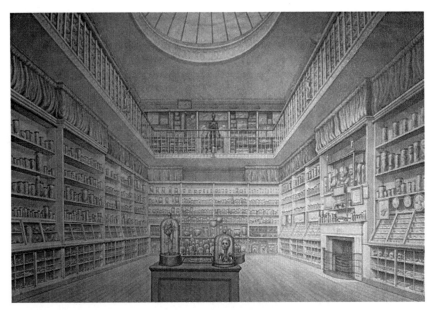

Fig. 3.3. Interior of John Heaviside's Anatomical Museum, by John Howship, 1814. Copyright the Royal College of Surgeons of England.

Francis Sandys, William Hewson, Magnus Falconer, and Andrew Blackall.[69] Upon the death of many medical collectors, their cabinets were purchased from their executors by their teaching partners at the private anatomy schools for hundreds or even thousands of pounds. This gave way to an even larger and more active network of collecting and sale in the nineteenth century, fuelled by the industrialized production of pathology, the post-mortem. John Heaviside's extensive collection (figure 3.3), for example, was largely based on the purchase of that of Henry Watson, surgeon to the Middlesex Hospital; the Middlesex in turn had to raise 350 guineas to purchase the accoucheur John Sweatman's collection upon his death in 1839.[70]

Many museums were especially active in purchasing acquisitions in the early century as they sought quickly to establish collections large enough for teaching. Such was the importance of a museum to the new University

[69] Chaplin, 'John Hunter'; Simmons and Hunter, *William Hunter*; Charles F. W. Illingworth, *The Story of William Hunter* (London: Livingstone, 1967).
[70] J. Kingston Fowler and J. B. Sutton, *A Descriptive Catalogue of the Pathological Museum of the Middlesex Hospital* (London: Churchill, 1884); John Heaviside, *Catalogue of the Museum of John Heaviside, Esq.* (London: Woodfall, 1818); C. E. Lakin, 'The Story of Our Museum and Some of Its Contents', *The Middlesex Hospital Journal* (1908), 84–98; George C. Peachey, *John Heaviside Surgeon* (London: St Martin's Press, 1931).

of London, for example, that faculty actively gathered specimens from Paris and Dublin to kick-start the collection.[71] But seeding a museum was a tricky business. In 1821 the Royal College of Surgeons of Edinburgh set about buying the Meckel collection, built up by three generations of anatomists in Halle and judged by the College to be 'considered to be without a rival in Europe', justifying the price of £5,000.[72] The sale fell through, however, leaving the curators to look elsewhere to build up the collection, and, as discussed in chapter 2, they eventually purchased Charles Bell's collection from Great Windmill Street, which arrived by sea in October 1825. Elsewhere, for £1,000 William Clark arranged for the University of Cambridge anatomy museum to purchase James Macartney's collection from Trinity College Dublin in the 1840s.[73] In between and after large purchases like these in their early years, medical museums tended to spend smaller amounts per annum, depending on the availability of purchase budgets. Guy's, for example, bought small portions of George Langstaff's popular collection in the mid century.[74] In Dublin, the Royal College of Surgeons paid £30 for an ankylosed skeleton that had been fragmented (in vain) by the sufferer's relatives in order to prevent the post-mortem theft of his remains.[75]

Some objects and collections, then, were sold directly to museums by a collector or his executors. Others were exchanged through that most curious of economic phenomena, the auction, which had become an important way of selling *objets curieux*, natural and anatomical items from the early eighteenth century.[76] Following Amsterdam and Paris,

---

[71] On Robert Carswell in Paris, see Maulitz, *Morbid Appearances*; on J. R. Bennett in Dublin, see Pauline M. H. Mazumdar, 'Anatomical Physiology and the Reform of Medical Education: London 1825–1835', *Bulletin of the History of Medicine*, 57 (1983), 230–46.

[72] Tansey and Mekie, *Museum of the Royal College*, 8; Matthew H. Kaufman, *Medical Teaching in Edinburgh During the 18th and 19th Centuries* (Edinburgh: Royal College of Surgeons of Edinburgh, 2003); Dawn Kemp with Sara Barnes, *Surgeon's Hall: A Museum Anthology* (Edinburgh: The Royal College of Surgeons of Edinburgh, 2009). Johann Friedrich Meckel ('The Elder' 1724–1774), Philipp Friedrich Theodore Meckel (1756–1803) and Johann Friedrich Meckel ('The Younger' 1781–1833) built what became known as *Die Meckelschen Sammlungen*, today at the Martin Luther University of Halle-Wittenberg in Halle.

[73] *Returns Relating to Medical Museums in the United Kingdom*, Parliamentary Papers 14 (London: House of Commons, 1857); Mark Weatherall, *Gentlemen, Scientists, and Doctors: Medicine at Cambridge, 1800–1940* (Woodbridge: Rochester, NY: Boydell, 2000).

[74] Habershon, *Pathological Catalogue*; Langstaff, *Catalogue of the Preparations*.

[75] Museum Committee Minutes 3 August 1838, Royal College of Surgeons in Ireland Archive RCSI/MUC/1; Charles Alexander Cameron, *A History of the Royal College of Surgeons in Ireland, and of the Irish Schools of Medicine* (2nd edn, Dublin: Fannin, 1916).

[76] On the history of auctioning, see J. M. Chalmers-Hunt (ed.), *Natural History Auctions 1700–1972: A Register of Sales in the British Isles* (London: Sotheby Parke Bernet, 1976); Bettina Dietz, 'Mobile Objects: The Space of Shells in Eighteenth-Century France', *British Journal for the History of Science*, 39 (2006), 363–82; Brian Learmount, *A History of the Auction* (Iver: Barnard and Learmount, 1985); Robin Myers, Michael Harris, and Giles

London had emerged as an important centre for auctioneers of various categories of things. There, anatomical preparations were bought and sold quite openly by the same houses as books and art in the broader exhibitionary complex; such sales were big news far beyond medical and naturalist circles, and were not cheap. Heaviside's collection (figure 3.3), for example—'one of the finest private collections of morbid anatomy in the kingdom'—raised £1,240 in 2,644 lots.[77]

Auctions were nodes in the networks of the medical marketplace, dramaturgical events in which extra-economic factors played powerful roles. Many of those present attended such sales and their previews simply to view the collections. The auction was a spectacular performance, with actors, a stage, props and a script; the catalogues acted as tickets of entry. Not only did the auctioneer and the bidders contribute to the resolution of value of the articles on sale, but so did the audience. The auction was thereby a social process that resolved ambiguities of classification and value—a public forum in which worth was established. Auctions come into their own when items for sale defy conventional forms of pricing, whether because they are old, used, unusual, or their ownership is in doubt. Unlike standard commodity exchange, the catalogues, the ballyhoo, the provenances, and the buyers all contributed to establishing the net worth of body parts on sale.

Auction houses puffed their sales shamelessly: 'The Medical Public [of Edinburgh in 1843] is respectfully informed that a Collection such as the Museum now offered for Sale by Maclachlan, Stewart, & Co., has never been brought before the Public in this country.'[78] Sales might last for weeks, and were often held on the premises of the collector. Institutional museums bid for whole collections wherever possible, especially in the formative years of the museum. Otherwise, the collection was dismantled. Collectors dreaded the posthumous break-up of their cabinets. John Barclay was desperate 'to prevent his Collection of Anatomical preparations from being scattered' and so arranged to have the whole collection

---

Mandelbrote (eds.), *Under the Hammer: Book Auctions since the Seventeenth Century* (London: British Library, 2001); Krzysztof Pomian, *Collectors and Curiosities: Paris and Venice, 1500–1800*, trans. Elizabeth Wiles-Portier (Cambridge: Polity, 1990); Charles W. Smith, *Auctions: The Social Construction of Value* (New York: Free Press, 1989); Stewart, *On Longing*; Cynthia Wall, 'The English Auction: Narratives of Dismantlings', *Eighteenth-Century Studies*, 31 (1997), 1–25. On medical specimens in particular, see Chaplin, 'John Hunter'; Richardson, *Death, Dissection and the Destitute*.

[77] William Wadd, *Nugæ Canoræ: Or, Epitaphian Mementos (in Stone-Cutters' Verse) of the Medici Family of Modern Times* (London: Nichols, 1827), cited in Peachey, *John Heaviside*, 22.

[78] MacLachlan and Stewart Booksellers, *Catalogue of an Extensive and Valuable Anatomical Museum* (Edinburgh: Thomson, 1843), inside cover.

'deposited with some learned and respectable Society or body of men who could estimate its value and render it useful to themselves and others'—namely, the Royal College of Surgeons of Edinburgh.[79] George Langstaff 'had long entertained the hope that [his] collection might be preserved entire', but in vain, for he 'was induced . . . to part with certain portions' and to auction the remainder.[80] The sale 'concluded most lamentably; for nearly 2,000 preparations, which he valued at £2,500, he did not realize £250 . . . the bottles would have sold for more if they had had neither spirit nor preparations in them.'[81] *The Times* lamented of another collection that was broken up, 'We could not help regretting once or twice, that so noble a collection was about to be scattered by the breath of an auctioneer.'[82] Similarly *The Lancet* reported a 'museum shattered to atoms . . . the dismembered fragments . . . sold at a frightful sacrifice, under the hammer of an auctioneer'.[83] The morbid body once again suffered the ignominy of fragmentation.

Take for example the sale of Joshua Brookes's museum, which he had painstakingly accumulated at his four-storey Blenheim Street School in London. It contained 6,000 items, including 'every description of Anatomical Preparation calculated for the elucidation of all parts of the human body and its diseases, both dried and in spirits, with a multitude of PATHOLOGICAL SUBJECTS, comprising Preparations, illustrative of Morbid Anatomy, on a very extensive scale', and allegedly took Brookes thirty years and £30,000 to compile.[84] The *Lancet* considered it 'second only to that of JOHN HUNTER' (as we have seen, a common claim).[85] Brookes was a renowned pedagogue, teaching some 5,000 students in his forty-year career. Upon his retirement in 1826, he offered his museum to the new University of London, but to no avail, and the first part of the collection was auctioned in 1828. For six days before the twenty-four-day sale, the museum was on view to anyone who purchased the 2s. 6d. catalogue. In this, the sale itself was an exhibition, a chance for public access to a renowned museum; an intermediate state in the already blurred

[79] The Deeds of Settlement and Catalogue of the Barcleian Museum, 1828, 3, Royal College of Surgeons in Edinburgh.

[80] *The Lancet*, 18 June 1842, 422.

[81] James Paget, *Memoirs and Letters of Sir James Paget*, ed. Stephen Paget (London: Longmans, Green 1901), 118.

[82] *The Times*, 14 July 1828, 2f.

[83] *The Lancet*, 19 January 1833, 544.

[84] George Robins, *A Catalogue of the Anatomical and Zoological Museum of Joshua Brookes, Esq.* (London: Taylor, 1828), 1, original emphasis.

[85] *The Lancet*, 19 January 1833, 544, original emphasis.

continuum between collection and showroom.[86] Up to 100 lots were sold in a day, clearing out the museum room by room, including the books and the furniture.

The remainder of Brookes's collection went under Wheatley and Adlards' hammer in 1830.[87] Benjamin Wheatley, formerly of Sotheby's, was one of the foremost auctioneers in London in the 1820s and 30s; his partner in bookselling and publishing was George Adlard, from a family of London printers.[88] In the late 1820s, the depression in the book trade led them to diversify into selling wine—and medical museums. 'The rooms were greatly crowded,' grumbled *The Times*, 'notwithstanding the unfavourable state of the weather, but, unfortunately, the model-room, which formed the great attraction [models and casts of Gravid uterus; foetal monsters, pathological "Fac Similes"; dissections of the brain], was so small, as not to contain more than a dozen persons at a time.'[89] By the time the sale opened, 'the crowd that had assembled was beyond even our sanguine expectation'.[90] Others were there in earnest, having studied the catalogues carefully, picked out their choices and decided upon maximum price.[91] Especially enthusiastic bidders could consult more substantial manuscript catalogues kept with the collection by the auction house.

'The sale was commenced with much spirit', reported *The Times,* 'the first lot was bought by the College of Surgeons, who are likely to be large purchasers; and there are agents from Berlin, Amsterdam, Vienna, Paris, Glasgow, &c.'[92] Representatives arrived from the University of Oxford, and from the Zoological Society. William Buckland was there; Robert Grant bid for the new museum at 'Godless Gower Street' (although the University of London turned down the opportunity to purchase the whole collection), and William Clift for the London Hunterian. Brooke's former student, the country doctor and budding physical anthropologist Joseph

---

[86] Jim Bennett, 'Knowing and Doing in the Sixteenth Century: What Were Instruments For?' *British Journal for the History of Science,* 36 (2003), 129–50; Tony Bennett, *The Birth of the Museum: History, Theory, Politics* (London: Routledge, 1995).

[87] Benjamin Wheatley and George Adlard, *Museum Brookesianum. A Descriptive and Historical Catalogue of the Remainder of the Anatomical and Zootomical Museum, of Joshua Brookes, Esq.* (London: Taylor, 1830).

[88] Marc Vaulbert de Chantilly, 'Property of a Distinguished Poisoner: Thomas Griffiths Wainewright and the Griffith Family Library', in Myers, Harris, and Mandelbrote, *Under the Hammer,* 111–42.

[89] *The Times* 14 July 1828, 2f; Robins, *Catalogue of the Anatomical and Zoological Museum,* 3.

[90] *The Times* 16 July 1828, 3e.

[91] See for example Wheatley and Adlard, *Museum Brookesianum* at the Wellcome Library and MacLachlan and Stewart, *Catalogue* at the Edinburgh University Library.

[92] *The Times* 16 July 1828, 3e.

Barnard Davis, purchased the human skulls for his personal collection. William Clark came up from Cambridge and spent £150.[93] Thomas Hodgkin may have been at the first sale, or at least an agent of the Guy's collection, for 44 specimens found their way to the hospital. The surgeon-geologist Gideon Mantell attended: 'Took Stutchbury [Samuel, naturalist] with me to Brooks [sic] Museum to select a few lots to purchase at the sale.' Clearly the break-up of the museum was devastating to Brookes, perched at Robins's elbow; as Mantell scoffed, 'Brooks was there—if ever very clever, his light has gone out—a great bore! Shall I come to this? No—I shall blow out before I am put in a save-all; at least I hope so.'[94]

And so a body part was given a price—between one and four shillings at the MacLachlan and Stewart sale in 1843.[95] Elsewhere prices ranged up to 20 shillings for an ordinary preparation. A better price could be had if the specimen retained details of the patient and case history. To obtain a collection was not only to purchase material culture, but also the documentation, provenances, and the very expertise and reputation of previous owners and collectors. In the context of pathological anatomy, as in other museological spheres, rarity increased monetary value (which is why John Hunter paid £500 for the remains of Charles Byrne, the 'Irish Giant'). For countless fragmented examples of other diseases, the advantage of the museum as a teaching tool rested on the availability of conditions that would rarely appear on the ward or in the dissection room. By the end of the century, however, this brought about the 'difficulty that certain types of specimen, which are genuine rarities within the limits of individual experience, become relatively common at such a centre as the museum'.[96]

It appears then that pathologized body parts became commodities. But to what extent *were* human remains commodified by their passage through this marketplace? Anthropologists who study exchange have unpacked the subtleties of the concept, and consider commodification not as a discrete event but as a process. Human remains, like other objects travelling to and from museums, may undergo a 'commodity phase' during their biographies, and as Margaret Lock argues, 'The commodity

[93] Adrian Desmond, *The Politics of Evolution: Morphology, Medicine and Reform in Radical London* (Chicago: University of Chicago Press, 1989); Helen MacDonald, *Human Remains*; Weatherall, *Gentlemen, Scientists, and Doctors*.

[94] *The Times* 16 July 1828, 3e; Gideon Algernon Mantell, *The Journal of Gideon Mantell, Surgeon and Geologist: Covering the Years 1818–1852*, ed. E. Cecil Curwen (London: Oxford University Press, 1940), 74.

[95] MacLachlan and Stewart, *Catalogue*; see also Chaplin, 'John Hunter'.

[96] Branson, 'Of the Museum', 24.

status of body parts is contestable, negotiable and mutable.'[97] And yet late modern Western attitudes to the human body render even the hint of commodification sensitive, and this tends to obliterate the subtleties of the exchange.[98] It carries with it echoes of the most disturbing form of commodifying living human bodies, slavery, which is anathema to twenty-first century readers and was becoming so in the early nineteenth century (Thomas Hodgkin was himself a fierce abolitionist). But because of the power relations around disease and death, and the nature of collections and collecting, payment for pathological specimens was not a pure market exchange. Neither are the more recent manifestations of the market of body parts, including organ sales, reproductive technologies and tissue cultures, all of which have prompted considerable ethical, legal, and cultural analyses.[99] The medical commodification of the body, dead or alive, is not a new phenomenon: but the debates that surround such practices, and the meanings of commodification, are culturally and historically contingent. For although scholars have observed similarities between then and now, especially in the connotation of market—harvesting the wards, mining or quarrying the body for tissues or specimens, and the 'treasures' or indeed 'spoils' to be found in museums—Duncan Wilson has argued that attitudes to body commodification are neither monolithic nor constant.[100] Rather, the nineteenth-century market for body parts imbued different values and meanings into human remains to those that inhere to modern organs and cell lines. The final parts of this chapter will address these meanings in light of relevant historical and anthropological scholarship.

---

[97] Margaret M. Lock, 'The Alienation of Body Tissue and the Biopolitics of Immortalized Cell Lines', in Scheper-Hughes and Wacquant, *Commodifying Bodies*, 63–92 at 71.

[98] For surveys, see Klaus Hoeyer, 'Person, Patent and Property: A Critique of the Commodification Hypothesis', *Biosocieties*, 2 (2007), 327–48; Lesley A. Sharp, 'The Commodification of the Body and Its Parts', *Annual Review of Anthropology*, 29 (2000), 287–328.

[99] Andrews and Nelkin, *Body Bazaar*; Mary Dixon-Woods, et al., 'Human Tissue and "The Public": The Case of Childhood Cancer Tumour Banking', *BioSocieties*, 3 (2008), 57–80; Fox and Swazey, *Spare Parts*; Parry and Gere, 'Contested Bodies'; Scheper-Hughes and Wacquant, *Commodifying Bodies*; Catherine Waldby and Robert Mitchell, *Tissue Economies: Blood, Organs and Cell Lines in Late Capitalism* (Durham, NC: Duke University Press, 2006); Stephen Wilkinson, *Bodies for Sale: Ethics and Exploitation in the Human Body Trade* (London: Routledge, 2003).

[100] Wilson, 'Whose Body (of Opinion) Is It Anyway?'; see also Ruth Richardson, 'Fearful Symmetry, Corpses for Anatomy: Organs for Transplantation', in Stuart J. Youngner, Renée C. Fox, and Lawrence O'Connell (eds.), *Organ Transplantation: Meanings and Realities* (Madison: University of Wisconsin Press, 1997), 66–100.

VESTIGES OF IDENTITY

Many of the circulating museum body parts were 'fungible', that is, they became interchangeable with other specimens. One ossified femur, one ulcerated oesophagus (figure 1.3), was in principle as good as another, regardless of the identity of the patient. And yet some specimens had particular value beyond the condition they illustrated. As both Ruth Richardson and Simon Chaplin have argued, they 'resonate with association'.[101] Sometimes this was because of the reputation of their originating person: Joseph Merrick's remains at the London Hospital Medical School Museum do much more than represent elephantiasis (his condition is in any case now diagnosed as Proteus syndrome).[102] Relics of the (in)famous, from medical celebrities to criminals, were to be found in medical museums throughout the century. Henry Wellcome, that most prominent of collectors, liked to collect the remains of people whose fame rivalled his own, including those of William Burke and Jeremy Bentham.[103] Like anthropologists of organ donation, the historian of medical museums can trace shreds of identity that travel with fragmented body parts; those meanings associated with people that did not become 'lost in the mix'.[104] Unlike donated organs, however, the association with the originating person is not always the most potent. Many specimens were afforded singularity by association with those through whose hands they subsequently passed. In stark contrast with the relics of saints, whose remains were 'empowered with means of identity', their 'division and distribution intended to maximize rather than to undermine its special status', for many morbid specimens the association with the original patient was obliterated by that of the collector.[105] It was possible in death, as anthropologist Lesley Sharp observes, for 'socially expendable categories of persons [to be] ironically transformed into valued objects through their involvement in medical research'—post-mortem body parts

---

[101] Ruth Richardson, 'Human Remains', in Ken Arnold and Danielle Olsen (eds.), *Medicine Man: The Forgotten Museum of Henry Wellcome* (London: British Museum Press, 2003), 319–45 at 342; Simon Chaplin, 'Emotion and Identity in John Hunter's Museum', in Karen Ingham, *Narrative Remains* (London: Royal College of Surgeons of England, 2009), 8–15.

[102] David Hevey, 'Beyond the Shadow of Merrick', in Richard Sandell, Jocelyn Dodd, and Rosemarie Garland-Thomson (eds.), *Re-Presenting Disability: Activism and Agency in the Museum* (Abingdon: Routledge, 2010), 79–91.

[103] Frances Larson, *An Infinity of Things: How Sir Henry Wellcome Collected the World* (Oxford: Oxford University Press, 2009).

[104] Fox and Swazey, *Spare Parts*; Rabinow, 'Severing the Ties'.

[105] Dacome, 'Resurrecting by Numbers', 104; Bynum, *Fragmentation and Redemption*.

could become highly prized, but not because of their originating person.[106] In the medical marketplace a body part could gain value as rarity and through association with particular practitioners, the dead part afforded greater value than the living patient had been.

The medical museum body was partible, and Marilyn Strathern has argued that partible persons are multi-authored; so too, as we shall explore in more detail in chapter 5, the conglomerate body in the pathology gallery had multiple identities wrapped around its parts.[107] Sharp asks of dismemberment and fragmentation 'how such processes may obscure, augment, or alter constructions of personhood and/or the social worth of human bodies' and 'how increasingly miniscule human parts may still embody persons'?[108] In the medical museum they did, but in subtle and often contradictory ways. Unlike transplanted organs, some gross morbid specimens were identified *only* with the anatomist or collector, and the patients' identity was entirely removed, subsumed by the practitioners'.[109] In its label and/or case history, the person-artefact carried with it varying elements of identification with each of these individuals, primarily the highest-status donor. And contrary to ostensibly absolute nature of the commodity exchange, such associations also endured with purchased specimens.

The imprint of the collector, as argued above, was most conspicuous for entire collections that retained the donor's name. William Hunter's fame was so strong that further additions to the Hunterian Museum in Glasgow were kept and catalogued separately for a century, and the founding specimens continue to be prized.[110] Prominent and generous donors' names lived on within other collections, as for example at the Royal College of Surgeons in Edinburgh, in which the [Charles] Bell and the [James] Wilson collections were discrete within the museum long after their purchase from the Great Windmill Street School.[111] Barclay had

[106] Sharp, 'Commodification of the Body', 296; Sharp, *Bodies, Commodities, and Biotechnologies*.

[107] Strathern, *Gender of the Gift*.

[108] Sharp, 'Commodification of the Body', 290, 310.

[109] Chaplin, 'John Hunter'; Patricia S. Gindhart, 'An Early Twentieth-Century Skeleton Collection', *Journal of Forensic Sciences*, 34 (1989), 887–93.

[110] For example the purchase of James Jeffray's collection in 1848. Allen Thomson, 'Collection of Anatomical Preparations Belonging to the Late Dr Jeffray', MS, *c*. 1848, Glasgow University Special Collections MR 41/6; Alice J. Marshall and J. A. G. Burton (eds.), *Catalogue of the Preparations of Dr. William Hunter, Sir William Macewen, Professor John H. Teacher, Professor J. A. G. Burton in the Museum of the Pathology Department, Glasgow Royal Infirmary* (Glasgow: University of Glasgow, 1962).

[111] Charles W. Cathcart, 'Some of the Older Schools of Anatomy Connected with the Royal College of Surgeons, Edinburgh', *Edinburgh Medical Journal*, 27 (1882), 769–81; Kemp with Barnes, *Surgeon's Hall*.

donated his collection on the condition 'that it should be associated with his name in perpetuity'.[112] And so not only donors but also sellers were recorded in documentation, their identities embedded into the textual component of the morbid body. In the St Bartholomew's collection, curators were enjoined to record 'the name of the person who gave it', but in practice prominent figures in the provenance of an item were recorded whether the specimen was sold or given.[113] These histories infused the collection with the reputations of previous owners regardless of the mode of exchange. In this, the traces of their collectors, human remains had much in common with other museum objects. Contrary to Shelton's claim that 'museums usually erase the identity of the collectors who have assembled their holdings', pathological preparations, like objects of art and ethnography, acquire a pedigree of collectors on their way to the gallery.[114] They gained value if they had been prepared, collected and displayed by a high-profile collector. They become biographical objects, but of the practitioner rather than the patient. Exploitative power relations were at play in these museological processes.

This chapter has concentrated on the formative decades of medical museums in the early nineteenth century. Later in the century, however, many of these resonances diminished. At Guy's, for example, it was decreed in 1888 that the 'name of the donor shall be omitted from the heading on the bottle, and only mentioned in the catalogue in connection with the references, except in the case of donations from outside the Hospital when the fact shall always be duly notified'.[115] In late Victorian catalogues, the histories and descriptions took up more space and the donor glorification less.[116] As one curator sneered,

> Museum shelves have many a curious tale to tell of how and why they acquired their furniture. This specimen because Mr. So-and-so cut it off; this because Mr. A. or B. gave it; this because, though a very ordinary thing, it came from some extra-ordinary man; this apparently that what there was to

[112] [William MacGillivray], *Catalogue of the Museum of the Royal College of Surgeons of Edinburgh* (Edinburgh: Neill, 1836); John Barclay to John Wishart, 3 July 1821, in Council Records Sederunt, 10 July 1821, cited in Tansey and Mekie, *Museum of the Royal College*, 5.

[113] St Bartholomew's Hospital Minutes of the Governors 23 June 1726, cited in Eve, 'Our Museum', 165.

[114] Anthony A. Shelton, 'Doubts Affirmations', in Anthony A. Shelton (ed.), *Collectors: Individuals and Institutions* (London: Horniman Museum, 2001), 13–22 at 19; see also Errington, 'What Became Authentic Primitive Art?'.

[115] Guy's Hospital Museum, Minute Book, 27 September 1888, 1, Gordon Museum Archive, King's College London.

[116] See for example Pitt, 'List of Specimens'; Samuel Wilks, *Pathological Catalogue of the Museum of Guy's Hospital* (London: MacKenzie, 1858).

show has long ceased to be appreciable; this because it is published some-
where, and so on.[117]

Over time, many specimens were entirely anonymized, on the shelf if not
in records—either because their identities were unknown to pathologists
or because they were purposefully left in the autopsy records and
not carried over to museum documentation; the identities of both patient
and collector were thereby discarded.[118] Purposefully or otherwise, many
specimens were avowedly biography-less as they became objects. They
were not individual, but dividual: which distinction—between the complete body of the originating person (alive or dead) and the composite,
multi-authored body in the museum, whose component parts originate
from different places—will be explored in more detail in chapter 5. Body
parts in this dividual were universalized, becoming metonymic for all
examples of a particular malady: like the votive fragments that Jessica
Hughes analyses, the corporeal fragment was the materialization of
illness.[119] They represented 'typical' structures of disease an important
museological practice across the natural sciences as type specimens came to
play a key part in taxonomy.[120] As Anita Guerrini reflects,

> Preparations and skeletons provided examples of the human body but not of
> the individual; the specific identity of the body part, including both whose
> body it came from and what body part it was, was often mysterious except to
> the anatomist. A preparation of a leg, for example, could be male or female,
> its age and other particulars erased. With its skin partly flayed and flared out
> in a varnished wing, it did not even look human but like some odd insect.
> The act of anatomy destabilized the idea of what was human and effaced the
> linkage between the part and the person as well as the function of the part,
> which could be either human or animal. The body's humanness receded as it
> was studied ever more deeply.[121]

---

[117] James F. Goodhart, 'List of Specimens Added to the Pathological Museum During
the Year 1882–83', *Guy's Hospital Reports*, 42 (1884), 101–8 at 102.

[118] Gindhart, 'Early Twentieth-Century Skeleton Collection'; Ruth Richardson, 'A
Potted History of Specimen-Taking', *The Lancet*, 11 March 2000, 935–6. See for example
Thomas Fawdington, *A Catalogue Descriptive Chiefly of the Morbid Preparations Contained
in the Museum of the Manchester Theatre of Anatomy and Medicine* (Manchester: Harrison
and Crosfield, 1833).

[119] Susan C. Lawrence and Kae Bendixen, 'His and Hers: Male and Female Anatomy
Texts for U.S. Medical Students, 1890–1989', *Social Science and Medicine*, 7 (1992),
925–34; Lawrence, 'Beyond the Grave'.

[120] William Aitken, 'On the Progress of Scientific Pathology', *British Medical Journal*,
2 (1888), 348–59; Alberti, 'The Status of Museums'; Lorraine Daston, 'Type Specimens
and Scientific Memory', *Critical Enquiry*, 31 (2004), 153–82.

[121] Anita Guerrini, 'Anatomists and Entrepreneurs in Early Eighteenth-Century London', *Journal of the History of Medicine and Allied Sciences*, 59 (2004), 219–39 at 231–2.

BODILY FRAGMENTS AS OBJECTS

Some body parts, then, were identified with particular people, others anonymised. All experienced a parallel and related process: a physical and conceptual transformation into material culture. They demonstrated, in Richardson's words, 'the capacity of the human body itself to become artefact'.[122] Like Erin O'Connor's exploration of Victorian physical deviance in the living, here we are concerned with

> a series of moments when diseased and deformed flesh merges metaphorically with other things—when the exigencies of the material body are explained as problems of material culture ... [for] nineteenth-century figurations of pathology constituted an elaborate meditation on the relationship between objects and persons: whether persons were objects; whether objects were subjects; and whether, and on what terms, there could be said to be any essential difference between the two.[123]

Further complicating matters, material culture is itself flexible and problematic as a category.[124] It is historically contingent, and was shaped in the late nineteenth century in and with museum collections. Similar conceptual and physical procedures to those enacted on ethnographic curios and archaeological finds in Victorian collections were applied to natural things—taxidermic mounts, herbarium sheets, even fossils—and anatomical preparations. They were all matter altered for use from some sort of raw material, be it stone, wood, or flesh. Like the unpacking of the gift—commodity distinction, it is helpful to view material culture as a process rather than a state: the way that museum things, be they organic or otherwise, underwent work on the way to the collection. Distinguishing anatomical specimens from other kinds of things, however, was the character of the raw material, the culturally specific attitudes to dead bodies (see chapter 6).

Anthropologists and archaeologists like to dissolve the traditional boundaries between person and things, and to acknowledge that the point of death was not the 'event horizon' at which a body becomes a thing—we have seen clearly in this chapter how anatomists began to objectify bodies of patients as they ailed. More broadly, living bodies

---

[122] Richardson, 'Human Remains', 323. See also Joanna R. Sofaer, *The Body as Material Culture: A Theoretical Archaeology* (Cambridge: Cambridge University Press, 2006).
[123] O'Connor, *Raw Material*, 15.
[124] Tim Ingold, 'Materials against Materiality', *Archaeological Dialogues*, 14 (2007), 1–16; Christopher Tilley, 'Materiality in Materials', *Archaeological Dialogues*, 14 (2007), 16–20.

were adapted and shaped and objectified, and conversely dead bodies
retained powerful traces of personhood.[125] However, the materiality of
the body was undeniably altered by death, and thereafter slowly changed
into entities of a different kind; from him or her to *it*. The practices
enacted upon human remains from the post-mortem examination onwards—not only the acquisition processes discussed here, but also the
preservation, bottling, arrangement, and inscription detailed in the next
chapter—wrapped new layers of meaning around the materiality of the
body that sometimes obscured, sometimes enhanced the living characteristics of the body part. As anthropologist Janet Hoskins observed of one
particular trophy head, 'Using the processual approach suggested in more
recent work on exchange, we can see that the head can be defined as a
particular type of "biographical object," one which was able to travel in
both directions from person to object and then from object back to
person.'[126] A pathological specimen, like a donated organ, could be the
remains of a person in one context, but raw material in another. In death,
as in life, the body was a 'culturally malleable category' that transgressed
the already blurred boundary between nature and artifice.[127]

Reversible or not, the journey to the museum was thereby a passage
from person to thing. Through processes of exchange and preparation, the
body was rendered material culture: like the twentieth- and twenty-first-
century human remains deployed in medical science, in Victorian museums fragmented human bodies were realized as biotechnological artefacts through complex and lengthy processes of exchange, re-invention,
and techniques that involve a complex web of patients, practitioners, and
publics.[128] These practices and audiences were of course markedly different to their descendants, as we shall see later: here it remains only to
discuss how they contributed to the objectification of the body part.

Bodies became objects not only through circulation and physical practices outlined in this and the following chapter but also by more subtle
processes of objectification. When thinking about the ways in which the
dead body is objectified, we can helpfully draw upon the study of objectification of the living—through slavery and pornography, for example.
Philosophers have untangled a number of ways that living persons can be
and are objectified, and many of them are applied to dead body parts on

---

[125] Sofaer, *Body as Material Culture*; Elizabeth Hallam, Jenny Hockey, and Glennys
Howarth, *Beyond the Body: Death and Social Identity* (London: Routledge, 1999); Elizabeth
Hallam and Jenny Hockey, *Death, Memory, and Material Culture* (Oxford: Berg, 2001).
[126] Janet Hoskins, 'On Losing and Getting a Head: Warfare, Exchange, and Alliance in
a Changing Sumba, 1888–1988', *American Ethnologist*, 16 (1989), 419–40 at 437.
[127] Sharp, 'Commodification of the Body', 313.
[128] Parry and Gere, 'Contested Bodies'.

their way to museums. Human remains, like the objectified living, are treated as instruments; they are fungible; they are violated and dismembered; and they are treated as property.[129] This latter is especially significant, for whatever the legal status of body parts, pathological specimens were in practice owned by collectors and institutions.[130] The authority of the medical practitioner was clearly demonstrated by the extent to which the specimen became the property of the collector or the hospital, just as organ and tissue trajectories in the twentieth century revealed the politics of biosociety. Power relations were as evident in this form of collecting human remains as they were in the colonial encounter during which Europeans appropriated countless indigenous human remains.[131] Anatomy collections played out not only racial hierarchies but also class relations; before and after the Anatomy Act of 1832, it was the bodies of the poor—stolen or unclaimed—that ended up on the anatomists' tables and in their collections.[132]

To objectify human remains is of course very different to objectifying living people. In part, medical practitioners from the eighteenth century onwards argued, it was a crucial element of medical education—such is the powerful resonance on the violability of the body, from their first encounter with a cadaver onwards, medical students learned to distance the dead from the living, as we shall see in chapter 6. Pathologists in particular objectified to help them cope with their day-to-day encounter with the corpse. It was easier to do so with a fragment than with a whole body, because in disintegration the body has been shucked of much of its personhood.

Objectification was rarely absolute. As we have seen, traces of identity inhered to many specimens, and even if these were not those of the patient, they hindered objectification. For not only if a body is still materially a person, but also if it still closely identified with a person, then the process of objectification is incomplete. Rather, the specimen betrayed complex relations between patient and practitioner, donor, and curator. The exchanges of ownership outlined here, their rituals and recording, contributed in complex ways to the symbolic value of human

---

[129] Martha Craven Nussbaum, *Sex and Social Justice* (New York: Oxford University Press, 1999); Wilkinson, *Bodies for Sale*.

[130] On the complexity of human body ownership, see Dickenson, *Body Shopping*; Anita Guerrini, 'Duverney's Skeletons', *Isis*, 94 (2003), 577–603; Lawrence, 'Beyond the Grave'; Paul Matthews, 'Whose Body? People as Property', *Current Legal Problems*, 36 (1983), 197–200; Parry and Gere, 'Contested Bodies'; Loane Skene, 'Who Owns Your Body? Legal Issues on the Ownership of Bodily Material', *Trends in Molecular Medicine*, 8 (2002), 48–9; Wilson, 'Whose Body (of Opinion) Is It Anyway?'.

[131] Fforde, *Collecting the Dead*.

[132] Richardson, *Death, Dissection and the Destitute*.

remains. Morbid fragments, fetishized or universalized, were wrapped in layers of meaning from pathological data to *memento mori*. Some were merely tank specimens, disposable, objectified; others were highly valued, medically, socially, and financially. As Margaret Lock writes of organ transplants,

> If less attention is paid to the objects themselves, and more to the systems and sequences of exchange—thus inserting a time dimension into the analysis—the shifting value of objects becomes evident as they change through time and space. At one moment objects may be understood as inalienable, even as sacred, but later they may gain commodity status and then occasionally return to their former status, or become only partially alienable under specific circumstances.[133]

The meanings of the specimens were fluid and contingent: in the next chapter, we turn from their epistemic instability to their physical instability—or rather, preparators' efforts to combat this.

---

[133] Lock, *Twice Dead*, 317.

4

Preserving Pathology

Craft and Technique in the Medical Museum

The previous chapter explored the conceptual and spatial processes that began the transformation of the dead body from subject to object, that rendered human flesh material culture. In this chapter we look closer at the physical element of the process of material culture, turning from how body parts were moved to how they were worked. As such, it is a history of *practice*, unpacking the processes involved in the 'black box' of the collection. After they arrive in the museum, but before they are seen by the visitors (if at all), what happened to objects behind the scenes?[1] What did anatomists, pathologists, curators, and technicians actually *do* on a day-to-day basis, and how did they learn to do it?

Studying museums in practice encourages us to look beyond exhibitions and texts to instruments, to specimens, and to methods. In doing so, we will find that particular skills gather around the very particular kinds of objects and we reveal the relationship between what John Pickstone calls

---

[1] The historiography of museum practice is expanding: see for example Samuel J. M. M. Alberti, *Nature and Culture: Objects, Disciplines and the Manchester Museum* (Manchester: Manchester University Press, 2009); Simon Chaplin, 'John Hunter and The "Museum Oeconomy", 1750–1800' (Ph.D. thesis, King's College London, 2009); Arthur MacGregor, *Curiosity and Enlightenment: Collectors and Collections from the Sixteenth to the Nineteenth Century* (New Haven, Conn.: Yale University Press, 2007); Robert M. Peck, 'Alcohol and Arsenic, Pepper, and Pitch: Brief Histories of Preservation Techniques', in Sue Ann Prince (ed.), *Stuffing Birds, Pressing Plants, Shaping Knowledge: Natural History in North America, 1730–1860* (Philadelphia: American Philosophical Society, 2003), 27–53. For earlier accounts by practitioners, see Francis Joseph Cole, 'History of the Anatomical Museum', in Oliver Elton (ed.), *A Miscellany Presented to John Macdonald Mackay* (Liverpool: Liverpool University Press, 1914), 302–17; Jessie Dobson, 'Some Eighteenth Century Experiments in Embalming', *Journal of the History of Medicine*, 8 (1953), 431–41; Rosina Down, '"Old" Preservative Methods', in Velson Horie (ed.), *Conservation of Natural History Specimens: Spirit Collections* (Manchester: Manchester University Press, 1989), 33–8; D. H. Tompsett, *Anatomical Techniques* (2nd edn, Edinburgh: Livingstone, 1970); and, especially, John James Edwards and M. J. Edwards, *Medical Museum Technology* (London: Oxford University Press, 1959), which is used throughout this chapter.

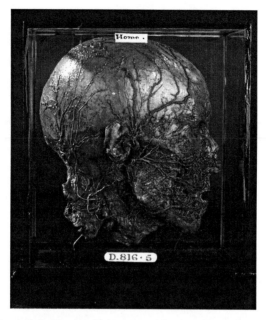

Fig. 4.1. The superficial nerves and arteries of the face and neck, by Joseph Swan, presented to the Royal College of Surgeons of England in 1865. Copyright the Hunterian Museum at the Royal College of Surgeons.

'ways of working' and 'ways of knowing'.[2] The latter relied heavily on the former. The Lincoln-based surgeon Joseph Swan, for example, who had trained at the Borough hospitals under Astley Cooper, was a pioneer in what we now call neurology, but his research depended upon a new method of drying preparations that he developed (see figure 4.1). 'A greater difficulty has been experienced in making preparations of the minute nerves than of any other part of the body,' he argued, 'and for this reason medical men have been less familiar with the anatomy of the nervous system than of many other parts, and consequently its physiology and pathology have remained in much obscurity.'[3] New techniques led to new knowledge, so that morbid anatomy was as dependent on preserving fluids as it was on theories of disease.

---

[2] John V. Pickstone, 'Working Knowledges before and after *circa* 1800: Practices and Disciplines in the History of Science, Technology and Medicine', *Isis*, 98 (2007), 489–516.
[3] Joseph Swan, *An Account of a New Method of Making Dried Anatomical Preparations* (2nd edn, Lincoln: Drury, 1820), v; Nicholas J. Barton and B. D. Smith, 'Joseph Swan (1791–1874): Pioneer of Research on Peripheral Nerves', *Journal of Hand Surgery (European Volume)*, 33E (2008), 252–9; Victor Plarr, *Lives of the Fellows of the Royal College of Surgeons of England*, 2 vols. (London: Royal College of Surgeons, 1930).

Unpacking these communities of practice surrounding these techniques deepens our understanding of both the medical community and the wider exhibitionary complex. Although most of this work was undertaken by the anatomists themselves, we also encounter the 'invisible technicians' who kept museums afloat: curators' assistants and conservators (or 'preservators'), even the too-often-overlooked porters.[4] Almost by definition, many of their practices were crafts, implicit skills that were reproduced by the transfer of tacit knowledge and never recorded, so the historian must look beyond the scant written traces to the outcomes of these practices: the preparations themselves. Museum products reveal much about museum processes, about the way in which practitioners invested energy and inscribed their identities upon these hybrid objects.

In the following chapter we encounter other products and media in the museum, especially wax and paper, but the focus here is upon organic preparations.[5] The preserved body part was for anatomists the next best thing to the living body, especially when fresh corpses were hard to come by. And as we established earlier there was a particular imperative to preserve diseased specimens, because many conditions were rare and students were unlikely to encounter them in the dissecting room or the clinic. 'Preparations serve two purposes chiefly,' argued William Hunter, 'to wit, the preservation of uncommon things, and the preservation of such things as required considerable labour to anatomise them, so as to shew their structure distinctly.'[6] William Henry Flower echoed him a century later: 'it is often desirable to preserve specimens for a considerable time or permanently, either on account of their intrinsic rarity, causing difficulties in procuring them when needed, or on account of the labour and skill which may have been expended upon their proper display, which it is desirable not to have wasted'.[7] Preparing specimens and later cleaning

---

[4] Steven Shapin, 'The Invisible Technician', *American Scientist*, 77 (1989), 554–63.

[5] For discussions of the production of other media, see for example Nick Hopwood, 'Artist Versus Anatomist, Models against Dissection: Paul Zeiller of Munich and the Revolution of 1848', *Medical History*, 51 (2007), 279–308; Anna Maerker, Model Experts: Wax Anatomies and Enlightenment in Florence and Vienna, 1775–1815 (Manchester: Manchester University Press, 2011); Michael Sappol, *A Traffic of Dead Bodies: Anatomy and Embodied Social Identity in Nineteenth-Century America* (Princeton: Princeton University Press, 2002). On the importance of organic remains, see for example Benjamin G. Babington and G. O. Rees, 'On the Preservation of Subjects for Anatomical Purposes', *Guy's Hospital Report*, 4 (1839), 442–7; Frederick John Knox, *The Anatomist's Instructor, and Museum Companion: Being Practical Directions for the Formation and Subsequent Management of Anatomical Museums* (Edinburgh: Black, 1836).

[6] William Hunter, *Two Introductory Lectures, Delivered by Dr. William Hunter, to His Last Course of Anatomical Lectures* (London: Johnson, 1784), 89.

[7] William Henry Flower, 'Museum Specimens for Teaching Purposes', *Nature*, 15 (1876–7), 144–6, 184–6, 204–6 at 144.

and maintaining them were ongoing and labour-intensive activities, as we shall see later in this chapter. Several thousand preparations evaporating and deteriorating, attracting mould, insects, and other pests, and generally responding to the entropic urge kept the museum staff on their toes. But they persevered in their efforts to prevent or retard the post-mortem senescence of the body—their quest to slow down time.[8]

THE PRESERVATOR'S PALETTE

The methods available to an Edwardian medical conservator were surprisingly similar to those employed a century earlier. They can be grouped into five categories: drying, storing in fluid, injecting, corroding, and articulating. All were intended to capture 'the organs themselves with all the physical properties they possessed at the moment of death'—that is, to 'preserve the tissues without altering the appearance of the flesh'.[9] They sought to maintain as far as possible the texture, colour, and size of the living part, and the success of each method was judged on its capacity to retain one or all of these aspects.

The oldest and simplest technique—but perhaps least satisfactory when judged by the criteria just laid out—was drying, or desiccation. Some mummies in ancient Egypt and South America were simply dried, of course, and for the most part this was the only method used in medieval and very early modern Europe. Specimens were stretched out, often with the blood left in for colour, with warmth supplied if necessary, sometimes briefly doused in alcohol, and simply left to dry. In the medical museum this suited some internal organs, calculi, and the skin (including gangrene and the ever-popular 'horny excrescences'). Its simplicity meant it was still in use in the nineteenth century, as for example by Allan Burns in

    [8] Harold J. Cook, 'Time's Bodies: Crafting the Preparation and Preservation of *Naturalia*', in Pamela H. Smith and Paula Findlen (eds.), *Merchants and Marvels: Commerce, Science and Art in Early Modern Europe* (New York: Routledge, 2002), 223–47.
    [9] Jean Nicolas Gannal, *History of Embalming, and Preparations in Anatomy, Pathology and Natural History*, ed. and trans. Richard Harlan (1838; Philedelphia: Dobson, 1840), 141; Frederick S. Eve, 'Our Museum and Its Associations', *St Bartholomew's Hospital Reports*, 17 (1881), 165–84 at 184. On the similarity of techniques at the beginning and end of the century, see Francis Joseph Cole, 'The History of Anatomical Injections', in Charles Singer (ed.), *Studies in the History and Method of Science*, 2 vols. (Oxford: Clarendon Press, 1921), ii. 285–343; Edwards and Edwards, *Medical Museum Technology*. Unless otherwise noted information for this section is drawn from these works, as well as Francis Joseph Cole, *A History of Comparative Anatomy: From Aristotle to the Eighteenth Century* (London: Macmillan, 1944); Cook, 'Time's Bodies'; Jessie Dobson, 'Historical Introduction', in Tompsett, *Anatomical Techniques*, xi-xvi; Robert Harrison, *The Dublin Dissector, or Manual of Anatomy* (5th edn, New York: Wood, 1854); MacGregor, *Curiosity and Enlightenment*.

Glasgow, and John Barclay in Edinburgh, who demonstrated the arterial and venous systems solely from dried preparations—to the disappointment of his students.[10] But it was cheap, and relatively easy.

The most prevalent technique involved more than a quick splash of alcohol. In 1660 Elias Ashmole is alleged to have shown King Charles II two abortions preserved by Dr Edward Warner for four years submerged entirely in spirits and glass; more certain is that two years later, having borrowed the idea from Robert Boyle (or vice versa), William Croone demonstrated to the Royal Society that puppies, soft parts and all, could be preserved in 'spirit of wine'. In 1663 Boyle committed the method to print, because 'it cannot but be a great help to the Student of Anatomy, to be able to preserve the parts of humane Bodies, and those of other Animals, especially such Monsters as are of a very singular or instructive Fabrick, so long that he may have recourse to them at pleasure'.[11] From the outset, then, preservative techniques were developed in order to retain rare, morbid, and minute specimens, and this practice expanded over the following centuries. By the end of the eighteenth century, 'wet' preservation was widespread, as the Quaker physician Thomas Pole revealed in 1790 in his popular *Anatomical Instructor*: 'Preparations of almost every part are . . . kept in spirits . . . more especially the diseased parts; as by this mode they undergo less change in appearance than by any other method of preservation, and consequently give the best idea of the natural or diseased appearance.'[12]

The University of Edinburgh anatomy museum was granted twelve gallons of whisky a year by the city in 1800.[13] The precise composition of

---

[10] Knox, *Anatomist's Instructor*; Ronald S. Wade, 'Medical Mummies: The History of the Burns Collection', *The Anatomical Record*, 253 (1998), 158–61.

[11] Robert Boyle, *Some Considerations Touching the Usefulnesse of Experimental Naturall Philosophy*, 2 vols. (Oxford: Hall, 1663), ii. 21.

[12] Thomas Pole, *The Anatomical Instructor; or, an Illustration of the Modern and Most Approved Methods of Preparing and Preserving the Different Parts of the Human Body* (2nd edn, London: Callow, 1813), 163; E. T. Wedmore, 'Thomas Pole', *Journal of the Friends' Historical Society*, supplement to volume 7 (1908), 1–53.

[13] Royal Commission on the Universities of Scotland, *Minutes of Evidence*, 4 vols., House of Commons Command Papers 92–55 (London: HMSO, 1837). For contemporary technical discussions of wet preservation, see J. W. Baggaley, 'Gelatin and Glycerine Spirit for Mounting Spirit Specimens', *Museums Journal*, 13 (1914), 272–3; John Green Crosse, 'A Memoir Upon the Method of Securely Closing Moist Anatomical Preparations, Preserved in Spirit', *Transactions of the Provincial Medical and Surgical Association*, 4 (1836), 284–305; S. H. Daukes, *The Medical Museum: Modern Developments, Organisation and Technical Methods Based on a New System of Visual Teaching* (London: Wellcome Institute, 1929); Flower, 'Museum Specimens'; James C. Laskey, *A General Account of the Hunterian Museum, Glasgow* (Glasgow: Smith, 1813); Alfred Tulk and Arthur Henfrey, *Anatomical Manipulation, or, the Methods of Pursuing Practical Investigations in Comparative Anatomy and Physiology* (London: Van Voorst, 1844); Alexander Watson, 'On Preserving Anatomical

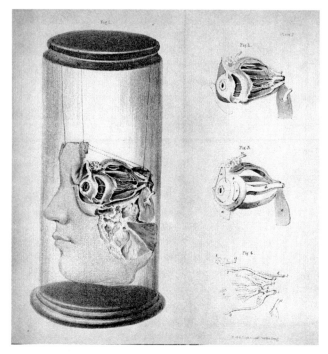

Fig. 4.2. Preparation of the nerves within the orbit, from John Green Crosse, 'A memoir upon the method of securely closing moist anatomical preparations, preserved in spirit', *Transactions of the Provincial Medical and Surgical Association*, 4 (1836), 284–305. Wellcome Library, London.

the preserving fluid was important: too strong, and the alcohol would corrugate the specimen; too weak, and it would putrefy. Practitioners complained about the cost of the liquor and the containers, which was slightly alleviated by the repeal of the glass tax in 1845 and the adoption in some quarters of methylated spirits. The shape of jars was vigorously debated, although most were cylindrical. Specimens were suspended within them with whalebone, hair, or dentists' silk (see figures 4.1 and 4.2); sometimes hung from hollow glass bulbs, perched on wax blocks, or even glued to the glass. Methods of sealing them varied, including bullock's bladder, lead, and tin foil. The Army Medical Museum had particular problems in this respect, as so many of its preparations arrived from

Preparations in Spirits', *Edinburgh Medical Journal*, 35 (1831), 328–31. For a brief discussion of jars see also Elizabeth Hallam, *Anatomy Museum. Death and the Body Displayed* (London: Reaktion, 2011).

warm climes; generally it was best to 'put up' the jars in summer, as jars sealed in the winter would loosen with warmer temperature.[14] Even more of a problem with these 'pots' was blanching. Astley Cooper had colour drawings made of all his specimens because 'he found it impossible, however well the spirits of wine in which his preparations were placed might preserve their form, size, or texture, to make them retain many characteristic appearance as to colour, consistency, and other important qualities'.[15]

And so whereas wet preservation was suited to demonstrating the shape of a body or an organ, other techniques such as embalming, which put fluid into the specimen rather than vice versa, were designed to reveal the inner workings. Most dissections, even those that were not to be kept, relied on a temporary injection of a preservative to reveal particular vessels and to prevent immediate putrefaction for however long it took to dissect (or was permitted by the Anatomy Act).[16] But pathologists demanded methods that would last in perpetuity, and this involved very particular substances 'thrown into' the specimen. Jan Swammerdam and Frederik Ruysch in Amsterdam (see chapter 1) had injected the blood and lymphatic vessels of corpses with a mixture of wax, talc, and pigments that set and endured. Eighteenth- and nineteenth-century anatomists were still using 'Swammerdam's syringe' to inject mixtures of varying proportions of wax, glue, size (sealing or stiffening liquids), isinglass (a pure form of gelatin), colouring, turpentine and/or varnish, and even quicksilver (that is, mercury—although this required special equipment).[17] Take for example the 'recipe' used at the Great Windmill Street School at the beginning of the century:

> Get, at the colour shops, a quantity of red lead, mixed up with linseed oil to a thicker consistence than is generally used for painting, and made more of the consistence in which white lead is kept. To this mixture of red lead and oil, add turpentine and varnish, until the composition is about the consistence of

[14] Army Medical Museum, *Catalogue of Preparations, &c. in Morbid, Natural, and Comparative Anatomy: Contained in the Museum of the Army Medical Department, Fort Pitt, Chatham* (London: Taylor, 1833).

[15] Bransby Blake Cooper, *The Life of Sir Astley Cooper, Bart.*, 2 vols. (London: Parker, 1843), ii. 109.

[16] As well as the general texts cited above, on injections in particular see temporary techniques, see Henry Goadby, 'An Account of a Chemico-Gelatinous Injection, with the Method of Employing It in Forming Anatomical Preparations', *The Lancet*, 10 March 1849, 287–9.

[17] For recipes, see for example Charles Bell, *A System of Dissections, Explaining the Anatomy of the Human Body, the Manner of Displaying the Parts, and Their Varieties in Disease*, 2 vols. (Edinburgh: Mundell, 1798–1803); Flower, 'Museum Specimens'; Knox, *Anatomist's Instructor*.

common thick oil; and also add a little spirits of turpentine, which makes it run better:—in this state the composition is injected. It is not possible to give, accurately, the proportions in which the different ingredients are to be mixed, as in the different shops the degree of fluidity of the turpentine varnish often varies; but the injection is so easily made, that there is no danger of going wrong:—immediately before injecting the composition, a little water should be sprinkled on it.[18]

Different recipes were used for coarse, fine and minute injections.

Like his successors at Windmill Street, William Hunter favoured injection as a method, especially in his preparations of the gravid uterus, and devoted four lectures in his course to injection techniques.[19] Once at the University of Glasgow, Hunter's preparations were complemented by intricate vascular injections by the embryologist and anatomist Allen Thomson in the anatomy department.[20] Back in London, Astley Cooper's exquisite injections demonstrating ligatures and aneurisms were renowned.[21] These preparations were striking to behold, as anatomists used different colours to accentuate different systems (commonly red for arteries, yellow for vessels). Even bones could be injected and rendered transparent to reveal their vascularity in the hands of William Hunter or Charles Bell. 'Injections may be of service as a means of making the parts more beautiful or natural,' claimed Bell, 'and more extensively useful, by unravelling that intricacy which so often occurs in wet preparations having no discrimination or colour. Even in organic affections of the heart, lungs, intestines, &c. injection gives a splendour and consequence which the real importance of these parts would perhaps claim in vain.'[22]

Even more dramatic results could be achieved if the surrounding flesh and organs were corroded, leaving only an impression of the vessels.[23]

---

[18] Pole, *Anatomical Instructor* (2nd edn), 2.
[19] [William Hewson], Manuscript catalogue of anatomical preparations in the Hunterian Museum, *c.* 1770, Glasgow University Special Collections Hunter 575 (S.4.20); William Hunter, *Anatomia Uteri Humani Gravidi Tabulis Illustrata* (Birmingham: Baskerville, 1774); Samuel Foart Simmons and John Hunter, *William Hunter, 1718–1783: A Memoir*, ed. C. Helen Brock (1783; East Kilbride: University of Glasgow Press, 1983).
[20] [Allen Thomson], Note of Dr Allen Thomson's collection of anatomical preparations, drawings, &c, MS, *c.* 1877, Glasgow University Special Collections MR 41/11.
[21] Astley Cooper, 'Case of Femoral Aneurism, for Which the Iliac Artery Was Tied by Sir A. Cooper, Bt. With an Account of the Prepartion of the Limb, Dissected at the Expiration of Eighteen Years', *Guy's Hospital Reports*, 1 (1836), 43–52.
[22] Bell, *System of Dissections*, vol. i. p. xi.
[23] This development of this technique had been incorrectly attributed to the physician Frank Nicholls, professor of anatomy at Oxford but it had been used before him by Govard Bidloo, William Cowper, and others at the turn of the seventeenth century. Cole, 'History of Anatomical Injections'. Anita Guerrini, 'Anatomists and Entrepreneurs in Early Eighteenth-Century London', *Journal of the History of Medicine and Allied Sciences*, 59 (2004),

This method—'the most elegant of all, requiring great care'—involved a very specific injection followed by immersion in an acid solution for several weeks, leaving only the intricate vascular system eerily isolated and fragile.[24] Corrosion casts were so fragile, however (they were commonly kept in vitrines), that practitioners criticized them as display for its own sake. Nevertheless (or as a result), they were popular in the later eighteenth century and still in use in the nineteenth. Thomas Hodgkin at Guy's, from example, used corrosion techniques he had witnessed in Bologna, involving the use of different colours to demonstrate dramatically the different circulatory systems: as for example a 'Corroded preparation of the Vessels of the Liver' in which the hepatic artery was coloured red, the 'Venæ Portæ, yellow; Venæ Cavæ Hepaticæ, black; and the Biliary Ducts, light green'.[25]

The final method in the medical museum arsenal, articulation, was of course applicable to skeletal mounts. They may seem to be the simplest to prepare, and yet, conservators argued, an osteological preparation required as much skill and care as any other. Ridding the bones of flesh without damaging them—'maceration'—was the first challenge: Vesalius had advised using lime and boiling water, but other options involved burying the bones, or even using insects to consume the flesh. Most simply left the carcass in water for weeks or months: initially changing the water periodically, resealing carefully afterwards, especially in London and other polluted areas. But this tended to leave the bones greasy and discoloured, so conservators used alum water or pearl ash to achieve the desired 'fine, white, ivory complexion'.[26] Once clean and bright, most bones were mounted individually, but if a full-body preparation was required, bones were joined with wires, tinplates, or skirt leather, using common carpentry and blacksmith's tools. This was the fate of the remains of individuals with systematic osteological conditions, including Joseph Merrick's supposed elephantiasis at the London Hospital and Charles Byrne's giganticism at the Hunterian. The most iconic preparations were based on the simplest methods.

219–39; Hunter, *Two Introductory Lectures*; Laskey, *General Account*; Simmons and Hunter, *William Hunter*.

[24] Bell, *System of Dissections*, vol. i. p. xi.

[25] Thomas Hodgkin, *A Catalogue of the Preparations in the Anatomical Museum of Guy's Hospital* (London: Watts, 1829), part ii, section vi, specimen 730; Amalie M. Kass and Edward H. Kass, *Perfecting the World: The Life and Times of Dr. Thomas Hodgkin 1798–1866* (Boston: Harcourt Brace Jovanovich, 1988).

[26] Pole, *Anatomical Instructor* (2nd edn), 99.

MANUAL METHODS AND METHOD MANUALS

Before, during, and after the nineteenth century, then, human remains were dried, submerged, injected, corroded, or macerated, flexible subjects made into (relatively) stable hybrid objects. The apparent continuity of these methods, however, obscures repeated attempts throughout the century to refine existing techniques and develop entirely new methods. Only at the turn of the century did the development of formalin mark a genuine qualitative change in medical museum technique. Before assessing the impact of this novel mode of preservation, however, we should first at least appreciate the earlier attempts to innovate, and, more significantly, address the quantitative expansion of preservation skills. Similar methods were being deployed, but on a much larger scale.

There were more anatomists in the nineteenth century than there had been, morbid or otherwise, and as we saw in chapter 2, more anatomists meant more collections. All needed to learn preservation techniques, and it seems most tried to improve them in one way or another. The holy grail of anatomical preparation was to find a cheaper alternative to alcohol for wet specimens. Already by 1844, 'many attempts [had] been made to obtain other antiseptic solutions. These attempts have but partially succeeded.'[27] Each anatomist in turn proposed his own new recipe, usually a solution of slightly different salts. Henry Goadby, later a prominent naturalist in Michigan, developed a popular recipe while he was a dissector at the Royal College of Surgeons in London, for example, whereas the physician Benjamin Babington's trial of pyroxilic acrid at Guy's was less successful.[28] In other techniques, isinglass, size, and 'Prussian blue' became more popular for injections and Joseph Swan dried specimens after injecting them with oxymuriate of mercury to retain their appearance.[29] Ultimately, however, simple dilute alcohol was difficult to beat. In 1929 staff at St Bartholomew's found that 'histological appearances were unexpectedly well preserved in many cases after as much as a century's immersion in spirit'.[30]

While basic principles of medical museum methods did not change significantly, anatomists' ways of communicating about them did. In the

[27] Tulk and Henfrey, *Anatomical Manipulation*, 72.
[28] Goadby, 'Account of a Chemico-Gelatinous Injection'; Babington and Rees, 'On the Preservation of Subjects'. See also *The Lancet* 6 August 1825, 153.
[29] Cole, 'History of Anatomical Injections'; Joseph Swan, *An Account of a New Method of Making Dried Anatomical Preparations* (London: Cox, 1815).
[30] Thomas Henry Gostwyck Shore, *A Descriptive Catalogue of the Pathological Museum of St Bartholomew's Hospital Medical College*, 2 vols. (London: Adlard, 1929), vol. i. p. vi.

late eighteenth century, Thomas Pole's *Anatomical Instructor*, first published in 1790, was one of only a few available texts detailing the minutiae of preservation practice, but he summarized existing methods rather than proposing anything especially new.[31] The popular anatomical vade mecums published in the early century (that is, handy guides, from the Latin 'carry with me') then re-capitulated Pole in their appendices.[32] Similarly, Charles Bell included a practical introduction to his *System of Dissections* (1798–1803).[33] Few others revealed their carefully guarded crafts. With the expansion of institutional collections in the 1820s and 1830s, however—'Now that museums of healthy and morbid anatomy are considered to be of so much importance'—a new cohort of practitioners provided a market for a new kind of handbook.[34]

Frederick John Knox may not have achieved the fame or notoriety of his brother, but his *The Anatomist's Instructor, and Museum Companion*, first published in 1836, was widely used, perhaps epitomizing a new wave of anatomical manuals.[35] Some disseminated Continental methods, including *Anatomical Manipulation* (1844) by the translator Alfred Tulk and the botanist Arthur Henfrey; and in Philadelphia, the comparative anatomist Richard Harlan translated the French chemist Jean Nicolas Gannal's *History of Embalming* (1840), with a host of contemporary techniques included.[36] Older expositions such as Thomas Pole's and Joseph Swan's were expanded and republished and techniques that had been guarded jealously were now published and circulated, as for example John Hunter's own preservative methods.[37] As medical periodical

---

[31] Thomas Pole, *The Anatomical Instructor; or, an Illustration of the Modern and Most Approved Methods of Preparing and Preserving the Different Parts of the Human Body* (London: Couchman and Fry, 1790).

[32] See for example Robert Harrison, *The Dublin Dissector: Or, Manual of Anatomy* (Dublin: Hodges and McArthur, 1827); Robert Hooper, *The Anatomist's Vade-Mecum* (London: Bell, 1797).

[33] Bell, *System of Dissections*.

[34] Watson, 'On Preserving', 328.

[35] Knox, *Anatomist's Instructor*; A. W. Beasley, 'The Other Brother—A Brief Account of the Life and Times of Frederick John Knox', *Journal of the Royal College of Surgeons of Edinburgh*, 46 (2001), 119–23; Matthew H. Kaufman, 'Frederick Knox, Younger Brother and Assistant of Dr Robert Knox: His Contribution to "Knox's Catalogues"', *Journal of the Royal College of Surgeons of Edinburgh*, 46 (2001), 44–56.

[36] Gannal, *History of Embalming*; Tulk and Henfrey, *Anatomical Manipulation*.

[37] Thomas Pole, *The Anatomical Instructor; or an Illustration of the Modern and Most Approved Methods of Preparing and Preserving the Different Parts of the Human Body* (3rd edn, London: Burgess and Hill, 1824); Joseph Swan, *A New Method of Making Anatomical Preparations: Particularly Those Relating to the Nervous System* (3rd edn, London: Longman, 1833); John Hunter, 'Directions for Preserving Animals and Parts of Animals for Anatomical Investigations; and Concerning Extraneous Fossils', in [William Clift] (ed.), *Invitation to Surgeons, and Naturalists, for Donations to the Museum of the Royal College of Surgeons in London* (London: Carpenter, 1826), 7–42, based on Hunter's notes from around 1785;

publishing expanded in the 1830s, new journals were employed as vehicles for disseminating techniques.[38] Periodicals and manuals alike were intended not only for instructors and preparators, but also for the students who used the collections—in the vain hope that a better understanding of the labour that went into the specimens might instil more respect for them (their failure in this regard is taken up in chapter 6).

The new manuals also reflected the take-up of pathological anatomy in Britain, if not as a distinct profession, as discussed in chapter 2, then as part of wider practice. Many volumes had dedicated sections on morbid preparations that had been absent in the eighteenth-century treatises. Knox, for example, devoted a large and distinct portion of his tome to 'the Modes of Preserving Diseased Structure Illustrative of Pathology', with techniques that were sensitive to the character of a range of conditions.[39] Gannal, too, claimed to be responding to the expansion of morbid anatomy in committing new techniques to print, criticizing desiccation as a method because it 'cannot be employed for specimens of pathological anatomy'.[40]

These early Victorian manuals reflected the importance of pathology as a distinct skill and material culture. Nevertheless, they were taking existing techniques and applying them to diseased specimens. Not until the end of the century can we discern genuine innovation applied to morbid preparations with the application of gelatine (for cystic and other soft specimens) and glycerine (for ophthalmic specimens).[41] Developments in glass

---

Simon Chaplin, 'Nature Dissected, or Dissection Naturalized? The Case of John Hunter's Museum', *Museum and Society*, 6 (2008), 135–51.

[38] Watson, 'On Preserving'; Crosse, 'Memoir Upon the Method'; Babington and Rees, 'On the Preservation of Subjects'. Medical museum technique would later be promulgated in the *Museums Journal* (1901–) and especially the *International Association of Medical Museums Bulletin* (1907–; later the *Journal of Technical Methods and Bulletin of the International Association of Medical Museums Bulletin*, still later *Laboratory Investigation*). See Robin A. Cooke (ed.), *Scientific Medicine in the Twentieth Century: A Commemoration of 100 Years of the International Association of Medical Museums and the International Academy of Pathology* (Augusta, Ga.: United States and Canadian Academy of Pathology, 2006); Daukes, *Medical Museum*.

[39] Knox, *Anatomist's Instructor*.

[40] Gannal, *History of Embalming*, 162.

[41] See for example H. Littlejohn, 'A New Method of Mounting Museum Specimens', *Journal of Pathology and Bacteriology*, 8 (1902), 369–73; Richard Thoma, 'The Preparation of Museum Specimens', *The Lancet*, 6 July 1891, 1270; Baggaley, 'Gelatin and Glycerine Spirit'; Henry Greenway Howse, 'On Embalming', *Guy's Hospital Report*, 32 (1872), 465–71; T. B. Johnston, 'The History of Guy's Hospital Medical School', in Leslie George Housden and Gordon Gould Cameron (eds.), *Guy's Hospital Gazette: Special Number in Commemoration of the Bicentenary of the Hospital and the Centenary of the Medical School, 1725–1925* (London: Ash, 1925), 64–78; Gunther von Hagens and Angelina Whalley (eds.), *Body Worlds—The Anatomical Exhibition of Real Human Bodies* (Heidelberg: Institut für Plastination, 2002).

technology allowed rectangular jars, with less distortion than the traditional cylinders (which nevertheless retained their utility thanks to the
strength of the jars and seals).[42] Large-scale freezing was more feasible,
remembered Ernest Shaw, then museum assistant at St Bartholomew's:

> For years after I went to the Museum [in 1884] all material for the histologi-
> cal section was frozen; the method of paraffin injection was not introduced
> until the middle nineties. After hardening in Müller's fluid the piece of tissue
> was immersed in gum solution, and frozen by means of an ice and salt
> mixture. I used to fetch the ice from the fishmongers.[43]

But one technique was more significant than all of these. 'In these days
museum specimens were more in spirit', continued Shaw: 'It was after the
appointment of Dr. Kanthack as pathologist that formalin came into use
for their preservation.'[44] The Brazilian-born Alfredo A. Kanthack headed
the pathological department at Barts in the 1890s before taking up the
chair of pathology in Cambridge (a tenure cut very short by his untimely
death in 1898). Kanthack introduced 'Formalin', a patented solution of
formaldehyde, to the hospital as a preservative. Industrial formaldehyde
had been available since the 1860s, but the German physician Ferdinand
Blum noticed the fixative properties of the solution while researching it as
an antiseptic in 1893; Kanthack and others in medical museums quickly
took it up.[45] In 1896 Johann Carl Kaiserling, a student of Virchow's,
published an especially effective formalin-based process. The Kaiserling
technique (as it became known) in particular and formalin generally was
evidently the ideal solution (in both senses) for wet specimens. It hardened
tissue far faster than alcohol, keeping the colour, and, crucially for the
increasing number of histopathologists, preserving the cellular structure of

---

[42] Andries J. van Dam, 'The Interactions of Preservative Fluid, Specimen Container,
and Sealant in a Fluid Collection', *Collection Forum*, 14 (2000), 78–92; Andries J. van
Dam, et al., 'The Warping and Cracking of Plexiglass™ Specimen Containers', *Collection
Forum*, 14 (2000), 47–56. See also Clemence M. Acland, 'An Improved Method of
Mounting Pathological Specimens in Flat Celluloid Cases', *Museums Journal*, 25 (1925),
111–14.

[43] Ernest H. Shaw, 'Pathology at Bart's in the Nineteenth Century', *St Bartholomew's
Hospital Journal*, 5 (1949), 75–8 at 77.

[44] Shaw, 'Pathology at Bart's', 77; *British Medical Journal*, 31 December 1898, 1941–2;
Alfredo Antunes Kanthack and Ernest H. Shaw, 'The Use of Formalin for the Preservation
of Museum Specimens', *Transactions of the Pathological Society of London*, 48 (1897),
282–8.

[45] F. Blum, 'Der Formaldehyd Als Härtungsmittel', *Zeitschrift für wissenschaftliche
Mikroskopie*, 10 (1893), 314–15; W. McAdam Eccles, 'Formic Aldehyde as a Rapid
Hardening Reagent for Animal Tissues', *British Medical Journal*, 26 May 1894, 1124;
Edwards and Edwards, *Medical Museum Technology*; E. M. Holmes, 'A New Preservative
Fluid', *Report of the Proceedings of the Museums Association*, 6 (1895), 30–6; Dobson,
'Historical Introduction'.

the specimen. It was non-flammable, and best of all, *cheap*. 'If this process should prove a permanent one', announced *The Lancet*, 'it will add very greatly to the value of our museum specimens.'[46] Kaiserling's method did prove itself, and was quickly taken up in Britain: new specimens were mounted in formalin, and old collections transferred.[47] 'These methods have given us, we may venture to say, beautiful results', proclaimed Kanthack, 'a museum specimen preserved in formalin affords a strange pleasure and a source of excusable pride to a curator.'[48]

Such was the expansion of pathological collections at the turn of the century, however, that the large-scale take-up of formalin complemented rather than banished older fluids, and medical institutions in Britain continued to use nearly 34,000 gallons of methylated spirits each year.[49] The craft of the Enlightenment morbid anatomy preparation had given way to an industrial system that manufactured pathology, which relied not only on the corpse as its raw material (see chapter 3) but also on chemicals. Like all factories, however, the pathology museum relied on its workers.

THE ROLE OF PREPARATION

If our goal is to understand the function of medical museums, it is as important to ask who was applying these methods as it is to describe them. Chapter 2 involved an assessment of the status of the morbid anatomists in relation to the medical realm generally, and chapter 3 followed by placing them within cultures of collecting. But to understand the production of museum objects, the next step in the trajectory of the specimens, we need to examine the role of different practitioners in relation to the collections. That is, we should examine the relationship between pathologists (and others) and material culture. Who undertook the work just outlined, the preservation and preparation of specimens? How did they pass on their methods?

---

[46] *The Lancet*, 26 September 1896, 897; Johan Carl Kaiserling, 'Über Die Conservirung Von Sammlungspräparaten Mit Erhaltung Der Natürlichen Farben', *Berliner Klinische Wochenschrift*, 33 (1896), 775–7.
[47] Sheridan Delépine, 'On the Arsenious Acid-Glycerin-Gelatin ("Arsenious Jelly") Method of Preserving and Mounting Pathological Specimens with Their Natural Colours, and on the Use of New Forms of Receptacles for Keeping Museum Specimens', *Museums Journal*, 13 (1914), 322–9; H. Campbell Thomson, *The Story of the Middlesex Hospital Medical School* (London: Murray, 1935); Victoria University of Manchester, *Victoria University of Manchester Medical School* (Manchester: Manchester University Press, 1908). For a detraction, see Hugh Galt, 'On a New Method of Preserving Museum Specimens', *The Lancet*, 16 November 1901, 1334–5.
[48] Kanthack and Shaw, 'The Use of Formalin', 286.
[49] Cole, 'History of the Anatomical Museum'.

In light of how unpleasant these tasks were (of which more below), it is surprising how often this work was undertaken by elite practitioners. In the early nineteenth century, the division of labour in medical collection stood in marked contrast to other kinds of museums. The work of natural history collections, for example, was undertaken by curators who were effectively glorified janitors, subject to the whims of a gaggle of elite honorary curators. But in the medical museum, preservation tended to be undertaken by the elite themselves. William Hunter had argued that 'injecting, macerating, corroding, boiling, distilling, in a word, every operation by which we endeavour to discover the structure and use of any part of the body, is anatomical'.[50] These techniques were an integral part of the construction of anatomical and pathological knowledge. Just as John Bell eschewed artists and illustrated his own work, so his brother Charles and other anatomists such as Astley Cooper insisted on putting up their own preparations. 'I am in the museum every morning betwixt six and seven', wrote Charles, '*doing up* my models.'[51] After a morning among the specimens, Bell and Cooper—knights of the realm—shrugged off their working aprons, donned their jackets and mixed with the great and the good.

Not just anyone could handle a medical collection, then. When assessing the staffing needs for the University of Edinburgh anatomy collection, Alexander Monro *tertius* argued that Robert Jameson in the natural history museum next door 'may easily obtain a Conservator who can stuff birds, and take charge of insects, &c.; but the Conservator of the Anatomical Museum must be a man who has been educated properly, who has gone through a complete Medical and Surgical education'.[52] Not all curators were so rarefied as the Bells and the Coopers, admittedly, but most were by necessity medically trained. In Edinburgh, thanks to the striking job-fixing we witnessed in the last chapter, the Royal College museum was managed by the surgeon Robert Knox, but for the day-to-day work of mounting specimens he employed his younger brother Frederick as his

[50] Hunter, *Two Introductory Lectures*, 3; Samuel J. M. M. Alberti, 'The Status of Museums: Authority, Identity and Material Culture', in David N. Livingstone and Charles W. J. Withers (eds.), *Geographies of Nineteenth-Century Science* (Chicago: University of Chicago Press, 2011).

[51] Charles Bell to Joseph George Bell, 1 June 1812, cited in Charles Bell (ed.), *Letters of Sir Charles Bell* (London: Murray, 1870), 200, original emphasis. John Bell, *Engravings, Explaining the Anatomy of the Bones, Muscles and Joints* (Edinburgh: Paterson, 1794); Cooper, *Life of Sir Astley Cooper*; Sappol, *Traffic of Dead Bodies*.

[52] Royal Commission, *Minutes of Evidence*, i. 273; Matthew H. Kaufman, *Medical Teaching in Edinburgh During the 18th and 19th Centuries* (Edinburgh: Royal College of Surgeons of Edinburgh, 2003).

assistant.[53] Knox Junior worked hard, preparing up to 300 preparations a year, for which he was well paid—his salary was greater than that paid by the College to Robert. (Frederick later used this experience to draft his *Anatomist's Instructor*, discussed above.) Crucially, he was well qualified in his own right, earning a fellowship of the college and operating a small surgical practice. He later emigrated to New Zealand, where he ran the free library and museum in Wellington.

The Edinburgh collection and other institutional anatomy museums in the early nineteenth century gradually employed more personnel, but the core practice was still undertaken by a surgeon-anatomist. The Royal of Surgeons in Ireland engaged porters to 'attend on the Curator in keeping his Laboratory clean, in assisting him in making preparations, in attending in the Museum, when so employed by the Curator, to receive Visitors, and keep the bottles + preparations in a proper state of order and cleanliness', but it was the curator himself—for example the respected anatomist John Houston—who had the principal responsibility for mounting the preparations.[54] Across town, James Macartney, doyen of the Dublin medical establishment, carefully prepared his own specimens.[55] Even the simplest of tasks were not to be left to assistants. Alexander Watson (Fellow of the Royal College of Surgeons of Edinburgh) complained, 'As the "tying-up", as it is called, of preparations in spirits, is generally left to be done by those who know very little about the matter, and care only so far as they are paid for their labour, they either cannot or will not improve upon the old, troublesome, and very inefficient way of doing it.'[56] Later in the century, the division of labour was somewhat more demarcated, especially in pathological institutes in which the collections were maintained by technicians. At the Dublin Royal College, the three museum porters were re-fashioned 'museum assistants', the most senior of whom 'had charge of the mechanical work of the Museum', and in Manchester, the anatomical department had two assistants for the museum.[57] Nevertheless, consultants and professors, those who managed these pathological factories, continued to get their

[53] Beasley, 'The Other Brother'; Kaufman, 'Frederick Knox'; Knox, *Anatomist's Instructor*; James A. Ross and Hugh W. Y. Taylor, 'Robert Knox's Catalogue', *Journal of the History of Medicine*, 10 (1955), 269–76.

[54] Museum Committee Minutes, 4 May 1833, Royal College of Surgeons in Ireland Archive RCSI/MUC/1. On the janitors at the University of Edinburgh, see Royal Commission, *Minutes of Evidence*, appendix.

[55] John Leonard Thornton, 'A Diary of James Macartney (1770–1843) with Notes on His Writings', *Medical History*, 12 (1968), 164–75.

[56] Watson, 'On Preserving', 328.

[57] Museum Committee Minutes, 16 November 1894 and 8 November 1887, Royal College of Surgeons in Ireland Archive RCSI/MUC/1.

hands dirty on the shop floor, and well into the twentieth century anatomy and pathology chairs were developing—or at least publishing—museum techniques.[58]

Whether or not such publications had any impact is a different question. The expanding market in technical literature did not and could not replace the hands-on nature of this work. The tacit skills involved in putting-up specimens were not be found on formal medical curricula at either end of the century. 'Though instructions may be given, to facilitate the acquisition of this art', conceded even Thomas Pole, author of one of the major handbooks on the subject, 'yet they will be found insufficient for the dextrous performance of its operations; a moderate share of experience can alone remove the difficulties, which result from the want of it.'[59] Like many aspects of clinical practice, anatomical preparation skills were learnt face-to-face, often as part of an apprenticeship William Hunter had learned how to put up specimens from his master Frank Nichols, and so in the nineteenth century John Crosse, for example, the Norfolk surgeon who proposed an innovative sealing technique for wet specimens (see figure 4.2), had learnt his craft directly from James Macartney in Dublin and Charles Bell in London.[60] The handbooks discussed above notwithstanding, travelling was often the only way to pick up the skills, and successive curators at the Royal College in Dublin would travel to the Edinburgh and London colleges to pick up the latest techniques.[61] (Fortunately for them they did not arrive during the tenure of one Hunterian prosector who is alleged to have locked himself in his lab for up to 30 hours to finish a preparation, and never revealed his methods.)[62]

PRESERVATION IN PRACTICE

This chapter has explored what preservative techniques were deployed, by whom, and when. By parity with the discussion in chapter 6 of the impact of medical museums on their visitors, their consumers, it is interesting here to discuss (insofar as it is recoverable) the experience of the producers,

---

[58] Delépine, 'On the Arsenious Acid-Glycerin-Gelatin'; C. Patten, 'A Suggested Method of Mounting Anatomical Specimens for Museum Purposes', *Museums Journal*, 4 (1905), 372–5; Owens College *Calendar* (1882–3), John Rylands University Library of Manchester Archives.

[59] Pole, *Anatomical Instructor* (2nd edn), 5.

[60] Crosse, 'Memoir Upon the Method'; Simmons and Hunter, *William Hunter*.

[61] Museum Committee Minutes, 24 September 1825; 5 October 1886, Royal College of Surgeons in Ireland Archive RCSI/MUC/1–2.

[62] Tompsett, *Anatomical Techniques*.

what it might have been like applying these techniques. Many obstacles had to be overcome, many hardships tolerated, but the sheer effort, the work involved, was closely wrapped up in the meaning and the value of the specimens.

To begin with, the places for these practices tended not to be very pleasant. We know from chapter 2 that museums were as close as possible to the sources of many of their objects, namely dissecting rooms and hospital wards. The interstitial space between these places that housed the specimen temporarily in its journey from person to shelf were often makeshift and usually cramped. Private collectors improvised in their homes—James Macartney put up specimens in his kitchen, for example—and institutional museums did not always fare better.[63] At Trinity College, the Professor of Anatomy complained in 1791 that there was no space 'for making or drying preparations but the common dissecting room to which all pupils have free access and where our preparations are liable to accidents from the giddiness or wantonness of young men'.[64] On the other side of Dublin, Royal College curators worked in a 'laboratory' beside the main gallery, and in the 1830s lobbied for extra rooms for drying and maceration; in the meantime, they dried specimens on the roof. The Council refused to build an extra storey above the laboratory, and instead fitted out a former stable in the College yard. Only in the 1880s did a new museum building include dedicated spaces for museum practice, in which 'The proximity of the work-room to the Curator's room will enable the Curator to exercise constant supervision over the work of the Porter'.[65]

Long hours were spent in these spaces. The considerable work that went into preparations, this 'labour bestowed upon them' as Frederick Knox put it, was then bound up in their meaning.[66] This was painstaking and intense labour, as those involved were quick to point out. Knox warned that collections 'can only be formed gradually, and require many years of hard labour, and much expense, to render them...fit to be consulted by any one'; Thomas Pole felt that the 'principal ingredients' of injections were 'time and patience, and not less so, an uniform fortitude against disappointments'; and the *Medical Times and Gazette* noted approvingly that Carmichael College had a 'rich and valuable

[63] Thornton, 'Diary of James Macartney'.
[64] James Cleghorn to an unidentified correspondent 29 January 1791, Trinity College Dublin Archive TCD/MUN/P/1/1972.
[65] Curator's report for the year ending 5 April 1886; Museum Committee Minutes 4 July 1833; 14 March 1835; 28 March 1835, Royal College of Surgeons in Ireland Archive RCSI/MUC/1–2
[66] Knox, *Anatomist's Instructor*, viii.

Museum of Pathology, the result of the labours of Professor Smith and other Surgeons of the Richmond Hospital'.[67] Under the bust of John Shekleton, the first curator of the Royal College of Surgeons in Ireland, were not celebrations of his intellectual achievements but rather admiration for his 'ardent zeal and unwearied industry'.[68] This zeal, we should remember, was not only in making the preparations but in sustaining them. Most specimens required topping-up due to evaporation, which was a complex and labour-intensive process, involving either piercing the lids or removing them altogether and re-tying them. William Flower argued that a collection 'requires continual and tender care', and he wrote of 'the cost and labour required to maintain it'.[69]

The tenderness Flower alluded to was especially apt for medical museums, given how intricate many of the objects were. 'Preparation-making is an art', he declared, 'which can only be acquired by labour and perseverance, superadded to some natural qualifications not possessed in an equal degree by all.' He expanded,

> To succeed in making a good anatomical preparation, much patience, neatness of hand, knowledge of the subject illustrated, and some artistic talent are required. No pains should be spared to make it tell the lesson it is intended to convey in the most attractive and pleasing manner. Everything should be displayed as definitively and clearly as in a drawing, and there should be no appearance of negligence or want of finish in any part.[70]

Knox likewise warned that 'Unless the conservator of a museum can himself perform every little manipulation in addition to that which is purely scientific, the work of the museum will never thrive in his hands'.[71] For preparators 'an aptness and dexterity of the hands is necessary', Charles Bell had argued, for the 'delicacy' required, which could only be 'acquired through practice'.[72]

Woe betide those collections that suffered through lack of skill, dexterity, or patience. Daybooks were littered with references to preparations

---

[67] Knox, *Anatomist's Instructor*, 131; Pole, *Anatomical Instructor* (2nd edn), 60; *Medical Times and Gazette*, 16 September 1854, 299.

[68] Museum Committee Minutes 11 April 1835, Royal College of Surgeons in Ireland Archive RCSI/MUC/1.

[69] William Henry Flower, *Essays on Museums and Other Subjects Connected with Natural History* (London: Macmillan, 1898), 13. On topping up and re-tying, see for example Allen Thomson, 'Report on Condition of Anatomical Preparations' MS, 1851, Glasgow University Special Collections MR 41/10; Commissioners for visiting the University of Glasgow, *Report* (London: HMSO, 1839); Watson, 'On Preserving'.

[70] Flower, 'Museum Specimens', 146, 204.

[71] Knox, *Anatomist's Instructor*, vii.

[72] Bell, *System of Dissections*, vol. i. pp. vii, xi.

'spoilt in preservation'.[73] Knox sneered at the specimen 'allowed to become half putrid, by lying amongst dirty spirits for days, and ultimately stuffed into a bottle, barely sufficient to hold it, with the view to saving some glass or two of whiskey'.[74] Indeed, lack of fluid in wet specimens was a common accusation—aimed for example at the Hunterian in Glasgow in the 1820s, which was also castigated for its crowded drawers and mouldy bones.[75] Allen Thomson later recommended that the deterioration of the vascular preparations in the university's collection was such that they should be burnt.[76] But few received as damning an indictment as the Royal College of Surgeons in Ireland museum:

> The condition of the spirit preparations was extremely bad. The fluid in which they were was in the majority of cases dirty and discoloured and when the bottles were opened the specimens generally required many changes of spirit before the latter remained clear. . . . a very large no. were found to be structureless and consequently worthless, owing to the fact that they had never been properly hardened and in consequence had macerated in the comparatively weak spirits in which they were put up.[77]

There was one apocryphal explanation for the lack or weakness of the preserving alcohol that recurs frequently enough for us to give it consideration. Staff of the wrong character were alleged to take advantage of the copious quantities of alcohol that passed through their hands. One of Astley Cooper's assistants 'fell into habits of drinking, so that he could never work without some stimulating beverage at his side', so Cooper dismissed him.[78] The Irish surgeons refused their curator's repeated request to construct a still in the museum, despite the money it would have saved them.[79] One sharp-witted Guy's student made a point of this, advertising for pathological donations: 'All wines, liqueurs, &c., will be tested free of charge, provided sufficient is sent for full analysis. Quart bottles are the most convenient size. . . . Dead meat must be placed in weak gin and water, the former unsweetened, and about a pint in a clean bottle must accompany it, to cover the loss from evaporation.'[80] Such loss

[73] See for example Guy's Hospital Museum Daybook 1893, Gordon Museum Archive, King's College London.

[74] Knox, *Anatomist's Instructor*, 129.

[75] James Coutts, *A History of the University of Glasgow* (Glasgow: Maclehose, 1909).

[76] Allen Thomson, 'Report on Condition'.

[77] Museum Committee Minutes 18 January 1907, Royal College of Surgeons in Ireland Archive RCSI/MUC/2.

[78] Cooper, *Life of Sir Astley Cooper*, ii. 110.

[79] Museum Committee Minutes, 2 November 1886, Royal College of Surgeons in Ireland Archive RCSI/MUC/2.

[80] [Nathaniel Burnett Ham], 'Our Special Pathologist', *The Guyoscope*, 2/18 (1898), 42.

was prevented by rendering the fluids non-potable by adding a noxious adulterant (such as the emetic introduced to the barrels en route to the US Army Medical Museum).[81]

Perhaps it is no wonder preparators were driven to drink, given their working environment. Even allowing for the 'necessary inhumanity' they may have developed (see chapter 6), the sensory experience is worth considering. James Macartney was probably not the only anatomist who had to fend off rats as he prepared specimens.[82] They may have been attracted by the maceration: 'the mass of offal, and the putrid vapours to which they give rise,' advised Tulk and Henry in their manual, 'will obviously need a separate apartment distinct from the private study of the anatomist'.[83] Take for example even so venerable a gaggle of institutions as the royal colleges of surgeons. In Edinburgh the curators were lucky enough to have a special macerating room in the basement, but their Irish counterparts originally had to make do with a shed, separate from the other work-rooms because of the 'foul smell'.[84] In London, Flower warned, 'The process of maceration is necessarily attended with disagreeable smells. As long as it continues the surface of the water slowly emits gases; but the worst is when the water is stirred up by pouring it off to remove the bones'—so he macerated outside.[85] No wonder then that Joseph Swan boasted that preparations dried by his new method were 'not offensive to smell, and may consequently be preserved in situations where other preparations could not be borne'.[86]

Smell was by no means the most severe threat. As Monro *tertius* cautioned, 'A Museum is composed of very combustible materials; we use a great deal of spirit of wine, wax and rosin, and oil of turpentine; and if a person were not always at hand, any trifling spark might lead to the destruction of the whole building.'[87] Joseph Towne, wax modeller for Guy's Hospital, had finished his final exquisite model for the museum after half a century working there when, 'Sad to relate, however, this work when just completed was destroyed by the ignition of some spirit which

[81] Michael G. Rhode and James Connor, 'Curating America's Army Medical Museum', in Amy Levin (ed.), *Defining Memory: Local Museums and the Construction of History in America's Changing Communities* (Lanham, Md.: AltaMira, 2007), 177–96.

[82] Thornton, 'Diary of James Macartney'.

[83] Tulk and Henfrey, *Anatomical Manipulation*, 2.

[84] Museum Committee Minutes 7 November 1839; Curator's report for the year ending 5 April 1886, Royal College of Surgeons in Ireland Archive RCSI/MUC/1–2; Violet Tansey and D. E. C. Mekie, *The Museum of the Royal College of Surgeons of Edinburgh* (Edinburgh: The Royal College of Surgeons of Edinburgh, 1982).

[85] Flower, 'Museum Specimens' 146.

[86] Swan, *Account of a New Method* (2nd edn), 4.

[87] Royal Commission, *Minutes of Evidence*, i. 274.

flowed out of an upset spirit bottle that was used at his work.'[88] The elimination of fire hazards was an constant concern for museum authorities across the century: the British Museum, after all, had had a fire engine and water main built into Montagu House before it opened.[89] Smoking was forbidden.

Anatomy was dangerous for your health. Headaches were a common problem for those who worked in the preparation room, and curators were generally ravaged by the various chemicals to which they were exposed. Thomas Wilkinson King, Thomas Hodgkin's successor at Guy's, was asthmatic: 'prematurely aged, emaciated by fits of coughing [he] laboured fruitfully in the Museum until his early death'.[90] At St Marks' Hospital, the surgeon Peter Gowlland blamed the high infection rate on the decaying state of the specimens in the pathological museum. Hodgkin himself was stricken down after dissecting a camel. John Shekleton's industry, mentioned above, was not rewarded: after only four years at Dublin Royal College museum, he died from an infection after pricking himself during a dissection, the same fate that met Edwards Stephens in Manchester. In 1823, a drayman had dropped a needle on his apron, which pierced it and infected him with a fatal infection; the surgeon performing the autopsy cut his finger and subsequently died himself.[91] Death and disease were not only the subject of anatomy and pathology, but also their unfortunate side effects.

THE ORGANIC COLLECTION

Dangerous or just smelly, tacitly acquired or book-learnt, the skill embedded in material is vital to the history (not to mention future) of museums. This work made pathological objects. In the last chapter we explored the

---

[88] Thomas Bryant, 'Joseph Towne, Modeller to the Hospital for Fifty-Three Years', *Guy's Hospital Journal*, 41 (1882), 1–12 at 7. Interleaved in the Gordon Museum Minute Book for 1911 (Gordon Museum Archive, King's College London) is a sign from the early twentieth century from Herbert L. Eason, noting that 'Smoking is strictly prohibited in the Gordon Museum'.

[89] *The Lancet*, 22 September 1866, 341; David M. Wilson, *The British Museum: A History* (London: British Museum Press, 2002).

[90] Hector Charles Cameron, *Mr. Guy's Hospital: 1726–1948* (London: Longmans, 1954), 288; Sheldon G. Cohen, 'Asthma among the Famous: British Physicians of the 18th–19th Centuries', *Allergy and Asthma Proceedings*, 17 (1996), 161–72; Babington and Rees, 'On the Preservation of Subjects'; Swan, *Account of a New Method* (2nd edn).

[91] Abraham Colles, 'Second Communication Relative to the Fatal Consequences Which Result from Slight Wounds Received in Dissection', *Dublin Hospital Report*, 4 (1827), 240–4; *The Lancet*, 19 October 1823, 94; Lindsay Granshaw, *St Mark's Hospital, London: A Social History of a Specialist Hospital* (London: King's Fund, 1985).

spatial processes that began the transformation of human flesh into museum pieces, yet the afterlife of a body part did not then cease when it reached the medical collection, and this chapter has been concerned with the practices that then rendered it as stable (and odour-free) as possible; practices that, as it turns out, remained surprisingly constant. At the heart of the medical museum, from elite cabinets to commercial anatomy shows, was the body part suspended in a solution. These intimate details have been the day-to-day concerns of museum personnel, consuming their time and attention as much as grand anatomical theories and wealthy patients.

Creating and maintaining things requires constant effort, and a study of collections must reflect this, the *work* of the museum. In doing so we can see the close relationship between communities of practice and the practices themselves. Medical curators relied not only on their education but also a set of very particular skills that were distinct from those in other museums and other parts of the medical establishment: and in the publications discussed above they fiercely guarded their social and material territory from those without these skills. Preparations were the material manifestation of the combination of this practical expertise and pathological knowledge. Like Michael Worboys, I see 'knowledge and practice being produced from social and material interactions'.[92] Morbid anatomy and its material culture was embedded not only in the institutions and communities that were the subject of chapter 2, but also in particular 'ways of working'.[93]

The medical museum was a dynamic, mutable assemblage, and one that required considerable labour to sustain it. The hybrid objects within them were listed, cleaned, dried, steeped, put up, immersed, and injected; they were later topped up, re-housed, and sometimes discarded and destroyed. Jars, syringes, mercury, alcohol, and formalin were the tools of the medical curator's trade, upon which modern pathology relied. For these techniques were all intended to render the body parts frozen in time, or at least to control change. In the following chapter we explore those practices that were intended to make them legible.

---

[92] Michael Worboys, *Spreading Germs: Disease Theories and Medical Practice in Britain, 1865–1900* (Cambridge: Cambridge University Press, 2000), 13. On disciplines, practices, and professional closure, see Thomas F. Gieryn, *Cultural Boundaries of Science: Credibility on the Line* (Chicago: University of Chicago Press, 1999); Hopwood, 'Artist Versus Anatomist'.

[93] Pickstone, 'Working Knowledges'.

5

Displaying Pathology

Maps of Morbidity

'Let us then,' William Hunter told his students, '*make* a man'.[1] Having addressed how Hunter and his successors rendered the post-mortem body partible, portable, and stable, the topic now at hand is how the specimens were re-assembled, how morbid anatomists arranged them in cases and on shelves: how they *made* the pathological body in the museum. But just as in previous chapters we have seen how the disciplinary territories and acquisition routes for different kinds of anatomy overlapped, so in the galleries morbid preparations sat alongside different anatomies (healthy, animal) and media (paper, wax, and catalogues). The premise of this chapter is that the pathological collection can be understood as a set of distinct but interlocking bodies that together framed and defined the morbid. Evident in classificatory schema, in catalogues and in jars, these constructed bodies overlaid and corresponded with each other in meaningful ways to generate pathological knowledge. Flesh and bone, human and animal, paper and wax, combined to produce an atlas of disease.

Atlases, whether literal or metaphorical, were essential components of a range of nineteenth-century scientific and medical fields, having spread from geography to astronomy and anatomy since the Renaissance. The anatomical vade mecums encountered in the previous chapter were tours around the human body, and, from Henry Gray's (and Henry Vandyke Carter's) *Anatomy* (1858) to Joseph Kahn's *Atlas of the Formation of the Human Body* (1852), medical texts were maps of the body.[2] So too

---

[1] William Hunter, *Two Introductory Lectures, Delivered by Dr. William Hunter, to His Last Course of Anatomical Lectures* (London: Johnson, 1784), 73, original emphasis.
[2] Joseph Kahn, *Atlas of the Formation of the Human Body* (London: Churchill, 1852); Lorraine Daston and Peter Galison, *Objectivity* (Boston: Zone, 2007); Roberta McGrath, *Seeing Her Sex: Medical Archives and the Female Body* (Manchester: Manchester University Press, 2002); Deanna Petherbridge, 'Art and Anatomy: The Meeting of Text and Image', in Deanna Petherbridge and Ludmilla J. Jordanova (eds.), *The Quick and the Dead: Artists and Anatomy* (London; Los Angeles: Hayward Gallery; University of California Press, 1997), 6–99; Ruth Richardson, *The Making of Mr. Gray's Anatomy* (Oxford: Oxford University

were the collections with which they were intimately associated (having been drawn from them and then serving as guides). Like a map, the museum collection combines word and image to depict, rationalize, and control—and, especially, to define territories. Nineteenth-century collecting was a profoundly cartographical enterprise, whether of natural history, art, artefacts, or body parts. As John Pickstone writes, pathological anatomists surveyed corpses to construct a 'new geography of the body'.[3] Thomas Hodgkin wanted the Guy's medical collection to be to the surgeon 'what an accurate chart is to the mariner steering his course on the most dangerous coast'; like other morbid anatomists he set out to find the site of disease in tissues—conceiving 'the form and relative situation of parts and of systems of organs as locally situated rather than chemically conditioned'.[4] To search for these locations they needed maps, which Hodgkin and other curators provided by way of exhaustive catalogues. 'From the visible operations of disease on the surface', he invited the reader in his 1829 catalogue, 'let the student proceed to the investigation of the derangement of the internal parts.'[5] The museum offered the opportunity to explore the interior of the body; the visitor's eye rehearsed the journey of the anatomist's knife, the human body rendered 'translucent'.[6]

This chapter therefore comprises a tour of the bodies displayed in medical collections. Two concepts—legends to our map—will help us to decipher this fleshly landscape, to understand how body parts were put back together and made legible: dividuality and intermediality. Underpinning both, it stands re-iterating that medical collections comprised body *parts*. Whole body mounts, although the focus of much contemporary and historical attention, comprised a tiny fraction of anatomy museums' holdings, and so most of the 'bodies' in them were made up of fragments from any number of living people, which has a significant impact upon their meanings. For even if it was anonymised, a complete corpse was

Press, 2008). On maps and museums as core components of modernity, see Eilean Hooper-Greenhill, *Museums and the Interpretation of Visual Culture* (London: Routledge, 2000).

[3] John V. Pickstone, *Ways of Knowing: A New History of Science, Technology and Medicine* (Manchester: Manchester University Press, 2000), 110.

[4] Thomas Hodgkin, *A Lecture Introductory to the Course on the Practice of Medicine Delivered at St Thomas's Hospital* (London: Watts, 1842), 19.

[5] Thomas Hodgkin, *A Catalogue of the Preparations in the Anatomical Museum of Guy's Hospital* (London: Watts, 1829), 13.

[6] J. Arthur Thomson, *Introduction to Science* (London: Williams and Norgate, 1911), cited in Elizabeth Hallam, 'Anatomy Display: Contemporary Debates and Collections in Scotland', in Andrew Patrizio and Dawn Kemp (eds.), *Anatomy Acts: How We Come to Know Ourselves* (Edinburgh: Birlinn, 2006), 119–38 at 129. This was an aspect especially emphasized by the popular anatomy showmen; see Maritha Rene Burmeister, 'Popular Anatomical Museums in Nineteenth-Century England' (Ph.D. thesis, Rutgers University, 2000).

clearly the remnant of a single person. By contrast, the pathological bodies in museums were (with a few exceptions) conglomerates of diseased parts: they were not individuals but dividuals. As we saw in the introduction, a dividual is a composite, multi-authored person, whose component parts originate from different places. Marilyn Strathern and other anthropologists have applied the concept to living communities, originally in contrast to Western notions of *in*dividuality (although more recently this polarization has been refined rather to better understand fluid states of personhood in different places).[7] Prehistorians subsequently found the concept useful in their studies of excavated human remains that clearly included a mixture of different originating people.[8] Like (some) Neolithic bones, nineteenth-century diseased specimens were partible and circulated before joining an assembly of remains—but in a collection rather than a barrow. Neither site commemorated a single person (even in eponymous collections like the Hunterian museums) but rather represented complex sets of relations between numerous people.

The historian of pathological collections, like an archaeologist, is 'concerned with the ways in which power was invested in human bodies, and how those bodies were represented—or more properly, materialised'.[9] But here dividuality is deployed as a heuristic device to frame the body parts themselves, to understand the consequences of amalgamation in the museum, rather than imputing anything about their former lives. *Morbid Curiosities* is concerned with post-mortem physical dividuality and its consequences, taking some of the interesting features of dividual personhood and applying them in quite a different context. Rather than inferring the personhood of prehistoric people, I seek to understand how human remains relate to each other on the shelves. I do not use dividuality to understand the construction of gender as Strathern has (although I do to address the particular place of the pathologized female body in the museum). I share the archaeologists' interest in the materiality of dividuality and the anthropologists' attention to the relationships between people; but in the medical collection this is a rather less subtle manifestation of partibility. One colleague complained to Strathern that 'he has never met a dividual'.[10] Perhaps he might visit a medical museum.

[7] Marilyn Strathern, *The Gender of the Gift: Problems with Women and Problems with Society in Melanesia* (Berkeley: University of California Press, 1988).

[8] Chris Fowler, *The Archaeology of Personhood: An Anthropological Approach* (London: Routledge, 2004); Julian Thomas, 'Death, Identity and the Body in Neolithic Britain', *Journal of the Royal Anthropological Institute*, 6 (2000), 653–68.

[9] Julian Thomas, *Understanding the Neolithic* (2nd edn, London: Routledge, 1999), 162.

[10] Dušan Borić, 'Arriving at a Good Description: Interview with Professor Dame Marilyn Strathern', *Journal of Social Archaeology*, 10 (2010), 280–96 at 286.

Re-constitution of scattered fragments was a common feature of nine-teenth-century collecting. General Pitt Rivers pieced together evolution-ary narratives about technology from the barest traces of tools; palaeontologists reconstructed antediluvian beasts from their little toes; and historic civilizations were re-assembled in the British Museum with scattered sculptural remnants.[11] In all these sites, the re-constituted entity reflected the approaches and intentions of the collectors and curators as much as it did the putative 'original'. And the re-assembled body/build-ing/culture need not be complete. Far from it: the antiquarianism that emerged as a central tenet of Romanticism was marked by the understand-ing of the previous whole from the surviving part. Like ruins, statues, and dinosaurs, pathological bodies were painstakingly pieced back together from that which survived, or could be preserved.

To compensate for this deficit, and for the lacklustre appearance of many specimens, partible morbid remains were juxtaposed with represen-tations of disease in other media. In her insightful studies of human remains in museums, Elizabeth Hallam deploys the concept of *intermedi-ality*. Visitors make sense of the corpse when it is juxtaposed with models and images, which 'converge to make visible and tangible the complex anatomy of the human body'. On the shelves of the museum 'we can detect processes of intermediality in the multiple relationships between anatomical images, objects, and texts that in their making and use, build upon and incorporate recurring features'.[12] This 'anatomical intermedi-ality', she argues, helps the anatomy student sensually to re-integrate the dismembered body. Likewise in pathological exhibits the deficiency of one form of specimen or representation was compensated by the benefits of another. Bone and bottle, watercolour and wax were often to be found next to each other on the shelf (see figure 5.1, in which glass, leather, and flesh are juxtaposed on shelf 'd'). Clinical illustrations and case history text were necessary to instruct the visitors how to *see* the preparations, and vice versa. Charts adorned museum walls, and students approached the speci-mens with catalogues in hand. Visitors to the Pine Street School anato-mical museum in Manchester, for example, found 'preparations exhibiting healthy and diseased states of various organs of the body; casts, in plaster and wax, illustrating both healthy and morbid conditions of the various

[11] See for example Chris Gosden and Frances Larson with Alison Petch, *Knowing Things: Exploring the Collections at the Pitt Rivers Museum 1884–1945* (Oxford: Oxford University Press, 2007); Nicolaas A. Rupke, *Richard Owen: Biology without Darwin* (2nd edn, Chicago: University of Chicago Press, 2009); Sophie Thomas, 'Assembling History: Fragments and Ruins', *European Romantic Review*, 14 (2003), 177–86.

[12] Hallam, 'Anatomy Display', 129.

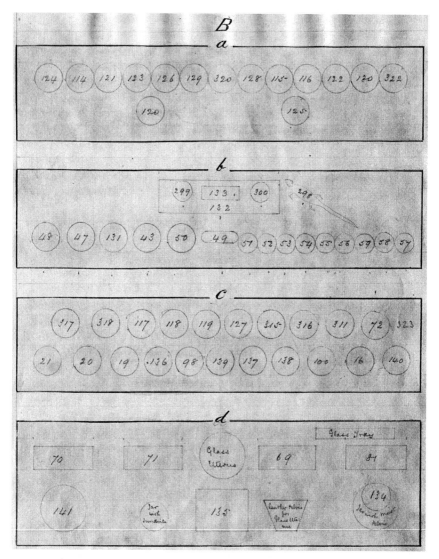

Fig. 5.1. Vitrine arrangement, showing glass, leather and flesh juxtaposed on shelf 'd'. From James Matthews Duncan, 'Catalogue of the Obstetric Museum of Dr Matthews Duncan', MS notebook, 70pp., 1868–1878. Copyright St Bartholomew's Hospital Archive, Barts and the London Hospital Trust Archives and Museums.

bones, organs and processes; and coloured drawings, engravings and diagrams of many singular cases'.[13]

The shelves of the medical museum were laden with body parts and cognate objects in various media from different sources, as we shall see in what follows. Specimens, labels, and models combined on the level of the shelf to provide an intermedial understanding of disease. Widen the focus and we can discern dividual bodies made up from the connections across the galleries. And wider still, the collection as a whole was a map of morbidity. But this pathological terrain rested on 'normal' anatomy, and so healthy bodies—male and female—are to be found at the first stop of our tour of the galleries of nineteenth-century medical museums.

THE HEALTHY BODY

Just as the normal and abnormal are co-definitive in other contexts, so we can only understand the pathological body in conjunction with the arrangement of healthy anatomy in the museum. Besides which, especially in the early century, most medical collections were in any case a combination of healthy and diseased (and, for that matter, animal) specimens. Modelled as many were on major collections such as the Hunterian in London, anatomy museums tended to be displayed in similar ways. As we saw in chapter 2, they were generally to be found in a tall rectangular room, something in the order of 70 by 30 feet, if possible with top-lighting and sometimes with upper-level balconies or galleries. Most objects were arranged on shelves lining the walls, or formed into bays; others were to be seen on tables in the centre of the room or in cases perched on the railing around the balcony (see figure 1.4).[14] In Dublin, for example, the Royal College of Surgeons ordered:

> Double Glass Case 10 feet long, 3 feet wide, with sash & front of Mahogany, all the rest of painted deal, best plated crown glass—no cross ties, plain turned legs—Depth of sash 10 inches in centre, and 7 in front, not more than one inch of a central division between sashes, to be made airtight—Height of frame 3 Inch, The Estimates to be furnished, as for either with, or without, Drawers.[15]

---

[13] 'A Relative', *Memoir of Thomas Turner, Esq.*, ed. David Bell (London: Simpkin, Marshall and Co., 1875), 153.

[14] Sophie Forgan, 'Bricks and Bones: Architecture and Science in Victorian Britain', in Peter Galison and Emily Thompson (eds.), *The Architecture of Science* (Cambridge, Mass.: MIT Press, 1999), 181–208; Hallam, 'Anatomy Display'.

[15] Museum Committee Minute Book, 21 February 1835, Royal College of Surgeons in Ireland Archive RCSI/MUC/1.

For those collections with a significant comparative anatomy proportion, the megafauna tended to be in the middle of the room (see figure 2.4). For larger items and delicate preparations or models, glass doors or vitrines were employed (especially later in the century, as we shall see in the following chapter). As well as size, the pragmatics of preservation often determined the arrangement of objects within the galleries and cases, so that bottled specimens were displayed separately from delicate dried and intricate injection preparations, even if they were morphologically similar—the Hunterian in Glasgow has a dedicated 'cabinet for dry anatomical preparations', for example.[16]

Most curators at least tried to introduce some system beyond these practicalities. For healthy human anatomy, the two most common approaches, both fundamentally cartographical, were by corporeal system (vascular, nervous, and so forth) or region (especially by specific organs). Hallam observes that Scottish anatomy museums in the twentieth century tended to be arranged according to the latter, through which 'spatial association of the body part and region . . . the body displayed in anatomy museums is kept "intact"'.[17] Looking further back, we see that in the original hall of anatomy at the Hunterian in Glasgow, the heart, lungs, kidney, and liver were displayed on the table in the middle of the room, with other organs and regions in 'presses' (shelved cupboards) around the perimeter: kidney on the east side, the brain on the west, et cetera.[18] Commercial museums tended likewise to have their specimens arranged regionally (better to emphasise the sexual organs, as we shall see in the following chapter). Visitors to J. W. Reimers's 'Gallery of All Nations' first

---

[16] Plan of the first floor of the Hunterian Museum, 1808, Glasgow University Special Collections MR 47/29. See also James C. Laskey, *A General Account of the Hunterian Museum, Glasgow* (Glasgow: Smith, 1813); MacLachlan and Stewart Booksellers, *Catalogue of an Extensive and Valuable Anatomical Museum* (Edinburgh: Thomson, 1843). For contemporary and later reflections on systems of arrangement and criticisms thereof, see Charles W. Cathcart, *Descriptive Catalogue of the Anatomical and Pathological Specimens in the Museum of the Royal College of Surgeons of Edinburgh* (Edinburgh: Thin, 1893); Simon Chaplin, 'John Hunter and The "Museum Oeconomy", 1750–1800' (Ph.D. thesis, King's College London, 2009); Lawrence Keppie, *William Hunter and the Hunterian Museum in Glasgow, 1807–2007* (Edinburgh: Edinburgh University Press, 2007); John H. Teacher, *Catalogue of the Anatomical and Pathological Preparations of Dr. William Hunter in the Hunterian Museum, University of Glasgow*, 2 vols. (Glasgow: MacLehose, 1900).

[17] Hallam, 'Anatomy Display', 128.

[18] William Hewson, 'Catalogue of anatomical preparations in William Hunter's Museum', *c*. 1770, MS Hunter 575; Matthew Baillie, MS appendix to the anatomical catalogue of William Hunter's museum, *c*. 1800, MR 41/1; plan of the first floor of the Hunterian Museum, 1808, MR 47/29, all in Glasgow University Special Collections; see also Laskey, *General Account*.

encountered the foetus, but then were presented with genitals, tongue, heart, and later lungs, kidneys and limbs.[19]

Those English curators more influenced by French pathological anatomists arranged their normal collections by system rather than by organ. In Paris, as Russell Maultiz explains, 'Bichat and Laënnec envisioned a sort of Russian-doll model of the body, a concentric affair in which tissue planes, enveloping and overlapping one another, invested the major organs of the thorax and abdomen.'[20] Hodgkin and others put this into practice in London's medical museums. The Guy's collection was arranged in 12 sections: first came the skeleton, working outwards from the spine; then the soft parts (muscles, tendons, etc.); the circulatory and nervous systems; the organs of speech, respiration and digestion; the urinary and generative organs.[21] At St Thomas's in the middle of the century, 'the preparations of the normal organs are disposed in physiological sections, each of which is well illustrated: for example, of the nervous system there are nearly sixty dissections from the principal classes'.[22] The surgeon George Langstaff was especially comprehensive in the arrangement of his private museum in London, in which he displayed the osseous, vascular, nervous, sensory, respiratory, digestive, urinary, and generative systems.[23] The specimens in the Army Medical Museum at Fort Pitt in Chatham were grouped into 'vital' functions (respiration, circulation); 'natural' functions (digestion, secretion, excretion); 'animal' functions (sensation, locomotion); and the ever-popular generative functions.[24]

The appeal of the generative displays will be explored in more detail in the following chapter; here it is important to appreciate how sexual difference was displayed in museums—which will handily take us from

---

[19] Charles V. Goulder (ed.), *Catalogue of J. W. Reimers's Gallery of All Nations and Anatomical Museum* (Leeds: Jackson and Asquith, 1853). See also Burmeister, 'Popular Anatomical Museums'; Joseph Kahn, *Catalogue of Dr. Kahn's Anatomical Museum, Now Exhibiting at 315, Oxford Street, near Regent Circus* (London: Golbourn, 1851); [Joseph T. Woodhead], *Descriptive Catalogue of the Liverpool Museum of Anatomy* (Liverpool: Matthews, 1877).

[20] Russell C. Maulitz, *Morbid Appearances: The Anatomy of Pathology in the Early Nineteenth Century* (Cambridge: Cambridge University Press, 1987), 177.

[21] Hodgkin, *Catalogue of the Preparations*, introduction.

[22] 'Dr'. Cormack and 'Dr.' Semple, 'The Hospitals of London. No. II', *London Medical Journal*, 3/26 (1851), 181–8 at 181. For a similar arrangement at Barts, see Anthony A. Bowlby, *A Descriptive Catalogue of the Anatomical and Pathological Museum of St Bartholomew's Hospital* (London: Churchill, 1884).

[23] George Langstaff, *Catalogue of the Preparations Illustrative of Normal, Abnormal, and Morbid Structure, Human and Comparative, Constituting the Anatomical Museum of George Langstaff* (London: Churchill, 1842); *The Lancet*, 18 June 1842, 422–4.

[24] Army Medical Museum, *Catalogue of Preparations, &c. in Morbid, Natural, and Comparative Anatomy: Contained in the Museum of the Army Medical Department, Fort Pitt, Chatham* (London: Taylor, 1833).

male normality to female pathology as we segue from healthy to morbid bodies. Since the late eighteenth century, anatomical atlases charted sexual difference in every part of the body, not only externally but also internally.[25] Male–female distinctions were becoming more acute in the nineteenth century. In Edinburgh, for example, John Barclay surveyed osteological sexual particularities in his *Anatomy of the Bones of the Human Body* (1829).[26] With skeletons, skulls, and other body parts, the museum was a key site in the construction of the nature of woman. In respectable museums as elsewhere, the generative system in particular featured prominently in anatomical displays. Female sexual organs were a perennial favourite of curators and visitors alike. The emergence of gynaecology as a distinct medical practice in the mid nineteenth century was reflected in the distinctions within medical exhibits, and here as elsewhere, as Roberta McGrath argues, 'Gynaecology quickly came to mean gynaecopathology.'[27] In William Hunter's collection, 'the series "*RR*. Gravid Uterus" comprised preparations illustrating not only the anatomy of the human gravid uterus and its contents, but also pathological conditions related to pregnancy and parturition'.[28] Male generative organs, by contrast, were more commonly to be found amongst the healthy anatomy—testicles in particular, which were especially amenable to injection. In three dimensions as in two, male anatomy was the norm against which female deviance was compared; anatomy museums exhibited what historians have dubbed 'misogynist corporeality'.[29]

---

[25] Katharine Park, *Secrets of Women: Gender, Generation and the Origins of Human Dissection* (New York: Zone, 2006); Londa Schiebinger, 'Skeletons in the Closet: The First Illustrations of the Female Skeleton in Eighteenth-Century Anatomy', in Catherine Gallagher and Thomas Laqueur (eds.), *The Making of the Modern Body: Sexuality and Society in the Nineteenth Century* (Berkeley: University of California Press, 1987), 42–82; Schiebinger, *The Mind Has No Sex? Women in the Origins of Modern Science* (Cambridge, Mass.: Harvard University Press, 1991) 42–82.

[26] John Barclay, *The Anatomy of the Bones in the Human Body*, ed. Robert Knox, 2 vols. (new edn, Edinburgh: MacLachlan and Stewart, 1829); see also [William MacGillivray], *Catalogue of the Museum of the Royal College of Surgeons of Edinburgh* (Edinburgh: Neill, 1836).

[27] McGrath, *Seeing Her Sex*, 34; Ornella Moscucci, *The Science of Woman: British Gynaecology 1849–1890* (Cambridge: Cambridge University Press, 1990). See for example Joseph Jordan, 'Catalogue of the Preparations of the Mount Street School Belonging to Joseph Jordan', MS ledger, 1824–37, Manchester Medical Collection, 23.1.58, John Rylands University Library of Manchester; Kahn, *Atlas*; see also Burmeister, 'Popular Anatomical Museums'; Jonathan Simon, 'The Theatre of Anatomy: The Anatomical Preparations of Honoré Fragonard', *Eighteenth-Century Studies*, 36 (2002), 63–79.

[28] Teacher, *Catalogue*, ii. 660.

[29] Susan C. Lawrence and Kae Bendixen, 'His and Hers: Male and Female Anatomy Texts for U.S. Medical Students, 1890–1989', *Social Science and Medicine*, 7 (1992), 925–34; Uli Linke, 'Touching the Corpse: The Unmaking of Memory in the Body Museum', *Anthropology Today*, 21 (2005), 13–19; Elizabeth Stephens, 'Anatomies of

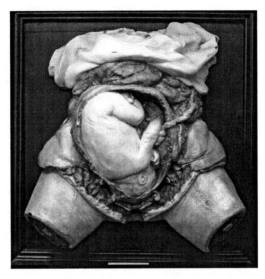

Fig. 5.2. Plaster cast 48.5 of female torso and foetus, Hunterian Anatomy Collection, University of Glasgow. Copyright Hunterian Museum and Art Gallery, University of Glasgow.

Misogynist or not, man-midwives wrenched the womb from the dead female body and disaggregated it in the displays (as part of a more general dislocation and isolation of internal organs on the shelves of museums). Following William Hunter's lead, anatomists took the pregnant body apart and displayed it, most commonly in model form, as for example in Hunter's famous plaster casts of the gravid uterus (see figure 5.2), which were closely related to the plates in *The Anatomy of the Gravid Uterus* (1774). By the middle of the nineteenth century, these models were at the nucleus of nearly 500 items illustrating pregnancy at the Hunterian—'the most valuable perhaps of any in the world'.[30] But even more (grimly)

Desire: Female Bodies in Fin-De-Siècle Anatomical Museums', in Peter Cryle and Chris Forth (eds.), *Fin De Siècle Sexuality: The Making of a Central Problem* (Newark: Delaware University Press, 2008), 25–41.

[30] Laskey, *General Account*, 51; William Hunter, *Anatomia Uteri Humani Gravidi Tabulis Illustrata* (Birmingham: Baskerville, 1774); Ludmilla J. Jordanova, 'Gender, Generation and Science: William Hunter's Obstetrical Atlas', in William F. Bynum and Roy Porter (eds.), *William Hunter and the Eighteenth-Century Medical World* (Cambridge: Cambridge University Press, 1985), 385–412; Ludmilla J. Jordanova, *Sexual Visions: Images of Gender in Science and Medicine between the Eighteenth and Twentieth Centuries* (Hemel Hempstead: Harvester Wheatsheaf, 1989); George Fordyce, David Pitcairn, and William [sic: Charles] Combe, *Catalogue of the Anatomical Preparations in the Hunterian Museum,*

prized by curators were organic preparations of mother and unborn child, as for example displayed in Desnoue's collection in London at the end of the eighteenth century.[31] As lying-in charities developed into maternity hospitals, institutional obstetric collections crystallized around the private cabinets of man-midwives and were put on display.[32] Pelvises of women who died in childbirth were sought after, evidence of sexual difference and the pathologies of pregnancy, and even the remains of healthy pregnant women were classified as pathology.[33] The embryo, meanwhile, was removed to a distinct part of the museum, leaving the womb—a dangerous, unsteady place—with the diseased organs. Hunter's model foetuses are lovingly rendered, tidy, and beautiful, in contrast to the butchered fragment of the mother, with transacted thighs emphasizing death and dissection. In industrial society, human reproduction became the manufacture of the infant; the faulty female machine taken apart and analysed on the shelves of the medical museum, to be contemplated by the visitor separately from the product of her labour. The female healthy body was not so healthy after all.

THE SICK BODY

As extensive as the (male and female) healthy anatomy displays just outlined were, the massive expansion in morbid anatomy in the second quarter of the nineteenth century meant that deviant bodies soon overwhelmed the normal on display in medical museums. 'This new labour', wrote Xavier Bichat as he set down his new science of pathology, 'was necessarily much more extensive than [healthy anatomy], in consequence of the multitude of different affections which the same tissue might

Glasgow (Glasgow: Richardson, 1841); N. A. McCulloch, D. Russell, and Stuart W. McDonald, 'William Hunter's Casts of the Gravid Uterus at the University of Glasgow', *Clinical Anatomy*, 14 (2001), 210–17; Elizabeth Stephens, 'Venus in the Archive: Anatomical Waxworks of the Pregnant Body', *Australian Feminist Studies*, 25 (2010), 133–45.

[31] Rackstrow's Museum, *A Brief Description of Those Curious and Excellent Figures of the Human Anatomy in Wax* (London: s.n., *c*. 1790).

[32] John G. Connor, *A Descriptive Catalogue of the Preparations, Drawings, Models, &c., Contained in the Museum of the Birmingham and Midland Counties Lying-in Hospital and Dispensary, for the Diseases of Women and Children* (Birmingham: Billing, 1847).

[33] John Williams and Charles Stonham, *Descriptive Catalogue of the Specimens Illustrating the Pathology of Gynaecology and Obstetric Medicine Contained in the Museum of University College, London* (London: University College, 1891); James Matthews Duncan, 'Catalogue of the Obstetric Museum of Dr Matthews Duncan', MS Notebook, 1878, St Bartholomew's Hospital Archive MU5.

exemplify.'[34] Every healthy organ had numerous abnormal counterparts. The collection at Guy's originally had around 2,000 specimens in each of its healthy and morbid sections, and while the former remained constant, the latter grew to more than 5,000 by 1880. By the end of the century the major catalogues listed only the pathological specimens.[35] Similarly at the Middlesex Hospital museum in the 1890s normal anatomy occupied only the tables in the museum, whereas pathology took up the floor-to-ceiling shelves.[36] In these and other collections, the healthy organ, reduced to a single type specimen, provided only the slimmest of guidelines to its swelling pathological counterpart.

How, then, to arrange this unruly mass of deviant material, to bring together body parts from countless individuals into a coherent whole? Pathologists' solutions to this, the spatial relationship between specimens on display, in principle reflected morbid anatomy as a conceptual enterprise. Some museums, such as at the Owens College in Manchester (see fig. 5.3), displayed the pathological specimens on the gallery above the normal and comparative anatomy below: the pathological body physically mapping over the healthy. In other museums, this correspondence was not so direct, but was nonetheless evident. 'As far as circumstances would admit,' Hodgkin pledged at Guy's, 'the same order has been adopted with the Special [healthy] and the Pathological Anatomy.'[37] His pathological arrangement was therefore by system, as it was for the normal anatomy, and this became an important exemplar for hospital collections in the capital. At St Thomas's, the leading pathologist Samuel Shattock set out the collection so that 'Each [pathological] series is preceded by a preparation of the normal organ to which it refers.'[38] Many other collections simply alternated their healthy and diseased specimens (whether individually or

[34] Xavier Bichat, *Physiological Researches on Life and Death*, trans. F. Gold (1799; London: Longman, Hunt, Rees, Orme and Browne, 1815), 16.

[35] Hodgkin, *Catalogue of the Preparations*; Lauriston E. Shaw, et al., *Descriptive Catalogue of the Pathological Specimens Contained in the Museum (Known since 1905 as the Gordon Museum) of Guy's Hospital*, 6 vols. (3rd edn, London: Churchill, 1894–1916). Pathology was similarly dominant in commercial anatomy museums, including for example Kahn, *Catalogue of Dr. Kahn's Anatomical Museum*; Goulder, *Catalogue of J. W. Reimers's Gallery*.

[36] J. Kingston Fowler and J. B. Sutton, *A Descriptive Catalogue of the Pathological Museum of the Middlesex Hospital* (London: Churchill, 1884); C. E. Lakin, 'The Story of Our Museum and Some of Its Contents', *The Middlesex Hospital Journal*, (1908), 84–98.

[37] Hodgkin, *Catalogue of the Preparations*.

[38] Samuel G. Shattock, *A Descriptive Catalogue of the Pathological Collection in the Museum of St Thomas's Hospital, London*, 4 vols. (2nd edn, London: Adlard, 1890–1894), vol. i. p. iii; A. E. Boycott, 'Shattock, Samuel George (1852–1924)', rev. Michael Worboys, *Oxford Dictionary of National Biography* (Oxford: Oxford University Press, 2004), www.oxforddnb.com/view/article/36043, accessed 29 Jan 2010. See also William Adams, 'Report of Work Done in the Museum of St Thomas's Hospital Since 1842', MS report, 23 August 1843, Wellcome Library WMS/PP/HO/D/B79.

by series), a more practical solution that allowed for expansion and adaptation.[39]

Taking morbid detours on the tour of the healthy body in this way, however, was not sustainable as more and more morbid specimens were manufactured and morbid taxonomies became more complex. If, as Georges Canguilhem argued, 'the morbid state of the living being is only a simply quantitative variation of the physiological phenomena which define the normal state of the corresponding function', then each healthy body part had numerous deviant counterparts.[40] Pathology wasn't the opposite of health, but rather a variation thereon; normality was simply the starting point in a spectrum of deviance. Curators soon found therefore that there were many ways in which a body part might be deviant, and establishing a coherent way to exhibit the fragments they were generating that seemed to correspond with clinical observation was no mean feat. As Hodgkin acknowledged:

> Every classification employed to facilitate an acquaintance with any of the various objects of Natural Science is necessarily artificial, rather then belonging to Nature herself. However scrupulously we may endeavour to be guided by those indications which she seems to afford us for making these divisions, the view which we present is like that which is gained by making a section of a compound solid mass. We may see the relations of some of the parts; but numerous other relations remain, which it requires fresh sections to expose. This observation is particularly applicable to Morbid Anatomy. Hence, for different purposes, different modes of arrangement are to be preferred. . . .
> To some, an arrangement founded on the basis of General Anatomy may be though the most desirable: others may prefer making their divisions correspond with different parts of the body: others may distribute them with reference to the functions of the parts preserved; and many systems might follow, grounded on Nosological Classifications.[41]

The solution to this proliferation of difference for many curators was to combine different arrangements within arrangements. Generally, this involved an overall schema on either a systemic or a regional basis, as

[39] Philip Bevan, *Descriptive Catalogue of the Anatomical and Pathological Museum of the Dublin School of Medicine, Peter-Street* (Dublin: Goodwin and Nethercott, 1847); [Mr MacKenzie], *Descriptive Catalogue of the Anatomical Museum of the University of Edinburgh* (Edinburgh: Whyte, 1829); Alice J. Marshall (ed.), *Catalogue of the Anatomical Preparations of Dr. William Hunter in the Museum of the Anatomy Department* (Glasgow: University of Glasgow, 1970); W. Mawhinney, *Anatomical & Physiological Description of the Late Signor Sarti's New Florentine Venus, Together with the Causes, Symptoms, and Treatment of the Diseases of the Principal Organs* (7th edn, London: Mallett, 1854); Teacher, *Catalogue*.

[40] Georges Canguilhem, *The Normal and the Pathological*, trans. Carolyn R. Fawcett (1943; 2nd edn, New York: Zone, 1989), 227.

[41] Hodgkin, *Catalogue of the Preparations*, viii–ix.

the healthy anatomy collections were, with further sub-classifications imposed within each series. The pathological characteristics could be found at a secondary or even tertiary arrangement within each section, so that each shelf became a self-contained guide to the diseases of a particular area. The Royal College collection in Dublin, for example, was to be arranged with 'The primary division to be into *series*, the principles on which this division is based being the same as in normal Human Anatomy [and the] sections to be divided into *sections* on general Pathological Principles.'[42] It was at this level, the sections of the exhibition detailing morbidity within the broader functional or regional arrangement, that Hodgkin was able to implement at Guy's the ideas of general pathological change he encountered while in Paris. And so, in principle at least, each of the systemic series was arranged according to 'deviations from the normal state', that is,

1. In Deficiency...
   a. The result of suspended development.
   b. Loss sustained or privation. . . .
2. In excess.
3. In form.
4. In appearances which may be regarded as the result of ordinary Inflammation.
5. In appearances which are the result of Scrofula.
6. Appearances from Malignant diseases (or structurally similar conditions): . . .
7. Hydatids in the organ in question
8. Accidental injury.[43]

In practice, Hodgkin also arranged pathological specimens according to their post-mortem identification, which he grouped into five classes: cadaveric; connected with last illness or death; adventitious; effects of chronic diseases; and congenital deformities. And in any case, these complex systems were always subject to brute practicalities, the spaces left on particular shelves, the position of pillars, and so forth.

Hodgkin, as we have seen, was an early exponent of pathological anatomy, and few other curators implemented such complex schemes in theory or practice in the first half of the century. Coincident with the disciplinary emergence of British pathology later in the century (see chapter 2), however, such systems became more evident elsewhere. The prominent surgeon

---

[42] Museum Committee Minute Book, 16 November 1886, original emphasis, Royal College of Surgeons in Ireland Archive RCSI/MUC/2. The plan was never realized.

[43] Hodgkin, *Catalogue of the Preparations*, xx.

Sir James Paget, whose first career step had been curating the museum at Barts, re-worked the extensive pathological sections of the Hunterian Museum in the early 1880s. He exhibited a selection of the morbid specimens to illustrate the general pathological changes (hyptertrophy, atrophy, repair and reproduction, inflammation, mortification, and tumours, which together accounted for some ten per cent of the collection), and cross-referenced them with the rest of the museum.[44] Under Paget's influence, his counterpart in Edinburgh, Charles Cathcart, also re-arranged the collection on the principles of general pathology, taking advantage of the recent developments in bacteriology and elsewhere, and seeking to present the specimens according to the cause rather than the effect of disease. He classified specimens in terms of their variation from healthy physiology in an initial general pathology series, and subsequently by system subdivided by condition.[45] In both royal colleges, the morbid sub-sections were far larger than the underlying systemic displays.

Meanwhile at Barts, although the 'anatomical grouping of the Series of Diseases and Injuries of the various Organs and Structures of the Body has not been materially altered', the specimens were rearranged so that 'in each Series the specimens have been arranged according to a uniform pathological classification'.[46] Perhaps the most rigorous system, however, was implemented in Manchester at the turn of the century (see figure 5.3) by the Owens College professor of pathology James Lorrain Smith. Each specimen was classified numerically, he explained: 'The *anatomical* description of the specimen is indicated by the numbers in front of the colon, and the nature of the *pathological* lesion or lesions illustrated, is given by the numbers following the colon'—so that within the area of the gallery, specimens were classified as for example ':40' (retrogressive disorders) or ':50' (inflammations).[47]

And so, while anatomy curators wrestled with function and form of the specimen, their pathological colleagues also tried to account for the way that the diseased part deviated from the norm in their arrangements of the specimen. The morbid body was a far more variegated entity than its healthy counterpart, and it was futile to seek to construct an idealized,

---

[44] James Paget, *Descriptive Catalogue of the Pathological Specimens Contained in the Museum of the Royal College of Surgeons of England*, 4 vols. (2nd edn, London: Churchill, 1882–1885).

[45] Cathcart, *Descriptive Catalogue*; Cathcart, 'Classification in Pathology', *Edinburgh Medical Journal*, 42 (1896), 37–46; 141–8.

[46] Frederick S. Eve, *A Descriptive Catalogue of the Anatomical and Pathological Museum of St Bartholomew's Hospital* (London: Churchill, 1882), v.

[47] James Lorrain Smith, *A Catalogue of the Pathological Museum of the University of Manchester* (Manchester: Manchester University Press, 1906), preface.

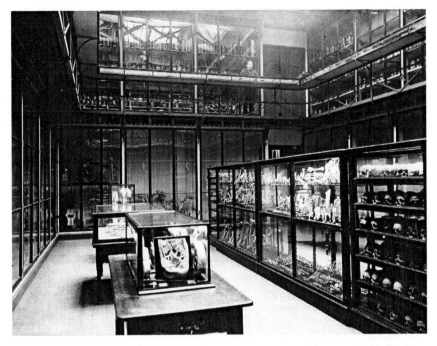

Fig. 5.3. Ground floor of the Victoria University of Manchester Medical School Anatomy Museum, *c.* 1894. Manchester Medical Collection, reproduced by courtesy of the University Librarian and Director, The John Rylands University Library, The University of Manchester.

universal body, a function that the healthy anatomical specimens on display arguably served. Daston and Galison's argument concerning pathological atlases thereby applies equally well to museums:

> 'characteristic' images [here read 'objects'] can be seen as a hybrid of the idealizing and naturalizing modes: although an individual object (rather than an imagined composite or corrected ideal) is depicted [here read 'displayed'], it is made to stand for a whole class of similar objects. It is no accident that pathological atlases were among the first to use characteristic images, for neither the *Typus* of the 'pure phenomenon' nor the ideal, with its venerable associations with health and normality, could properly encompass the diseased organ.[48]

The pathological body evident in the nineteenth-century medical museum was a complex and multi-layered entity comprising singular elements

---

[48] Daston and Galison, *Objectivity*, 82.

from diverse sources. For although specimens from the same person sometimes did appear in different parts of the same collection—at the Mount Street School in Manchester, specimen 406, 'Stomach of a soldier inflated & dryed [was] taken from the same subject as intestines, no. 426'—the vast majority of organic preparations were taken from different patients in different places at different times.[49] The body that pathologists materialized on the shelves, bays, and galleries was a multi-authored, amalgamated composite: the morbid dividual.

THE ILLUSTRATED BODY

It appears, then, that the core question at the heart of this book has been addressed—how the dividual, pathological body was constructed in medical museum displays with preserved body parts. And yet these human remains were not alone on the shelves. To account for the fate of organic specimens is to tell only part of the story: pathological bodies were composed not only of flesh and bone, but also of paper, words, and wax, and the remainder of this chapter is devoted to this pathological intermediality.

Two-dimensional representations were a common feature of pathological collections as they were of other museums, and the story of medical museology is closely tied to the rich history of anatomical art, from the atlases mentioned already to clinical photography. Among the earliest avowedly pathological museum projects in Britain, Robert Carswell's plans for the collection at the University of London, was based on splendid colour delineations (see figure 5.4). As we saw in chapter 2, Carswell was dispatched to Paris by the Edinburgh military surgeon John Thomson to compile a collection of images of morbid cases directly from dissected bodies.[50] He delayed his appointment to the chair in London to remain in France to complete this work. Returning to the UK he published this collection as *Pathological Anatomy. Illustrations of the Elementary Forms of Disease* (1838), modelled on the great French pathological atlases; but the tome contained only a fraction of the 1,000 delineations he made, which were displayed as an integral part of the morbid anatomy collection at University College.

---

[49] Jordan, 'Catalogue of the Preparations'.

[50] Hugh Hale Bellot, *University College London 1826–1926* (London: University of London Press, 1929); Robert Carswell, *Pathological Anatomy. Illustrations of the Elementary Forms of Disease*. (London: Longman, Orme, Brown, Green and Longman, 1838); L. Stephen Jacyna, 'Robert Carswell and William Thomson at the Hôtel-Dieu of Lyons: Scottish Views of French Medicine', in Roger French and Andrew Wear (eds.), *British Medicine in an Age of Reform* (Abingdon: Routledge, 1991), 110–35.

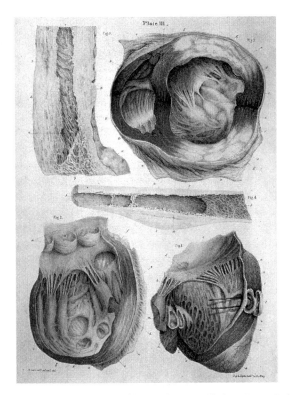

Fig. 5.4. Hypertrophy: aneurism of heart, diseases of tibia. From Robert Carswell, *Pathological Anatomy. Illustrations of the Elementary Forms of Disease* (London: Longman, Orme, Brown, Green and Longman, 1838). Wellcome Library, London.

Carswell's images made up for what specimens lacked. Crucially, they recorded the immediate post-mortem appearance of the body part—especially colour—which could then be used in the preparation of the specimen. Charles Bell advised the would-be pathologist, 'In preparing morbid parts, there are often appearances, curious and important, which cannot be preserved. Often, in examining the parts, the colour is the only criterion by which the nature of the disease is to be determined; and this is often impossible to preserve. Recourse must be had to painting, to give the lively tints which alone remain of the disease'.[51] Accordingly, at the

[51] Charles Bell, *A System of Dissections, Explaining the Anatomy of the Human Body, the Manner of Displaying the Parts, and Their Varieties in Disease*, 2 vols. (Edinburgh: Mundell, 1798–1803), vol. i. p. xi.

Marsden Street Theatre of Anatomy in Manchester, the morbid anatomist Thomas Fawdington showed coloured drawings of the pathological specimens 'should any of the specimens appear to be obscure, and seem to require illustration'.[52] Barts, Guy's, and George's hospitals all compiled large drawing collections, and at Trinity College Dublin and Marischal College in Aberdeen, giant anatomical diagrams to illustrate lectures were kept in the museum in the late nineteenth century.[53]

The largest images were most commonly to be found on the walls; in Cooper's cabinet and elsewhere, smaller pictures were kept in special cupboards, others bound in thick volumes, in which their arrangement corresponded to that of the flesh collection. Others, especially later in the century, were directly juxtaposed with the specimens, displaying the most immediate anatomical intermediality. At Barts, 'The arrangement of the [dermatological] drawings is made to correspond with the classification of the museum specimens', and a distinct catalogue of the illustrations was published.[54] In Edinburgh, 'In many cases published drawings of the patients from whom the specimens were taken have been copied by photography and placed beside the specimens they illustrate.'[55] In isolation (especially when published) such images might act as 'proxy specimens', and were exchanged between collections as such.[56] But their utility was most potent when immediately juxtaposed with specimens and models (see figure 5.5).

These bodies of illustration were not only composed of paper: glass lantern slides for teaching purposes were often taken from specimens, or in any case stored in museums. So too photographs. Clinical photography emerged soon after the spread of the Daguerrotype in the mid nineteenth century, as clinicians captured morbid conditions to extend and complement pathological atlases.[57] They soon came to play a role in the museum,

[52] Thomas Fawdington, *A Catalogue Descriptive Chiefly of the Morbid Preparations Contained in the Museum of the Manchester Theatre of Anatomy and Medicine* (Manchester: Harrison and Crosfield, 1833), v.

[53] Anatomical diagram collection, Trinity College Dublin Archives; Elizabeth Hallam, *Anatomy Museum. Death and the Body Displayed* (London: Reaktion, 2011).

[54] *The Lancet*, 9 November 1867, 590–1; St Bartholomew's Hospital Museum, *A Descriptive Catalogue of the Drawings and Photographs of Diseased or Injured Parts (Series LVII) in the Museum of St Bartholomew's Hospital* (2nd edn, London: Skipper, 1893).

[55] Cathcart, *Descriptive Catalogue*, xiii.

[56] On proxy specimens, see Martin J. S. Rudwick, *Bursting the Limits of Time: The Reconstruction of Geohistory in the Age of Revolution* (Chicago: University of Chicago Press, 2005); Martin J. S. Rudwick, *Worlds before Adam: The Reconstruction of Geohistory in the Age of Reform* (Chicago: University of Chicago Press, 2008).

[57] Daniel M. Fox and Christopher Lawrence, *Photographing Medicine: Images and Power in Britain and America since 1840* (New York: Greenwood, 1988); Larissa N. Heinrich, *The Afterlife of Images: Translating the Pathological Body between China and the West*

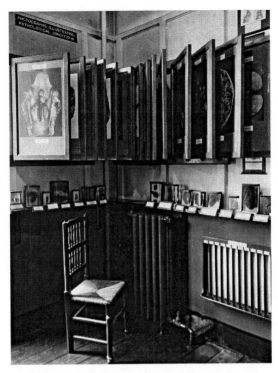

Fig. 5.5. A display on the upper ground floor of the Wellcome Building, Euston Road, London, showing photographs and specimens illustrating pathological conditions. Mid twentieth century. Wellcome Library, London.

often housed and exhibited with pathological collections, and used, circulated, and sold much as specimens were. Like preparations, they attracted censure for titillation while at the same time garnering praise for their educational and clinical utility. Nevertheless, photographs were donated alongside specimens—the Glasgow surgeon Sir William Macewen, for example, built up a large collection of specimens, slides,

(Durham, NC: Duke University Press, 2008); Nora Jones, 'The Mütter Museum: The Body as Spectacle, Specimen, and Art' (Ph.D. thesis, Temple University, 2002); Andreas-Holger Maehle, 'The Search for Objective Communication: Medical Photography in the Nineteenth Century', in Renato G. Mazzolini (ed.), *Non-Verbal Communication in Science Prior to 1900* (Firenze: Olschki, 1993), 235–78. On the construction of the behavioural abnormality with composite photography, see Francis Galton, *Inquiries into Human Faculty and It Development* (New York: Macmillan, 1883); Dario Gamboni, *Potential Images: Ambiguity and Indeterminancy in Modern Art* (London: Reaktion, 2002); Stephen Jay Gould, *The Mismeasure of Man* (2nd edn, Norton, 1996).

drawings, and photographs he had taken himself.[58] Barts Hospital employed a 'pathological draughtsman', Thomas Godart, as a photographer in the 1880s, and he was based in the pathology museum. Godart generated hundreds of photographs of the specimens that were published as a catalogue to accompany the collection.[59]

Whether of behavioural or physical deviance, however, photography had disadvantages. Often the details were indecipherable, especially of the all-important texture. And so throughout the century, pathologists continued to utilize other modes of illustration, including engravings, oils, pastels, and watercolours, but especially lithography. *The Lancet* reckoned that 'Lithographic drawing appears to be peculiarly adapted to the representation of morbid conditions of the soft parts of the body; but there is wanting, withal, that great desideratum in the portraiture of abnormal structure—colour'; nevertheless lithographers were in high demand, developing hatching and shading conventions to depict texture.[60] Like photographs, these illustrations were to be found on display in the pathological collection. Despite the rich literature on the history of medical art, few acknowledge this interplay between specimen and illustration in the museum.[61] Just as naturalists accumulated 'paper museums', so anatomists collected elaborate depictions of the dead body and its interior. And like organic specimens, these images were often of body *parts* from different sources, isolated and fragmented.[62] But spread out across the galleries, the net result was to present to the visitor another dividual body; the illustrated body corresponding to its organic counterpart.

[58] Paula Summerly, 'A Case Study in the History of Clinical Photography in Scotland' (Ph.D. thesis, University of Glasgow, 2003).

[59] St Bartholomew's, *Descriptive Catalogue*; John Leonard Thornton, 'Books', in Victor Cornelius Medvei and Thornton (eds.), *The Royal Hospital of Saint Bartholomew 1123–1973* (London: Saint Bartholomew's Hospital, 1974), 308–31; A. F. Wallace, 'The Early History of Clinical Photography for Burns, Plastic and Reconstructive Surgery', *British Journal of Plastic Surgery*, 28 (1985), 451–65; A. F. Wallace, '"Look under My Sink"', *Bart's Journal*, 18/2 (1994), 6.

[60] *The Lancet*, 26 October 1850, 478; see Army Medical Museum, *Anatomical Drawings, Selected from the Collection of Morbid Anatomy in the Army Medical Museum, Chatham*, 5 fasciculi vols. (London: Longman, 1824–1850).

[61] See for example Andrea Carlino, *Paper Bodies: A Catalogue of Anatomical Fugitive Sheets, 1538–1687*, trans. Noga Arikha, *Medical History* Supplement 19 (London: Wellcome Institute for the History of Medicine, 1999); Sander L. Gilman, *Health and Illness: Images of Difference* (London: Reaktion, 1995); Benjamin Rifkin, Michael J. Ackerman, and Judy Folkenberg, *Human Anatomy: Depicting the Body from the Renaissance to Today* (London: Thames and Hudson, 2006).

[62] Michael Sappol, *Dream Anatomy* (Bethesda Md.: National Library of Medicine, 2006).

THE MODEL BODY

Illustrations also came in three dimensions: models were as striking as the specimens on the shelves of the medical museum, often more so. They merited detailed entries in the catalogues, and they were commonly the bases for two-dimensional representations.[63] They were to be found in plaster, glass, papier maché, and even leather. The medium most suited to anatomy (especially of the interior), however, was wax. The construction of detailed anatomical *ceroplastica* had been pioneered in eighteenth-century Italy and arguably perfected in the German states in the nine-teenth, and like their European counterparts, British curators and collec-tors gathered large numbers of (often expensive) models and casts to complement or even replace specimens and illustrations. The medical museum relied on this, the model body.

Most collections had at least a handful of waxes.[64] Private anatomy shows boasted of their glorious full-body 'anatomical Venuses' based on

---

[63] Hunter, *Anatomia Uteri*; Kahn, *Atlas*. On modelling in the sciences generally, see Soraya de Chadarevian and Nick Hopwood (eds.), *Models: The Third Dimension in Science* (Stanford: Stanford University Press, 2004); Lorraine Daston (ed.), *Things That Talk: Object Lessons from Art and Science* (New York: Zone, 2004). Other materials used in medical models included ivory, plaster, leather, calico, wood and papier mâché. Hallam, *Anatomy Museum*; John James Edwards and M. J. Edwards, *Medical Museum Technology* (London: Oxford University Press, 1959); Mark Dreyfuss, 'The Anatomical Models of Dr. Auzoux', *Medical Heritage*, 2/1 (1986), 60–2; B. W. J. Grob, *The Anatomical Models of Dr. Louis Auzoux* (Leiden: Museum Boerhaave, 2004); Thomas N. Haviland and Lawrence Charles Parish, 'A Brief Account of the Use of Wax Models in the Study of Medicine', *Journal of the History of Medicine and Allied Sciences*, 25 (1970), 52–75; Arthur MacGregor, *Curiosity and Enlightenment: Collectors and Collections from the Sixteenth to the Nineteenth Century* (New Haven, Conn.: Yale University Press, 2007); Renato G. Mazzolini, 'Plastic Anatomies and Artificial Dissections', in Chadarevian and Hopwood, *Models*, 43–70; Roberta Panzanelli (ed.), *Ephemeral Bodies: Wax Sculpture and the Human Figure* (Los Angeles, Calif.: Getty Research Institute, 2008); Marta Poggesi, 'The Wax Figure Collec-tion in "La Specola" in Florence', in Monika von Düring, Georges Didi-Huberman, and Marta Poggesi (eds.), *Encyclopaedia Anatomica: A Complete Collection of Anatomical Waxes* (Köln: Taschen, 1999), 6–25; Kenneth Fitzpatrick Russell, 'Ivory Anatomical Manikins', *Medical History*, 16 (1972), 131–42. For brief survey of the literature on medical waxes, see Samuel J. M. M. Alberti, 'Wax Bodies: Art and Anatomy in Victorian Medical Museums', *Museum History Journal*, 2 (2009), 7–35.

[64] Alan W. Bates, 'Dr Kahn's Museum: Obscene Anatomy in Victorian London', *Journal of the Royal Society of Medicine*, 99 (2006), 618–24; Alan W. Bates, ' "Indecent and Demoralising Representations": Public Anatomy Museums in Mid-Victorian England', *Medical History*, 52 (2008), 1–22; Burmeister, 'Popular Anatomical Museums'; Claire E. Fox and Saretta Berlin, 'Abraham Chovet (1704–1790): The "Perfect Original" ', *Transactions and Studies of the College of Physicians of Philadelphia*, 38 (1970–1), 221–30; Anna Maerker, *Model Experts: Wax Anatomies and Enlightenment in Florence and Vienna, 1775–1815* (Manchester: Manchester University Press, 2011); E. J. Pyke, *A Biographical Dictionary of Wax Modellers* (Oxford: Clarendon Press, 1973); Thomas Schnalke, *Diseases in Wax: The History of the Medical Moulage*,

those crafted in late eighteenth-century Florence and Bologna, and in the early century several such Venuses were on display in London. The Paris-trained anatomist, surgeon, and modeller Abraham Chovet—who intro-duced glass vessels with fluid blood into his models—worked and dis-played in London before he emigrated to Philadelphia to build up a renowned collection there; some of his models were later displayed in London at Rackstrow's Museum. Charles Bell's hand-crafted models were among the choice items that led the Royal College of Surgeons in Edinburgh to purchase his collection. A handful of British curators, practitioners and artists turned their hands to anatomical modelling in the following century—Charles Cathcart in Edinburgh, for example, was a skilled wax artist.

These notable exceptions notwithstanding, British modellers were a rare breed, and medical curators therefore looked elsewhere for their *ceroplastica*. The Earl of Shelbourne bought waxes by the renowned Parisian surgeon Guillamme Desnoues and gave them to Trinity College Dublin.[65] The Cambridge anatomist William Clark, later to buy James Macartney's collec-tion from Dublin, travelled in Europe between 1818 and 1820, taking home a series of wax anatomical models from Bologna and Florence; the surgeon John Hutchinson (depicted third from the right, with the beard, in figure 3.2) also imported models at considerable expense.[66] When Hugh Percy, Duke of Northumberland, Lord Lieutenant of Ireland, gave the Dublin Royal College of Surgeons £500 to enrich the museum, the Committee used it to commission wax models from Jacques Talrich in Paris and to build a new room for the 'Northumberland Museum'.[67]

Most of these famous (and expensive) waxes on display in the early part of the century were of idealized, normalized healthy anatomy—it is alleged that some of the waxes at La Specola were based on up to 200 dissections. (On a humbler scale, William Hunter used a small wax

trans. Kathy Spatschek (Chicago: Quintessence, 1995); Violet Tansey and D. E. C. Mekie, *The Museum of the Royal College of Surgeons of Edinburgh* (Edinburgh: The Royal College of Surgeons of Edinburgh, 1982).

[65] George Newenham Wright, *An Historical Guide to the City of Dublin* (2nd edn, London: Baldwin, Cradock, and Joy, 1825). They also passed through the hands of the showman Benjamin Rackstrow in London.

[66] Herbert Hutchinson, *Jonathan Hutchinson, Life and Letters* (London: Heinemann, 1946); Mark Weatherall, *Gentlemen, Scientists, and Doctors: Medicine at Cambridge, 1800–1940* (Woodbridge; Rochester, NY: Boydell, 2000).

[67] Museum Committee Minute Book, 9 March 1825–16 November 1840, Royal College of Surgeons in Ireland Archive RCSI/MUC/1; T. Clive Lee and Elizabeth Allen, 'Anatomical Wax Modelling and the Northumberland Museum of the Royal College of Surgeons in Ireland', *Journal of the Irish Colleges of Physicians and Surgeons*, 21 (1992), 213–18; T. Clive Lee, *Catalogue of the Northumberland Museum of the Royal College of Surgeons in Ireland* (Dublin: Royal College of Surgeons in Ireland, 1992).

'perfect man', a flayed figure showing muscle groups, for his teaching.)[68]
For every stunning whole body model, however, there were dozens of
smaller fragments—the body dismembered in effigy. And by the middle
of century, anatomists and wax artists also began to expand their repertoire
beyond healthy anatomy. By 1853, the Inspectors of Anatomy noted that
wax was more commonly used to teach pathology than anatomy, and
models of normal anatomy fell from favour in some quarters—by 1842,
even the elaborate anatomical waxes at Trinity College Dublin 'possess
[ed] little interest'.[69] Museums concentrated rather on morbidity as the
subject of models.

Take for example the work of one of the few British artists in this genre,
Joseph Towne, the modeller employed at Guy's Hospital for half a century.[70] He may have crafted 200 justifiably renowned models of 'normal'
anatomy, but he also generated nearly 800 pieces illustrating morbid conditions. Like other nineteenth-century preparators and craftsmen, in creating these models and casts Towne formed close working relationships with
medical practitioners such as Thomas Hodgkin and John Hilton—they as
author and Towne as illustrator of a material 'publication'.[71] He crafted
tumours, aneurisms, various lesions, and afflictions of all the major organs.
Artificial as well as natural complaints were represented: some models
demonstrated the effects of poison, and marks of violence on the body.

But of all the fragmented morbid organs, the skin appealed most to
Towne as it did to many later nineteenth-century ceroplasticians (see for
example figure 5.6). Over 500 of his works were 'moulages' cast from the
faces of patients (or based on those of his assistant). Working in concert

[68] Hunterian Museum and Art Gallery William Hunter collections, catalogue number
GLAHM C.6; Martin Kemp, *Dr William Hunter at the Royal Academy of Art* (Glasgow:
University of Glasgow Press, 1975).

[69] Robert Harrison, *Catalogue of the Preparations Contained in the Museum of the Medical
School of Trinity College, Dublin* (Dublin: The University, 1842), 41; see also John Green
Crosse, 'A Memoir Upon the Method of Securely Closing Moist Anatomical Preparations,
Preserved in Spirit', *Transactions of the Provincial Medical and Surgical Association*, 4 (1836),
284–305; Frederick John Knox, *The Anatomist's Instructor, and Museum Companion: Being
Practical Directions for the Formation and Subsequent Management of Anatomical Museums*
(Edinburgh: Black, 1836).

[70] Alberti, 'Wax Bodies'; John Maynard, 'Towne, Joseph (1806–1879)', *Oxford Dictionary of National Biography* (Oxford: Oxford University Press, 2004), www.oxforddnb.com/
view/article/27600, accessed 19 Feb 2008; Schnalke, *Diseases in Wax*.

[71] Nick Hopwood, *Embryos in Wax: Models from the Ziegler Studio* (Cambridge: Whipple Museum of the History of Science, 2002); Hopwood, 'Plastic Publishing in Embryolo-
gy', in Chadarevian and Hopwood, *Models*, 170–206; Hopwood, 'Artist Versus Anatomist,
Models against Dissection: Paul Zeiller of Munich and the Revolution of 1848', *Medical
History*, 51 (2007), 279–308; Anna Maerker, ' "Turpentine Hides Everything": Autonomy
and Organization in Anatomical Model Production for the State in Late Eighteenth-
Century Florence', *History of Science*, 45 (2007), 257–86.

with Joseph Addison, Towne built up what Thomas Schnalke has dubbed 'the complete spectrum of contemporary dermatology'.[72] As the (admittedly partisan) Guy's Medical School's *Prospectus* boasted, 'A most important and valuable branch of the pathological museum is that showing disease of the skin by a series of wax models . . . wonderful for their exactness in the representations of the disease, and for the skill with which the part of the body affected is placed life-like before the observer.'[73] Elsewhere, important collections were gathered and crafted by the dermatologist Erasmus Wilson and the Liverpool modeller Robert William MacKenna.[74]

In the Guy's museum, Towne's models were 'arranged in good light, and with sufficient intervals between them to allow of them being conveniently studied'.[75] Whether of skin diseases or embryos (another popular subject for waxwork), models were crucial in teaching students how to think in three dimensions, how to *see*. When successive works were juxtaposed in a developmental series, this lent a temporal element to the displays, showing the development of the disease or of the foetus. And they were especially potent when in intermedial juxtaposition with paper representations; image and model drew from each other in style and in content. Whereas the waxes of La Specola were flamboyantly beautiful, seemingly alive and beautiful, moulages and other pathological waxes brutally represented the ugly facts of agony, death, and bodily invasion. They combined the exquisite aesthetic of the Florentine studio with the tradition of unflinching realism in anatomical art encountered in William Hunter's obstetrical images and the work of John Bell in whose illustrations the paraphernalia of dissection, the wedges and pulleys, are still evident.[76] This style would later give way to a different kind of

---

[72] Schnalke, *Diseases in Wax*, 64. See also Thomas Hodgkin, 'Illustrations of the Museum', *Guy's Hospital Reports*, 1 (1836), interleaved; C. Hilton Fagge, *Catalogue of the Models of Diseases of the Skin in the Museum of Guy's Hospital* (London: Churchill, 1876); [Samuel Wilks], 'Description of Some New Wax Models, Illustrating a Peculiar Atrophy of the Skin', *Guy's Hospital Reports*, 22 (1861), 297–312.

[73] Guy's Hospital Medical School, *Prospectus 1881–2* (London: Ash, 1882), 34–5.

[74] Lawrence Charles Parish, et al., 'Wax Models in Dermatology', *Transactions and Studies of the College of Physicians of Philadelphia*, 13/1 (1991), 29–74; D'Arcy Power, 'Wilson, Sir (William James) Erasmus (1809–1884)', rev. Geoffrey L. Asherson, *Oxford Dictionary of National Biography* (Oxford: Oxford University Press, 2004), www.oxforddnb.com/view/article/29702, accessed 19 Feb 2008; Augustus Ravogli, 'Far Echoes from the XVII International Congress of Medicine in London', *Journal of Cutaneous Diseases Including Syphilis*, 32 (1914), 28–9.

[75] Guy's Hospital, *Prospectus*, 32.

[76] John Bell, *Engravings, Explaining the Anatomy of the Bones, Muscles and Joints* (Edinburgh: Paterson, 1794); Hunter, *Anatomia Uteri*; Martin Kemp, *Bodyscapes: Images of Human Anatomy from the Collections of St Andrews* (St Andrews: Crawford Arts Centre, 1995). On different kinds of realism in anatomical representation, see Sappol, *Dream Anatomy*; for a discussion of realism and hyper-realism in waxes and artwork, see Jordanova,

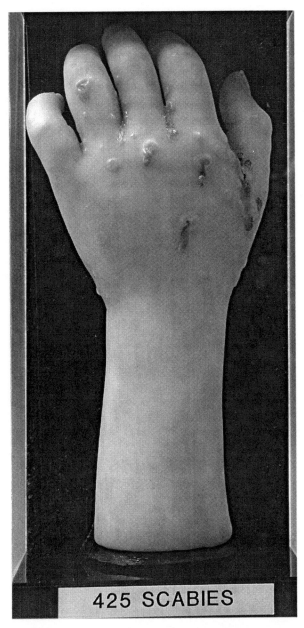

425 SCABIES

Fig. 5.6. Joseph Towne, dermatological moulage of scabies, *c.* 1850, from Guy's Hospital Museum. Courtesy of the Gordon Museum, King's College London.

realism—the stark, normalized 'remorsely sober woodcuts' of Henry Gray's *Anatomy* and later, as we have seen, to clinical photography.[77] Morbid waxes were similarly warts and all, fashioned with such meticulous verisimilitude that they became *hyper-real*; that is, the facsimile became more real than the corroded, decaying original.

There were commonalities between representations on paper and wax—but it was the tensions between them, their differing strengths and weaknesses, that led to the intermediality prevalent in museum displays. To their advocates, models had undeniable advantages; one Guy's curator chose not to include figures in his descriptions of Towne's models because they would not do the waxes justice.[78] Waxes were often life-size, or larger, whereas paper representations of the complete body tended not to be so after the demise of the grand folio in the nineteenth century.[79] One model could represent a complex system that would take many drawings to reproduce. The student gained far greater intimacy with the model than they could with an image, ceroplasticians claimed, and they could be viewed from all angles and even touched and manipulated.[80] In representing depth and texture, paper images sacrificed faith in the original colour with shading.[81] Hodgkin was never in doubt that models, like preparations, had the advantage over drawings, for they were not only 'visible' but 'tangible', and the models were 'representing real causes with a fidelity and minuteness not to be observed in drawings and plates'.[82] Paper always had the edge, however, by virtue of convenience: images and books were easily stored, and even before various Victorian print

Sexual Visions; on pain in bodily representation, see Lucy Bending, *The Representation of Bodily Pain in Late Nineteenth-Century English Culture* (Oxford: Clarendon Press, 2000); James Elkins, *Pictures of the Body: Pain and Metamorphosis* (Stanford: Stanford University Press, 1999).

[77] Martin Kemp and Marina Wallace, *Spectacular Bodies: The Art and Science of the Human Body from Leonardo to Now* (London; Berkeley: Hayward Gallery; University of California Press, 2000), 32. On Gray, see Richardson, *Making of Mr. Gray's Anatomy*; on hyperrealism, Umberto Eco, *Travels in Hyperreality: Essays* (London: Picador, 1987); David Freedberg, *The Power of Images: Studies in the History and Theory of Response* (Chicago: University of Chicago Press, 1989); Jordanova, *Sexual Visions*; Marina Warner, 'Waxworks and Wonderlands', in Lynne Cooke and Peter Wollen (eds.), *Visual Display: Culture Beyond Appearances* (Seattle: Bay, 1995), 179–201.

[78] [Samuel Wilks], 'Remarks on the Wax Models in Guy's Museum Representing *Roseola Cholerica* and *Roseola Variolosa*', *Guy's Hospital Reports*, 18 (1857), 341–50.

[79] Kemp and Wallace, *Spectacular Bodies*.

[80] Nick Hopwood and Soraya de Chadarevian, 'Dimensions of Modelling', in Chadarevian and Hopwood, *Models*, 1–15.

[81] Jay F. Schamberg and J. Frank Wallis, 'Wax Models—Their Preparation and Uses', *University of Pennsylvania Medical Bulletin*, 14 (1901), 262–4.

[82] Hodgkin, *Catalogue of the Preparations*, x; Thomas Hodgkin, 'Illustrations of the Museum', *Guy's Hospital Reports*, 1 (1836), interleaved, facing p. 188.

innovations, easier to reproduce than models (which as we shall see was an important virtue of catalogues). Paper representations of the body were more adaptable—especially in diagrammatic form, which was arguably better suited to late nineteenth-century medical education.

In a sense, models competed with other modes of displaying the human body, with two-dimensional images on the one hand, and real specimens on the other. 'Physicians and students', argued two *fin-de-siècle* mouleurs, 'would doubtless evince more interest in and derive more instruction from a collection of well-executed wax models of pathological specimens than from the rows of jars containing shrunken and decolourised specimens so frequently encountered.'[83] As one Guy's student wrote of the organic specimens, 'Colour is not a safe thing to go on, as it seems to come out a bit in the wash.'[84] From the early nineteenth century, thanks to the wax mixing techniques of Charles Bell and others, models retained their original colours even more faithfully.[85] Preserved remains also lost size, texture and detail—whereas waxes could represent more faithfully, and while fragile were nonetheless durable.[86] Again, the Guy's *Prospectus* proclaimed, 'Mr. Towne has added elaborate models of those organs and structures which cannot be preserved in the recent state'. They were therefore especially useful before the development of formaldehyde preservation in the later century, discussed in the previous chapter. And given the risks taken by anatomists also outlined there, it was helpful that models were clean, dry, and uncontaminated. Furthermore, as we saw in chapter 3, obtaining an organic specimen depended on its incidence in the hospital ward—models could represent rare conditions regardless, and thereby 'give the student constant opportunities of becoming familiar with the diagnosis of pathological conditions which the wards of any hospital show only on rare occasions'.[87] 'These reproductions', argued turn of the century mouleurs, 'serve not only as substitutes for clinical teaching, but they may be used for the faithful presentation of visual changes observed in rare cases or diseases.'[88]

At the end of the century, waxes remained a vital component of the morbid body in the museum. Moulages especially were still highly valued,

[83] Schamberg and Wallis, 'Wax Models', 264.

[84] [Nathaniel Burnett Ham], 'Guide to the Pathological Museum', *The Guyoscope*, 2/18 (1898), 69–70 at 70.

[85] Lakin, 'The Story of Our Museum'.

[86] Hortense P. A. Douglas, 'The Reproduction of Pathological Specimens by the Use of the Wax Moulage', *Journal of Technical Methods and Bulletin of the International Association of Medical Museums*, 12 (1929), 52–5.

[87] Guy's Hospital, *Prospectus*, 34, 35.

[88] Schamberg and Wallis, 'Wax Models', 263.

their utility cemented with exhibitions at world congresses. Fewer waxes were made as the twentieth century progressed, however, and many existing collections fell into disuse in the inter-war period. As we shall see in chapter 7, their fortunes thereby mirrored that of the medical museum generally. For a century and a half until that time, however, the wax model was an integral part of the medical museum, an instrument of education, a clinical tool, and a work of art. And as I have argued throughout this chapter, the value of this wax body stemmed from the way it was juxtaposed with other media: with specimen, picture, and, finally, with text.

THE TEXTUAL BODY

Images and preparations meant little without words. To render the diseased body legible, morbid anatomists also had frequent recourse to text, whether on display or in voluminous catalogues. Most body parts arrived at the museum with considerable accompanying documentation, including case histories and details of previous owners and donors. These descriptions became integral and valued parts of the collections, whether royal college museum or private anatomy show. Medical curators thereby accumulated a textual body to go alongside the organic body, without which the other media lost much of their value. As Samuel Wilks complained (somewhat unfairly) in 1857, 'those who know our London Museums best are aware that, until late years, they have been little better than show-rooms, there being no history to explain the meaning of the bare fact in the bottle before us'.[89] Rather, curators should gather text to accompany the preparations, so that each 'specimen is accompanied, wherever possible, by a short clinical account', as John Fawcett of Guy's prescribed, 'in order that the student might acquire a mental picture of the patient and so a more vivid impression that would be the case from a description of so much dead matter.'[90] *With* the proper documentation the specimen was no longer a sensational exhibit, but rather a serious

---

[89] Samuel Wilks, 'Remarks Upon Some of the Specimens of Disease of the Bone Contained in Guy's Museum, Especially Those Syled Osteosarcona and Myeloid, with Reference to the Question of Malignancy', *Guy's Hospital Reports,* 18 (1857), 143–78 at 145. See also George Langstaff, *Catalogue of the Preparations Illustrative of Normal, Abnormal, and Morbid Structure, Human and Comparative, Constituting the Anatomical Museum of George Langstaff* (London: Churchill, 1842).
[90] John Fawcett, 'In Memoriam: Lauriston E. Shaw, M.D., F.R.C.P., Consulting Physician to Guy's Hospital', *Guy's Hospital Reports,* 75 (1925), 5–19 at 6. See also Guy's Hospital Minutes of the Court of Committees, 18 May 1831, London Metropolitan Archives H09/GY/A/003/006/001.

clinical and educational tool. Ideally each specimen would have a comprehensive history and clinical description extracted from post-mortem reports or from donors' accounts. Related correspondence stayed with the preparation if possible, and these texts became part of the collection.[91] Whether as labels, loose-leaf slip files, or published catalogues, these words were as valued by curators as specimens and images. Laid out, like the museum, by region and system, descriptions and case histories assembled to form a multi-authored, partible, textual body corresponding with the other bodies described above.

Sometimes such case histories were kept with the specimen to act as a label, for example on small cards.[92] For the most part, however, labels took the form of small slips of coloured paper stuck directly to the jar or to the stand on which a preparation was mounted. Information was pared down as far as possible—whether to include anatomical location, condition, and species (if non-human), or simply the catalogue number of the specimen (see figure 1.3). Slips of paper were fragile and easily lost, and curators dreaded the dislocation of text and object. (In Glasgow, the solution was to carve the number of the specimen onto the glass jar with a diamond.[93]) For a museum object in isolation was considered useless—it either had no meaning, or, worse, the visitor was too free to afford it their own meaning. 'A museum without labels', concluded the British Association committee convened on the subject, 'is like an index torn out of a book; it might be amusing, but it teaches very little.' More than any other exhibitionary device, labels rendered collections accessible, shaped audiences, and extracted particular kinds of information from objects. 'Effective labelling is an art to be studied;' proclaimed the committee, 'it is like a style in literature ... The reader grasps the thought with the least possible effort.'[94]

The brevity of most labels meant that the bulk of the textual body was to be found not on the shelf, however, but in the museum catalogue.[95] Human remains were displayed there in print, whether to be used on the

[91] See for example Hunterian Museum donation letters 1808–1893, Glasgow University Special Collections MR50/1–59.

[92] John Houston, *Descriptive Catalogue of the Preparations of the Museum of the Royal College of Surgeons in Ireland*, 2 vols. (Dublin: Hodges and Smith, 1834–40).

[93] Commissioners for visiting the University of Glasgow, *Report* (London: HMSO, 1839); Alice J. Marshall and J. A. G. Burton (eds.), *Catalogue of the Preparations of Dr. William Hunter, Sir William Macewen, Professor John H. Teacher, Professor J. A. G. Burton in the Museum of the Pathology Department, Glasgow Royal Infirmary* (Glasgow: University of Glasgow, 1962).

[94] *Report of the British Association for the Advancement of Science*, 57 (1887), 127.

[95] Museum Committee Minutes, 16 November 1886, Royal College of Surgeons in Ireland Archive RCSI/MUC/1.

galleries or circulated more widely, and their importance is indicated by the care taken over them. Charles Cathcart in Edinburgh elucidated the form of the catalogue common across medical museums in the nineteenth century: 'Each specimen is furnished with its Series-number, followed in smaller type by its own number within the Series. These numbers are of course repeated in the Catalogue.' Following the Cambridge pathology museum and that of Guy's hospital, Cathcart gave

> each specimen a general heading in bold type... followed in the same paragraph by a statement of what the specimen is, and by an account of how it has been prepared and mounted. Next comes the clinical history in small print. Every effort has been made to obtain these histories of the specimens... In addition, every available clue has been followed that promised to lead to a clinical account of any of the specimens, whether in the old Infirmary records, or in the published writings of the donors of the specimens... In natural sequence after this paragraph follow, in larger type, the descriptions of the specimens in their recent state (when obtainable), and as they are permanently seen in the Museum.[96]

Most catalogue entries included a numerical classification, a brief description by way of a heading, a longer description in prose including the specimen's history (in a smaller font), and finally, for some specimens, details of the donor or acquisition route. They referenced other documentation, especially in the journal of the parent institution, which became de facto extensions of the catalogues.[97] Their form was markedly consistent across different sites. This is no surprise among elite collections such as those of the royal colleges, which explicitly shared practices; what is more striking is the extent to which smaller collections in proprietary medical schools, commercial anatomy shows, and even auction houses were catalogued in similar ways.

As much as the scalpel, the preserving jar, and the specimen itself, the catalogue was an essential working tool of museum practice. When Hodgkin arrived at St Thomas's for a brief tenure in 1842, second only to 'Glass & spirit' in his list of necessary equipment was 'A Guy's museum

---

[96] Cathcart, *Descriptive Catalogue*, xiv. See also George Murray Humphry, *Descriptive Catalogue of the Surgical Specimens in the Pathological Museum of the University of Cambridge* (Cambridge: The University Press, 1890); Samuel Wilks, *Catalogue of the Pathological Preparations in the Museum of Guy's Hospital* (London: MacKenzie, 1863); Matthew H. Kaufman, 'Frederick Knox, Younger Brother and Assistant of Dr Robert Knox: His Contribution To "Knox's Catalogues"', *Journal of the Royal College of Surgeons of Edinburgh*, 46 (2001), 44–56; James A. Ross and Hugh W. Y. Taylor, 'Robert Knox's Catalogue', *Journal of the History of Medicine*, 10 (1955), 269–76; James Paget, 'Suggestions for the Making of Pathological Catalogues', *British Medical Journal*, 11 December 1880, 911–12.

[97] Especially *Guy's Hospital Reports* and *St Bartholomew's Hospital Journal*. Periodic updates to the museums, and acquisitions per annum, were published in such periodicals.

catalogue interleaved for the use of curators.'[98] Those for use in-house
were often interleaved with blank pages, and James Lorrain Smith had the
University of Manchester pathological catalogue printed without page
numbers and with punch holes so that curators and other readers could
add to it; it was accompanied by a fold-out chart of the classification to aid
navigation.[99] Smith's and other catalogues were staggering undertakings
of many years' work. The third edition of Guy's—nearly 2,000 pages in
six volumes—took over twenty years to complete.[100] Nevertheless, the
curator's headache was that the catalogue was redundant even before it was
complete. In a satirical guide to the museum, one Guy's man noted dryly
'it is well to start in the South Room, for there the student will have the
advantage of the new catalogue, which is up to date. Doubtless by the time
he has completely mastered the contents of the South Room the catalogue
will have been revised for the whole collection.'[101]

Organic specimens could be reproduced in images, as we have seen
above, and in wax, as we shall see below. So too the textual body could be
reproduced. Great effort and expense was devoted to publishing catalogues, in order to spread the fame and worth of the collection. The
'museum of any large hospital', wrote James Goodhart of Guy's, 'is a
part, and a very important part, of the records of medicine'—and the
catalogue was its emissary.[102] 'The value of a museum catalogue,' echoed
The Lancet,

> is not limited to the halls in which the preparations are preserved, it is at all
> times and in every situation a trustworthy register of practical existences;
> hypothesis and imagination are unsuited to its pages. In the catalogues of
> museums we have the eloquent representatives of the museums themselves
> available at the instant to aid us in research and inquiry. With what gratifi-
> cation must no the practitioner survey his collection of museum catalogues,
> they almost make him possessor of the collections which they illustrate.[103]

Of the St George's collection, the *Edinburgh Medical Journal* proclaimed,
'Not only is the Museum, by their labours, rendered available for scientific
study to all who have access to it, but even pathologists at a distance may
consult the Catalogue with advantage.'[104] Curators went to lengths to

---

[98] Hodgkin, *Lecture Introductory*, 2.

[99] Smith, *A Catalogue of the Pathological Museum*; James Lorrain Smith, *University of Manchester Pathological Museum Classification* (Manchester: Sherratt and Hughes, 1906).

[100] Shaw, et al., *Descriptive Catalogue*.

[101] [Ham], 'Guide to the Pathological Museum',69.

[102] James F. Goodhart, 'List of Specimens Added to the Pathological Museum During the Year 1882–83', *Guy's Hospital Reports*, 42 (1884), 101–8 at 101.

[103] *The Lancet*, 18 June 1842, 422–3.

[104] *Edinburgh Medical Journal*, 14 (1868), 86.

make certain that such 'pathologists at a distance' would have access to the catalogue, funding print runs in the hundreds, and distributed to other members of staff, to libraries of major institutions, to medical societies, and to other museums, acting as ambassadors for the collection and textbooks in their own right.[105] The exchange of catalogues followed and expanded the networks discussed in chapter 3, and like the exchanges of specimens, they generated and regenerated the identity of the individuals, collections, and institutions.

Although many of their physical and textual qualities are evident across the century, there was considerable quantitative change in production over time. Anatomy museum catalogues were published in three loose waves that echoed the development of pathology in the UK over the century. The first batch were published around 1830 as British curators began to implement Parisian notions of pathological anatomy. Notable among them was Hodgkin's catalogue of Guy's and Edward Stanley's of Barts.[106] There followed a steady output of catalogues that were either dedicated specifically to morbid anatomy, or which differentiated pathology within multi-volume sets. Over the next three decades, most institutional museums published at least a one-volume catalogue, and some (like Guy's and the Hunterian in London) published their second editions, heavily reworked. Gradually the textual body became disarticulated, as individual catalogues became more specialized.[107]

But the golden age of the pathological catalogue was the final decades of the nineteenth century. Following the lead of Barts and the Hunterian in the early 1880s, many medical museums, huge by this time, published exhaustive catalogues—first in London and then in other centres.[108] They

---

[105] At the Royal College of Surgeons in Ireland, for example, the Museum Committee arranged for copies to be sent to Sir Astley Cooper, James Macartney, the museums of the Army Medical Department, the Royal College of Surgeons of England and Trinity College; specially bound copies were to be presented to the Duke of Northumberland (a former beneficiary) and the Lord Lieutenant. Museum Committee Minute Book, 20 December 1834, Royal College of Surgeons in Ireland Archive RCSI/MUC/1. On catalogues as textbooks, see Cathcart, 'Classification in Pathology'; Hodgkin, 'Illustrations of the Museum'; Kahn, *Atlas*; P. H. Pye-Smith, *Catalogue of the Preparations of Comparative Anatomy in the Museum of Guy's Hospital* (London: Ash, 1874); Teacher, *Catalogue*. The Guy's catalogue was worth of note in the *Sunday Times* (17 January 1830, p 2., col. 6).

[106] Hodgkin, *Catalogue of the Preparations*; Edward Stanley, *A Description of the Preparations Contained in the Museum of St Bartholomew's Hospital* (London: Wix, 1831). See also Army Medical Museum, *Catalogue of Preparations*; [MacKenzie], *Descriptive Catalogue*; Fawdington, *Catalogue Descriptive*; Houston, *Descriptive Catalogue*.

[107] See for example Joseph Toynbee, *A Descriptive Catalogue of the Preparations Illustrative of the Diseases of the Ear, in the Museum of Joseph Toynbee, F.R.S.* (London: Churchill, 1857).

[108] Eve, *Descriptive Catalogue* [Barts]; Paget, *Descriptive Catalogue* [RCS]. See also Marcus Beck, S. G. Shattock, and Charles Stonham, *Descriptive Catalogue of the Specimens Illustrating Surgical and Medical Pathology in the Museum of University College, London*,

signalled the disciplinary maturity of British pathology, as discussed in chapter 2. As the *Lancet* noted in 1891,

> It is obvious too that a good catalogue is indispensable to a museum; and we note with satisfaction that of late year many of the London hospitals have followed the example set by the older institutions, and issued such works from the press. The advantage to the student is very great, whilst to the investigator no less valuable: and it may be noted that, since the plan pursued is mainly the same at all the hospitals, there is great facility given for the comparison of specimens and the collation of facts of morbid anatomy.[109]

Another *Lancet* reviewer, in assessing the value of one catalogue, commented that 'the foregoing observations form rather a review of the museum, than of the catalogue; the latter *being necessarily so connected with the former*, that it would be neither practicable nor desirable to notice it otherwise'.[110] Catalogue and collection were presented as seamlessly co-constitutive. The words taught the eye how to see things. Tony Bennett's account of the importance of labels in Victorian museums also applies to other associated texts: 'No matter how much things were said to be able to speak for themselves, however, there was, in museums, an incessant effort to provide a written supplement that would help anchor their meaning.'[111] Imposing they may have been, circulatable and reproducible they were, but catalogues were nevertheless anchored by the material specimens, and were used in conjunction with images (their own lack of illustrations is marked). Like labels, they were keys to the two- and three-dimensional maps of morbidity. Text, illustration, and specimen worked together in the medical museum to form maps of morbidity.

3 vols. (London: Taylor and Francis, 1881–1890); Fowler and Sutton, *A Descriptive Catalogue* [Middlesex]; John H. Morgan, *A Descriptive Catalogue of the Pathological Museum of Charing Cross Hospital* (London: Harrison, 1888); F. Charlewood Turner, Frederick S. Eve, and T. H. Openshaw (eds.), *A Descriptive Catalogue of the Pathological Museum of the London Hospital* (London: Taylor and Francis, 1890); Humphry, *Descriptive Catalogue* [Cambridge]; Shattock, *A Descriptive Catalogue*; J. Jackson Clarke, *Descriptive Catalogue of the Pathological Museum of St Mary's Hospital* (London: Morton and Burt, 1891); Williams and Stonham, *Descriptive Catalogue* [UCL]; Cathcart, *Descriptive Catalogue* [RCSEd]; Shaw, et al., *Descriptive Catalogue* [Guy's]; Teacher, *Catalogue* [Hunterian Glasgow]; Smith, *Catalogue of the Pathological Museum* [Manchester].

[109] *The Lancet*, 17 January 1891, 148.
[110] *The Lancet*, 19 December 1829, 482, emphasis added.
[111] Tony Bennett, 'Pedagogic Objects, Clean Eyes, and Popular Instruction: On Sensory Regimes and Museum Didactics', *Configurations*, 6 (1998), 345–71 at 361.

PATHOLOGICAL INTERMEDIALITY

The body is a cultural phenomenon as well as a biological entity, and it has a history. Somatic knowledge is generated through interactions between people and objects in particular sites. Literary, cultural, and medical historians have accordingly contributed to a rich literature in this respect over the last three decades. In studying museums, we can add a material dimension to these analyses. The objects, illustrations, and texts described here were anatomical and pathological 'facts': flexible, contingent entities that nonetheless had a considerable physical presence in the collection.

These facts, in flesh, bone, paper, and wax, came together from different places to form dividual bodies in the medical museum. As archaeologist Chris Fowler observes, 'The materiality of death is ... closely bound up with the practices and principles structuring personhood', but in the medical museum, as we saw in chapter 3, the identities of the patients, the raw material from which these facts were manufactured, were obscured by those of the collectors and curators.[112] Case histories and details—the textual body—may have provided links with the living, but these objects in different media were multi-authored by the patient, practitioner, artist, and others. These pathological bodies represented not individuals, but disease(s). In this respect the bodies in the medical museum were successors to the Renaissance 'wound man', suffering every conceivable ailment simultaneously (see figure 5.7). They were sacrificed in effigy for medical education, so that others might recover from such torment: not as a single Frankensteinian entity, but rather as dividual bodies displayed on the gallery by region, by system, or condition. For alongside multiple authorship, partibility is a key element of dividuality, and the fragmentations of the carcasses allowed for these different arrangements.

The objects on the shelves, then, had complex associations with others in the collection. One preserved organ was related to all the other organs elsewhere in the museum with the same condition; to similar organs demonstrating different diseases; and most intimately to the model next to it showing how it should appear, and the text on the jar and in the catalogue describing its symptoms and provenance. Historians of medical images have identified the 'dynamic conversation between medical texts ... and the images that illuminate them', but the museum added the crucial third dimension.[113] Innovative ocular technologies in the nineteenth century came not only in brass and glass, but in spirits and wax, and the function

---

[112] Fowler, *Archaeology of Personhood*, 92.
[113] Heinrich, *Afterlife of Images*, 9.

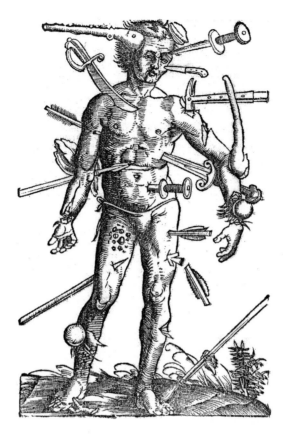

Fig. 5.7. 'Wound-man' woodcut, from Hans von Gersdorff, *Feldtbůch Der Wundartzney: Newlich Getruckt Und Gebessert* (Strassburg: Hans Schotten zům Thyergarten, 1528). Wellcome Library, London.

of the medical museum—the efficacy of which is explored in the next chapter—depended on this pathological intermediality. Dismembered en route, pathological bodies were re-integrated with different media on these shelves. Like other collections, then, the medical museum was a relational assemblage, the specimens' individual biographies combining to generate an entity even more complex than its constituent parts.[114]

[114] Hallam, *Anatomy Museum*; Anita Herle, Mark Elliott, and Rebecca Empson, *Assembling Bodies: Art, Science and Imagination* (Cambridge: University of Cambridge Museum of Archaeology and Anthropology, 2009); Bruno Latour and Peter Weibel (eds.), *Making Things Public: Atmospheres of Democracy* (Cambridge, Mass.: MIT Press, 2005); Robert Louis Welsch, 'One Time, One Place, Three Collections: Colonial Processes and the Shaping of Some

Curators intended this complex entity to be nothing less than a complete tour of disease, the material basis for a cartographical physic. The museum was an atlas of the pathological body, a confluence of three great modernist projects—medicine, museology, and mapping.[115] This could only be achieved by drawing on this range of media, and by juxtaposing morbid anatomy with comparative and normal—the pathological body explicated by the healthy and the animal. To collect, possess, and present specimens was to construct a natural history of illness, their materiality accompanied by their collected case histories, advertising the efficacy and experience of hospital staff. To visit the museum was to see in a single setting the sum of pathological knowledge laid out on the shelves, a panorama of disease, above and below the surface. The morbid body was dissected, invaded, turned inside out for visitors. The powerful responses they then elicited are the subject of the following chapter.

Museum Collections from German New Guinea', in Michael O'Hanlon and Robert Louis Welsch (eds.), *Hunting the Gatherers: Ethnographic Collectors, Agents and Agency in Melanesia, 1870s–1930s* (New York: Berghahn, 2000), 155–180.

[115] Benedict Anderson, *Imagined Communities: Reflections on the Origin and Spread of Nationalism* (rev. edn, London: Verso, 2006); Hooper-Greenhill, *Museums*.

6

Viewing Pathology

Medical Museums and their Visitors

Morbid Curiosities has so far been concerned with the ways in which dead bodies were fragmented, preserved, and re-assembled in medical museums. The (living) people featured have therefore been medical practitioners, collectors, curators, and artists. But a history of museum production is hamstrung without the corresponding history of museum consumption, an account of those who viewed, handled, and otherwise used pathological collections. Having explored what, where, why, and how bodies were constructed in medical museums, we now ask, for whom?

The would-be historian of museum visitors is faced with a problem, however: while professionals and curators (if not craftsmen and artists) leave bounteous records and of course the objects themselves, visitors leave few traces, if any.[1] We should not take from this absence that museum visitors were a passive audience, however—rather, they were active participants in the construction of meaning. This chapter therefore addresses not only the intended use and visitor constituency but also as far as possible the ways in which visitors experienced and responded to the collections. It will come as no surprise that the former and latter did not always tally, and my aim is to explore the tension between visitors' appropriation of the material, sensory, and epistemological experience of the objects and the explicit aims of the museums themselves. The preserved corpse was contested and debated terrain. Medical specimens, like

---

[1] For a brief survey of the history of museum visiting, and a rehearsal of some of the ideas presented here, see Samuel J. M. M. Alberti, 'The Museum Affect: Visiting Collections of Anatomy and Natural History', in Aileen Fyfe and Bernard Lightman (eds.), *Science in the Marketplace: Nineteenth-Century Sites and Experiences* (Chicago: University of Chicago Press, 2007), 371–403. For recent works that include the history of visiting in their analyses, see for example Anna Maerker *Model Experts: Wax Anatomies and Enlightenment in Florence and Vienna, 1775–1815* (Manchester: Manchester University Press, 2011); Christopher Whitehead, *Museums and the Construction of Disciplines: Art and Archaeology in Nineteenth-Century Britain* (London: Duckworth, 2009).

all museum objects, are polysemic, and even among the different communities of visitors (medical students being an important constituency here) we should not assume a homogeneity of interpretation. Different visitors could take from any or none of the carefully constructed bodies discerned in the previous chapter.

This chapter thereby shifts the narrative of this book from the movement of things on their way to the museum and the museological processes enacted upon them to their use and audiences. Having assessed acquisition and display, this is the third and final phase in the career of the specimens. It opens with an outline of the role of specimens in medical education, the ostensible aim of most of the museums explored earlier in the book. This leads on to an assessment of access to these museums, for medical students and others, and thereby the intended audience constituency, paying particular attention to the restriction in access towards the end of the century that belied the move to inclusivity in other parts of the museums sector. Having situated these visitors in the museum and laid out the curators' intentions for their engagement, we turn to how they experienced the collections. This history incorporates not only sight but also the other senses (the title of this chapter, 'Viewing pathology' is a conscious misnomer). Finally we encounter the rich spectrum of responses to pathological collections, from wonder through disgust to anger—many of which were remote from the curatorial intentions with which this account of the history of the use and abuse of the Victorian medical museum begins.

THE OBJECT OF MEDICAL EDUCATION

'It is only by accurate and careful comparison of what you have noted at the bedside, with what is disclosed (anatomically speaking) after death,' the morbid anatomist Thomas Fawdington told his students in Manchester, 'that you can ever hope to become good Pathologists.'[2] The principal stated reason for displaying morbid anatomy of the institutions and individuals of concern here was to educate. The imagined visitor, their addressee, was the medical student, formally enrolled or otherwise. From the Royal College of Surgeons to Kahn's Anatomical Museum and Gallery of All Nations, curators trumpeted the didactic potential of their collections.

---

[2] Thomas Fawdington, *A Catalogue Descriptive Chiefly of the Morbid Preparations Contained in the Museum of the Manchester Theatre of Anatomy and Medicine* (Manchester: Harrison and Crosfield, 1833), iii–iv.

The preparation became central to medical education at the turn of the eighteenth century with the emergence of pathological anatomy, the increasing reliance on practical training, and the dominance of institutions in medical instruction, and it remained an important tool of formal and informal curricula until the inter-war period.[3] We have seen how medical education in late Georgian Britain was provided by an array of institutions, led by the London hospitals and the Scottish Universities, all of which began to gather extensive collections. Corpses, models, and images were then essential components alongside living patients of the practical anatomical education that underpinned nineteenth-century medical and surgical training. Lectures and books would not suffice. Furthermore, after significant changes in British medical education in the first decades of the nineteenth century, morbid anatomy in particular was part of the raft of practical sciences that gained prominence on medical syllabuses, the bridge between clinical work and scientific disease frameworks. Historians of medicine have examined in some detail how successive legislation through the century increased the significance of laboratory sciences in medical education.[4] Less attention has been paid to the importance of the museum.

This is surprising, given that the regulation of medical training over the course of the nineteenth century incrementally rendered morbid collections more significant, and accordingly more numerous. The royal colleges placed heavy emphases on the hands-on study of anatomy, and those who wished to satisfy their requirements needed exposure to collections. The 1815 Apothecaries Act gave the Society of Apothecaries licensing power and made formal courses of lectures compulsory, stimulating the growth of the provincial medical schools. We have seen that preparations were key to these courses, and that the schools therefore absorbed and developed considerable collections. In 1821, for example, the Society recognized Joseph Jordan's courses in Manchester, and in 1827 his rival

[3] Simon Chaplin, 'John Hunter and The "Museum Oeconomy", 1750–1800' (Ph.D. thesis, King's College London, 2009). For careful studies of the history of British medical education see Matthew H. Kaufman, *Medical Teaching in Edinburgh During the 18th and 19th Centuries* (Edinburgh: Royal College of Surgeons of Edinburgh, 2003); Susan C. Lawrence, *Charitable Knowledge: Hospital Pupils and Practitioners in Eighteenth-Century London* (Cambridge: Cambridge University Press, 1996); Vivian Nutton and Roy Porter (eds.), *The History of Medical Education in Britain* (Amsterdam: Rodopi, 1995); Keir Waddington, *Medical Education at St Bartholomew's Hospital, 1123–1995* (Woodbridge, Suffolk: Boydell, 2003).
[4] On the laboratory in medical education, Thomas Neville Bonner, *Becoming a Physician: Medical Education in Great Britain, France, Germany and the United States 1750–1945* (New York: Oxford University Press, 1995); Andrew Cunningham and Perry Williams (eds.), *The Laboratory Revolution in Medicine* (Cambridge: Cambridge University Press, 1992).

Thomas Turner also gained the Society's recognition. Morbid specimens in particular became more important to the schools' courses in the 1830s when the Society recommended the study of morbid anatomy.[5]

In London, meanwhile, the extensive collections were integral to the training provided by the teaching hospitals. In the mid century, however, reforms of the General Medical Council shifted the locus of medical education from hospital to university, and the ownership of medical museums reflected this, as we saw in chapter 2. The 1858 Medical (Registration) Act stipulated that all medical students must study anatomy for two years, and by this time most training organizations included morbid anatomy or pathology in their syllabuses. The Scottish universities, which had strong museums from the early century, also continued to expand their collections apace, and morbid sections especially, for example after the 1861 ordinances for the Glasgow MB demanded three months of lectures in pathological anatomy. The professor of anatomy John Cleland encapsulated the significance of morbid specimens in their curricula:

> They are the means of furnishing permanent and accessible records of remarkable phenomena, and are even more useful in affording comparison of different stages and varieties of disease one with another. There are no doubt certain matters connected with the general appearance of morbid textures which are better observed in recent condition; but there is much more which cannot be seen to advantage, nor indeed studied at all, except in carefully designed preparations permanently preserved.[6]

In England and Ireland, too, by the end of the century pathology was a key component of medical degrees. The Victoria University in Manchester was by no means the only institution to demand that candidates recognize microscopical and gross specimens in their final MB exam.[7] (See also figure 3.2.)

The medical museum, then, was a fundamental element in nineteenth-century formal medical training, providing a crucial material resource to complement and underpin the laboratory and clinic.[8] Lectures especially relied on specimens and models, as evidenced by the great lengths to

[5] Bonner, *Becoming a Physician*; F. W. Jordan, *Life of Joseph Jordan, Surgeon, and an Account of the Rise and Progress of Medical Schools in Manchester, with Some Particulars of the Life of Dr Edward Stephens* (London: Sherratt and Hughes, 1904); Russell C. Maulitz, *Morbid Appearances: The Anatomy of Pathology in the Early Nineteenth Century* (Cambridge: Cambridge University Press, 1987).

[6] John Cleland, *Truth, Pathology, and the Public* (Glasgow: Maclehose, 1880), 17.

[7] Helen K. Valiér, 'Between Science and Clinical Practice: A History of Pathology in Manchester, C.1870–1905' (M.Sc. thesis, University of Manchester, 1997).

[8] Elizabeth Hallam, *Anatomy Museum. Death and the Body Displayed* (London: Reaktion, 2011); Jonathan Reinarz, 'The Age of Museum Medicine: The Rise and Fall of the Medical Museum of Birmingham's School of Medicine', *Social History of Medicine*, 18 (2005), 419–37.

which medical teachers would go to illustrate their sessions. 'There was no chemical laboratory, no museum', remembered Edward Stephens of the medical school in Pine Street, Manchester:

> Each lecturer had to send to his own house for such preparations as were wanted to illustrate his lecture, and afterwards to convey them home again; even the most simple things such as bones, etc. This wretched state of things continued even for some years after I jointed [sic] the staff of the Pine Street School, which was in the Session 1834–5. I was continually, at our meetings, urging the necessity of building a room for a museum, because the preparations were seriously damaged by carrying them backwards and forwards. Both Mr. Turner and I went to considerable expense to provide large cupboards to lock-up and preserve the preparations.[9]

Collections were heavily used throughout the country, although perhaps none more so than the University of London's during its confused early years, when multiple staff claimed dominion over anatomy teaching: 'three certainly were lecturing in the same class-room, on the same subjects, and with the same preparations put upon the table three successive times in the same day'.[10] Overuse was an endemic problem: the Royal College of Surgeons in Ireland refused repeated requests to borrow specimens for teaching, but some museums like that of Glasgow University had a dedicated 'class collection'.[11]

The use of pathological specimens for educational purposes in formal sites such as medical schools and universities will come as little surprise—but it is also important to acknowledge that education was also the stated purpose of less orthodox collections. Joseph Woodhead claimed that his anatomical museum in Liverpool (figure 6.1), for example, was 'An Intellectual Study!! And a Public Advantage!!!'[12] Together with Joseph Kahn, Woodhead purported to offer the visitor from any walk of life a chance to 'know thyself', to democratize anatomical knowledge. But this education came with unsubtle moral overtones. Kahn's intention in displaying models of 'the terrible effects of debauchery under the form of

---

[9] Jordan, *Life of Joseph Jordan*, 103, 109.

[10] 'Mr. Bell's Letter to His Pupils of the London University, On Taking Leave of Them', *London Medical Gazette* 7 (1830), 308–11 at 309.

[11] Museum Committee Minutes, 9 November 1833; 1 August 1835, Royal College of Surgeons in Ireland Archive RCSI/MUC/1; [Allen Thomson], 'Note of Dr Allen Thomson's Collection of Anatomical Preparations, Drawings, &c.', MS, *c.* 1877, Glasgow University Special Collections MR 41/11.

[12] [Joseph T. Woodhead], *Descriptive Catalogue of the Liverpool Museum of Anatomy* (Liverpool: Matthews, 1877), back cover. Alan W. Bates, '"Indecent and Demoralising Representations": Public Anatomy Museums in Mid-Victorian England', *Medical History*, 52 (2008), 1–22; Maritha Rene Burmeister, 'Popular Anatomical Museums in Nineteenth-Century England' (Ph.D. thesis, Rutgers University, 2000).

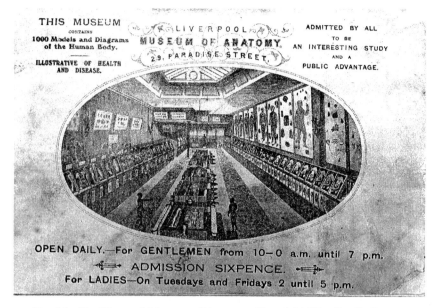

THIS MUSEUM
CONTAINS
1000 Models and Diagrams
of the Human Body.

ILLUSTRATIVE OF HEALTH
AND DISEASE.

LIVERPOOL
MUSEUM OF ANATOMY,
29, PARADISE STREET.

ADMITTED BY ALL
TO BE
AN INTERESTING STUDY
AND A
PUBLIC ADVANTAGE.

OPEN DAILY.—For GENTLEMEN from 10—0 a.m. until 7 p.m.
ADMISSION SIXPENCE.
For LADIES—On Tuesdays and Fridays 2 until 5 p.m.

Fig. 6.1. The Liverpool Museum of Anatomy. [Joseph T. Woodhead], *Descriptive Catalogue of the Liverpool Museum of Anatomy* (Liverpool: Matthews, 1877). Wellcome Library, London.

Syphilis' was 'not to gratify a prurient curiosity, but to present the scientific observer with a general and correct view of the perfect and wonderful structure of the body, and to point out the dreadful consequences attending any departure from the unerring and beneficent laws ordained by the great Creator of the Universe for the government and propagation of the human race'.[13] In his 'Gallery of All Nations and Anatomical Museum', J.W. Reimers was one of several showmen who demonstrated the terrible effects of tight-laced corsets:

Model of a young female, a resident and native of Munich, who was rendered pregnant by seduction. With the intention of concealment, she laced her waist very tightly with the stays: this terrible abuse of the body exercised its injurious influence over the circulation of the blood, and she became a victim to poplexy [sic] one evening whilst immoderately dancing at a ball, where she suddenly fell senseless in the arms of her companion. Knowing that it was impossible to save the female, they endeavoured at once to recover the offspring, which upon dissection was discovered in this

---

[13] Joseph Kahn, *Catalogue of Dr. Kahn's Anatomical Museum, Now Exhibiting at 315, Oxford Street, near Regent Circus* (London: Golbourn, 1851), iii.

emaciated condition, it is distorted, and its entrails forced out through the anus.[14]

Another popular topic was danger of self-abuse, including the terrible condition dubbed 'Spermatorrhœa'.[15] The sincerity of the proprietors' insistence on the didactic function was somewhat undermined, however, by the practice of selling cures to these conditions at the exhibitions.[16] But as we shall see below, regardless of what their motives were, visitors arrived with their own intentions and left with their own impressions.

ACCESSING COLLECTIONS

From their inception, then, those training in anatomy, medicine, and surgery comprised a significant visiting constituency for medical museums. Even private collections had considerable audiences, as renowned teachers including Astley Cooper and Charles White opened their cabinets for educational purposes. 'Have you been to Dr. Hunter[']s Museum in Windmill Street'? asked one father of his medical student son at the beginning of the century, 'it is worth seeing... it is to be seen gratis'.[17] After it was transferred to Glasgow, Hunter's collection was accessible to students enrolled in the courses of the trustees (that is, the medical faculty) during term time.[18] Advanced students from elsewhere, with suitable references, could gain access for a three month period, and could even open the presses.[19] Across town, the anatomical collection at Anderson's University was

[14] Charles V. Goulder (ed.), *Catalogue of J. W. Reimers's Gallery of All Nations and Anatomical Museum* (Leeds: Jackson and Asquith, 1853), 27; see also [Woodhead], *Descriptive Catalogue*, item 259.

[15] See for example Joseph Kahn, *The Shoals and Quicksands of Youth, Being the Latest Researches in Physiology and Chemistry, as Applied to the Diseases of the Urinary and Generative Organs, and the Nervous Weakness, Debility, and Mental Imbecility, Arising from the Abuses of the Same* (London: privately published, 1856). Ellen Bayuk Rosenman, 'Body Doubles: The Spermatorrhea Panic', *Journal of the History of Sexuality*, 12 (2003), 365–99; Elizabeth Stephens, 'Anatomies of Desire: Female Bodies in Fin-De-Siècle Anatomical Museums', in Peter Cryle and Chris Forth (eds.), *Fin De Siècle Sexuality: The Making of a Central Problem* (Newark: Delaware University Press, 2008), 25–41.

[16] Bates, '"Indecent and Demoralising Representations"'; William H. Helfand, *Quack, Quack, Quack: The Sellers of Nostrums in Prints, Posters, Ephemera, and Books* (New York: Grolier Club, 2002).

[17] Richard Weekes to Hampton Weekes, 3 January 1803, in John M. T. Ford, *A Medical Student at St Thomas's Hospital, 1801–1802: The Weekes Family Letters, Medical History* Supplement 7 (London: Wellcome Institute for the History of Medicine, 1987), 249.

[18] From the 1810 regulations. Lawrence Keppie, *William Hunter and the Hunterian Museum in Glasgow, 1807–2007* (Edinburgh: Edinburgh University Press, 2007).

[19] Commissioners for Visiting the University of Glasgow, *Report* (London: HMSO, 1839).

also freely open to medical students, as was the Royal College of Surgeons museum in Edinburgh.[20] At the University of Edinburgh, by contrast, each student was charged a guinea 'for the support of the Anatomical Museum'; on the grounds that

> it being at the same time understood, that if he pays this money at his first matriculation at the university, he shall be entitled to free entrance to the museum during the whole course of his studies ... no other student shall be compelled to contribute to the museum, but ... tickets of admission shall be issued to all who wish for them at 7s. for the season, and that none but students of [Alexander Monro *Tertius*'s] class shall be admitted to the museum' without such tickets.[21]

Elsewhere, students could use and study collections by virtue of matriculation. Some gained especially privileged access to the collection, as for example the members of the famous Guy's Hospital Physical Society, who met weekly for an evening of discussion that often centred around specimens.[22]

By whatever means, the volume of student visitors was significant, especially in Scotland, where large numbers of British doctors and surgeons trained.[23] By 1815 there were 820 medical students at the University of Edinburgh; Robert Knox alone used the Barclay collection to teach over 500 in 1828. These figures would be dwarfed, however, with the expansion of medical education in the later nineteenth century. By 1890, there were over 2,000 medical students at the University of Edinburgh and 800 in Glasgow. Even the relatively modest Victoria University of Manchester medical faculty, for example, more than doubled its enrolment from 134 in 1872 to 380 in 1888. It seems likely that most of the 947 visitors to Royal College of Surgeons of Ireland Museum in 1885–6

---

[20] John Butt, *John Anderson's Legacy: The University of Strathclyde and Its Antecedents 1796–1996* (East Linton: Tuckwell, 1996); Frederick John Knox, *The Anatomist's Instructor, and Museum Companion: Being Practical Directions for the Formation and Subsequent Management of Anatomical Museums* (Edinburgh: Black, 1836); [Mr MacKenzie], *Descriptive Catalogue of the Anatomical Museum of the University of Edinburgh* (Edinburgh: Whyte, 1829).

[21] Royal Commission on the Universities of Scotland, *Minutes of Evidence*, 4 vols. (House of Commons Command Papers 92–5; London: HMSO, 1837), appendix, 168.

[22] Susan C. Lawrence, '"Desirous of Improvements in Medicine": Pupils and Practitioners in the Medical Societies at Guy's and St Bartholomew's Hospitals, 1795–1815', *Bulletin of the History of Medicine*, 59 (1985), 89–104.

[23] For trends and specific data on student numbers, see David Hamilton, *The Healers: A History of Medicine in Scotland* (2nd edn, Edinburgh: Mercat, 2003); 'Report of the Medical Section of the Senate Concerning Additional Accommodation, &c., required in the Department of Medicine', 1889, Manchester Medical Collection MMC/5/7/3/5, John Rylands University Library of Manchester; Museum Committee Minute Book, Curator's Report for the year ending 5 April 1886; Curator's Report for the Year ending 5 April 1890, Royal College of Surgeons in Ireland Archive RCSI/MUC/2.

were medical students; four years later there were 1,218. Elsewhere in the medical museum sector, Joseph Woodhead claimed that 'hundreds of thousands' had visited his Museum of Anatomy in Liverpool. Many of these would have taken advantage of the opportunity to visit in the evening after work, whereas college and hospital collections had far more restricted opening hours.[24]

But these opening hours were not only for students. From their inception, medical museums attracted a range of other visitors, usually for a fee. With a little persuasion and a letter or two, the elite could gain access to Enlightenment collections. The surgeon Peter Clare reported that Hunter's 'grand anatomical museum' on Windmill Street was 'shewn to the inquisitive and learned of every nation [by Hunter's assistants or servants] with the utmost affability and condescension'.[25] These curious folk came from near and far to see the collection, as for example the Yale chemist Benjamin Silliman who perused 'diseased parts, and monstrous productions... the preserved remains of thousands of our fellow mortals [which] exhibit, in melancholy array, the host of ills that "flesh is heir to"'.[26] John Hunter's museum, meanwhile, was open to the 'public' (narrowly construed) for two months of the year. Among the elite visitors to Charles White's collection in Manchester was a young Thomas de Quincey.[27]

Once in Glasgow, the Hunterian collection, like the Cambridge University Anatomy collection, was originally open one hour a day for 'strangers', Hunter having stipulated that 'for the sake of the public... any of the Books or other articles in my said library and museum may be examined'; after the numbers became so great that they distracted from the appropriate studious use of the museum a ticketing system was introduced (first one shilling, later two), but waived for academics, clergy, officers and donors to the museum.[28] By the 1820s, admission receipts

---

[24] [Woodhead], *Descriptive Catalogue*, back page; Helfand, *Quack, Quack, Quack*. On opening hours of individual museums, see Keppie, *William Hunter*; Reinarz, 'The Age of Museum Medicine'; Royal Commission, *Minutes of Evidence*, appendix, 168; *Returns Relating to Medical Museums in the United Kingdom*, Parliamentary Papers 14 (London: House of Commons, 1857); Museum Committee Minutes, 26 July 1887, Royal College of Surgeons in Ireland Archive RCSI/MUC/2.

[25] Peter Clare, *A New and Easy Method of Curing the Lues Venerea* (3rd edn, London: Cadell, 1780), xx–xxi, cited in Keppie, *William Hunter*, 26. See also Samuel Foart Simmons and John Hunter, *William Hunter, 1718–1783: A Memoir*, ed. C. Helen Brock (1783; East Kilbride: University of Glasgow Press, 1983).

[26] Benjamin Silliman, *A Journal of Travels in England, Holland and Scotland*, 2 vols. (2nd edn, New Haven, Conn.: Converse, 1812), ii. 75; Keppie, *William Hunter*.

[27] Thomas De Quincey, *Autobiographic Sketches 1790–1803* (Edinburgh: Black, 1862).

[28] From the 1822 regulations. William Thomson (ed.), *Deeds Instituting Bursaries, Scholarships, and Other Foundations, in the College and University of Glasgow* (Glasgow:

totalled around £200 per annum from up to 4,000 visitors; later they dwindled, so that it became unknown to the townsfolk 'save by repute'. In Edinburgh, the University Anatomy Museum sold tickets for seven shillings for the season. Elsewhere, students were sometimes permitted to grant access to others, as in Glasgow and at the opening of Thomas Turner's course in Manchester in 1840, when 'The attendance of the students and their friends was large...they were invited to take a hasty glance at the now very large, valuable and highly interesting museum of human and comparative anatomy'.[29]

Although the University of Glasgow made it clear in 1822 that those wearing 'working clothes' were not to be admitted, towards the middle of the century those who ran medical collections, like their peers in other museums, began to turn their attention to the lower orders of society. Partly this was prompted by a wider move to 'rational recreation' for the working classes provided by the haute bourgeoisie; partly no doubt orthodox medical collections were aware of the emerging appeal of commercial anatomy shows. On the days when it was open to the townsfolk, the Anderson University Museum in Glasgow attracted up to 1,000 visitors; and in the first five years after the Royal College of Surgeons Museum in Edinburgh opened to the wider public in 1832, it attracted some 50,000 visitors:

> of which three-fourths have been non-professional, of both sexes and of all classes. None have [sic] been refused admittance, excepting a very few (not more than five) persons in a state of intoxication. There has never been a disturbance in the Museum. Although upwards of 2,000 preparations have been exposed on open shelves, none of them has received injury from visitors.... There is reason to believe that the privilege of admission to the Museum is highly valued by the public at large, and something has been done in this quarter towards reconciling the minds of the lower orders to the necessity and advantages of anatomical and pathological investigations.[30]

Later in the century other museums including those in Birmingham and Aberdeen followed suit by inviting non-medical visitors, especially working men, to visit.[31]

Maitland Club, 1850), 242; Keppie, *William Hunter*; Mark Weatherall, *Gentlemen, Scientists, and Doctors: Medicine at Cambridge, 1800–1940* (Woodbridge; Rochester, NY: Boydell, 2000).

[29] 'A Relative', *Memoir of Thomas Turner, Esq.*, intr. David Bell (London: Simpkin, Marshall and Co., 1875), 153. For the specific data on visitors and visiting these sites, see University of Glasgow Minutes of Senate 95, 22 November 1877, Glasgow University Archives; [MacKenzie], *Descriptive Catalogue*.

[30] William MacGillivray, Unidentified journal clipping, 21 November 1837, Royal College of Surgeons of Edinburgh Archive; Butt, *John Anderson's Legacy*.

[31] Hallam, *Anatomy Museum*; Reinarz, 'Age of Museum Medicine'.

Providing access to a female audience was more complicated. Women were of course excluded from formal medical education for most of the century, ostensibly on the grounds that the study of anatomy—or some parts of it—was grossly indelicate; many medical museum doors remained closed to laywomen for the same reason. In the first half of the century, however, medical showmen and some of their more orthodox colleagues found a way round this by differentiating access to men and women, either by separating the space (for example with curtains or in cupboards), the time of entry, or both.[32] 'The preparations illustrative of healthy and morbid structure of the male and female organs of reproduction' in Glasgow were 'stowed away in presses with closed wooden doors' because it was 'proper to keep [them] out of sight.'[33] Female visitors to the Lying-In Hospital in Manchester could inspect the collection initiated by Charles White in the morning, accompanied by the matron, whereas their male counterparts could visit in the afternoons with the porter.[34] Joseph Kahn and some of his peers employed female lecturers exclusively to address women, as his eighteenth-century predecessor Benjamn Rackstrow had done—and Joseph Woodhead pointed out the obstetric section as of particular interest 'to the female sex'.[35] 'Man know thyself' insisted the showmen; woman could, too, under the right circumstances; although William MacGillivray noted a tendency among middle-class women to 'merely walk through the room without looking at the object particularly'.[36]

The accessibility of medical collections to women was not to last. As many civic museums were rendered more inclusive after the mid-century museum acts, access to many medical collections became more restrictive. Public access to the commercial shows was severely curtailed after the medical profession—that had once lauded them—closed ranks. Proprietors were condemned as quacks and in some cases sued for obscenity;

---

[32] See for example Museum Committee Minutes, 8 July 1833, Royal College of Surgeons in Ireland Archive RCSI/MUC/1; *Manchester Guardian*, 29 October 1851, 1b; *The Lancet*, 24 June 1854, 654; Joseph Kahn, *Catalogue of Dr. Kahn's Anatomical and Pathological Museum, 4 Coventry Street, Leicester Square* (London: private, 1856); [Woodhead], *Descriptive Catalogue*; see also Hallam, *Anatomy Museum*.

[33] Commissioners for Visiting the University of Glasgow, *Report*, 87.

[34] Peter Mohr and Bill Jackson, 'The University of Manchester Medical School Museum: Collection of Old Instruments or Historical Archive?' *Bulletin of the John Rylands University Library of Manchester*, 87 (2005), 209–23.

[35] Richard D. Altick, *The Shows of London: A Panoramic History of Exhibitions, 1600–1862* (Cambridge, Mass.: Belknap, 1978); [Woodhead], *Descriptive Catalogue*, 24.

[36] William MacGillivray, Unidentified journal clipping, 21 November 1837, Royal College of Surgeons of Edinburgh Archive.

by the 1870s there were very few commercial exhibitions remaining.[37] Experiments in access to orthodox museums such as that of the Royal College of Surgeons in Edinburgh were discontinued, ostensibly due to costs and risk to the specimens. As civic museums opened their doors in the late nineteenth century, those of medical museums were closed. Which is not to say that the elite could not still gain admittance: the Guy's Hospital museum visitor books in the late century include the autographs of the Duke of Devonshire (twice), Lord Bowingdon, Mungo Park the African explorer, the Duke of Wellington, Lord Brougham, and on one notable occasion a Chinese 'minister' and his entourage, likely to have been the general and statesman Li Hung-Chang.[38] But for the most part, the dismembered body and its representations disappeared into the museum, removed from the public sphere. A telling detail is the response of the Royal College of Surgeons in Ireland to a questionnaire from the British Association for the Advancement of Science requesting information on public museums. After some debate, the Council refused on the grounds that their collection did not fit in this category.[39]

Rather, the medical museum was re-framed as a serious medical tool— not only for education, but now for pathological research and diagnosis. The latter use had always been evident, as 'members of the medical profession in general' were enjoined to consult collections alongside the students who hoped to join them.[40] The clinical utility of pathology collections in particular was central to the expansion and re-housing of such museums in the decades around 1900, as described in chapter 2. Clinicians engaged very differently with the collection as a whole than students and lay visitors, and demanded exclusive and undisturbed access. As other kinds of collections became more inclusive in the twentieth century, audiences for (most) medical museums were gradually but firmly restricted.

[37] Bates, '"Indecent and Demoralising Representations"'; Burmeister, 'Popular Anatomical Museums'; Michael Mason, *The Making of Victorian Sexuality* (Oxford: Oxford University Press, 1994). Joseph Woodhead's Museum of Anatomy in Liverpool was a notable survivor.

[38] Guy's Hospital Museum, Visitor Book 1829–1862; Visitor Book 1862–1900, Gordon Museum Archive, King's College London. On visitor books as historical resources, see Sharon Macdonald, 'Accessing Audiences: Visiting Visitor Books', *Museum and Society*, 3 (2006), 119–36; Lisbet Nys, 'The Public's Signatures: Visitors' Books in Nineteenth-Century Museums', *Museum History Journal*, 2 (2009), 163–80.

[39] Museum Committee Minutes 22 March 1887; 17 May 1887; 6 December 1887, Royal College of Surgeons in Ireland Archive RCSI/MUC/2.

[40] Royal Commission, *Minutes of Evidence*, appendix.

MORBID SENSESCAPES

Whether research pathologist or visiting dignitary, visitors not only looked but also touched, listened, and smelled. Like other kinds of collections, pathological objects engaged with the full gamut of visitors' senses, even as museum professionals across the disciplinary range of the nineteenth-century exhibitionary complex sought to reduce the visiting experience solely to a visual engagement. Museologists, historians, and anthropologists have shown that by studying the traces that remain of visitors' experiences it is possible to discern these diverse 'sensescapes' of the nineteenth-century medical museum.[41]

As reflected in the ocularcentric title of this chapter, however, the first sense associated with the museum visit is the visual, especially during the nineteenth century as the museum became so firmly part of the 'empires of sight'.[42] Theorists of visual culture have posited historically contingent 'scopic regimes' and have characterized the high Victorian era as an age of panoramic spectacle. But medical museums with their macabre contents were in danger of exposing the dark underbelly of this panorama. In *Our Mutual Friend*, the ghoulish taxidermist Mr Venus greets Mr Wegg, who has come into Venus's macabre place of business seeking the remains of his own leg:

'You're casting your eye round the shop, Mr. Wegg. Let me show you a light.... Bones, warious. Skulls, warious. Preserved Indian baby. African ditto. Bottled preparations, warious. Everything within reach of your hand, in good preservation. The mouldy ones a-top. What's in those hampers over

---

[41] Constance Classen and David Howes, 'The Museum as Sensescape: Western Sensibilities and Indigenous Artefacts', in Elizabeth Edwards, Chris Gosden, and Ruth Phillips (eds.), *Sensible Objects: Colonialism, Museums and Material Culture* (Oxford: Berg, 2006), 199–222; Constance Classen, 'Museum Manners: The Sensory Life of the Early Museum', *Journal of Social History*, 40 (2007), 895–914; Steve Sturdy, 'Making Sense in the Pathology Museum', in Andrew Patrizio and Dawn Kemp (eds.), *Anatomy Acts: How We Come to Know Ourselves* (Edinburgh: Birlinn, 2006), 109–17. For medical historians' treatment of the senses, see William F. Bynum and Roy Porter (eds.), *Medicine and the Five Senses* (Cambridge: Cambridge University Press, 1993).

[42] Richard Bellon, 'Science at the Crystal Focus of the World', in Fyfe and Lightman, *Science in the Marketplace*, 301–35; Teresa Brennan and Martin Jay (eds.), *Vision in Context: Historical and Contemporary Perspectives on Sight* (London: Routledge, 1996); Jonathan Crary, *Techniques of the Observer: On Vision and Modernity in the Nineteenth Century* (Cambridge, Mass.: MIT Press, 1990); David Howes (ed.), *Empire of the Senses: The Sensual Culture Reader* (Oxford: Berg, 2004); Ralph Hyde, *Panoramania! The Art and Entertainment of The 'All-Embracing' View* (London: Trefoil, 1988); Susan Stewart, 'From the Museum of Touch', in Marius Kwint, Christopher Breward, and Jeremy Aynsley (eds.), *Material Memories: Design and Evocation* (New York: Berg, 1999), 17–36.

them again, I don't quite remember. Say human warious. Cats. Articulated English baby.... Glass eyes, warious. Mummied bird. Dried cuticle, warious. Oh, dear me! That's the general panoramic view.'[43]

Dickens's parody indicates the prevalence of human remains in an exhibitionary complex that incorporated freak shows and circuses. Museums were intended to contrast brightly with such heterodox sites, and were chastised when they failed. The Middlesex Hospital museum was condemned as 'a tiny room' with 'a motley collection of specimens...a conglomeration of jars crowded with specimens with which no one could keep pace'.[44] In Glasgow 'preparations on the shelves are much more crowded than is compatible with their proper exhibition, for, instead of free spaces being left between them, as in every properly accommodated collection, they may be said to jostle one another';[45] and at Guy's, 'The man who for the first time in his life makes an attempt at going over the museum,' wrote a student with a sharp pen, 'is apt to be somewhat disconcerted by the number of specimens he will have to look.'[46]

Nevertheless, medical museums were intended to be books of the body, clear and ordered. If the untrained eye could not see this, the untrained eye needed help. Anatomists provided this assistance with a variety of technologies designed to regulate the morbid spectacle. The textual body we explored in the previous chapter was a way of guiding the visitor's eye: the anatomical vade mecum, which as we have seen shared a common format with the museum catalogue, was designed to be taken around the museum, a guidebook to the fleshy terrain.[47] Word and object informed each other as part of this pathological intermediality—in the Trinity College Dublin museum 'a full catalogue remains in the room for the information of visitors, and short printed catalogues are distributed among the students'.[48] Whether or not visitors availed themselves of this opportunity is another matter—after all, as Charles Bell exclaimed of the Windmill Street Museum, 'It would require a month to go round the museum with a book in your hand.'[49] Other, speedier techniques to

[43] Charles Dickens, *Our Mutual Friend*, ed. Adrian Poole (1864–5; London: Penguin, 1997), 52–3.

[44] H. Campbell Thomson, *The Story of the Middlesex Hospital Medical School* (London: Murray, 1935), 83–4.

[45] Commissioners for Visiting the University of Glasgow, *Report*, 87.

[46] [Nathaniel Burnett Ham], 'Guide to the Pathological Museum', *The Guyoscope*, 2/18 (1898), 69–70 at, 69.

[47] See for example Robert Harrison, *The Dublin Dissector, or Manual of Anatomy* (5th edn, New York: Wood, 1854); see also Hallam, *Anatomy Museum*.

[48] *Returns Relating to Medical Museums*, 57.

[49] Charles Bell to Joseph George Bell 1 June 1812, in Charles Bell (ed.), *Letters of Sir Charles Bell* (London: Murray, 1870), 200.

regulate looking were not paper but brass and glass. Optical technologies for viewing specimens became more elaborate in the later century, including not only the omnipresent microscopes in the museum but also magic lanterns and epidiascopes in the lecture room.[50] The pathology museum was an atlas of disease, and atlases were ways to train the scientific eye.

Part of the privileging of the visual in the museum over the course of the nineteenth century was the removal of other sensory stimuli. And there were plenty to remove. Whether from personal tours, organized talks, or simply the noisy bustle of the audience, the visit remained an aural as well as a visual experience. Like other exhibitionary sites, the medical museum was a sociable space (see figure 6.2): following John Hunter's example, anatomists such as John Heaviside held soirées within or using their

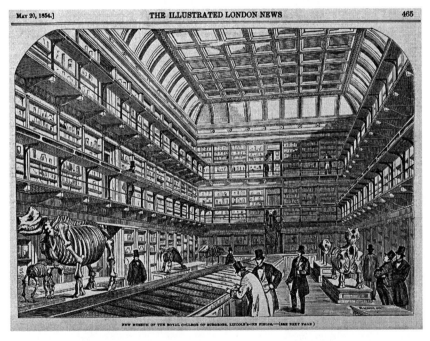

Fig. 6.2. The sociable museum: the Royal College of Surgeons Museum from the *Illustrated London News*, 20 May 1854. Wellcome Library, London.

---

[50] Victoria University of Manchester, *Victoria University of Manchester Medical School* (Manchester: Manchester University Press, 1908); Anne Secord, 'Botany on a Plate: Pleasure and the Power of Pictures in Promoting Early Nineteenth-Century Scientific Knowledge', *Isis*, 93 (2002), 28–57.

collections.[51] During such *conversazioni*, social equals conversed with the collector; later, visitors were talked *at* in the museum. In commercial anatomy shows in particular, the exhibits must have resounded with the ballyhoo of the proprietor as he touted for business, and the exchanges of the visitors as they encountered the curious, the titillating and the diseased. Admission to such establishments, in common with many other museums, involved a museum lecture.

Although such lectures and talking guides continued throughout the century, gradually those who ran the collections sought to eradicate other noise. The museum, like other ritual sites in the public sphere, was intended to be a silent place for quiet contemplation.[52] As the journalist Frederick Knight Hunt reflected approvingly of entering the Hunterian Museum in London: 'Without, we left an atmosphere of life and living bustle; within, we find a stiller, calmer company. We walk amidst an abundant harvest yielded by death to teach the lesson of how life continues... Now all are quiet in the serene dignity of death.'[53] But curators' efforts (including polite notices such as that seen in figure 6.3) tell as much of their failures as their successes in this endeavour. In hospital and college museums, for instance, the presence of medical students, a notoriously rowdy body, rendered silence unlikely. 'On entering [the museum] it is well to get together a few stools', advised the cynical Guy's student, '(not necessarily to sit on, but as a guarantee of hard work) which should be dragged along the galleries, not carried. This will impress any junior man, which may be reading anatomy in the lower regions, with your importance as a pathologist.'[54]

If these aural experiences have too often been ignored in the history of museums, more attention has recently been paid to the tactile realm. It is clear that the twenty-first century emphasis on touch in museums has

[51] Samuel J. M. M. Alberti, 'Conversaziones and the Experience of Science in Victorian England', *Journal of Victorian Culture*, 8 (2003), 208–30; Chaplin, 'John Hunter'; Classen, 'Museum Manners'; Paula Findlen, *Possessing Nature: Museums, Collecting, and Scientific Culture in Early Modern Italy* (Berkeley: University of California Press, 1994); George C. Peachey, *John Heaviside Surgeon* (London: St Martin's Press, 1931).

[52] Simon Gunn, 'The Sublime and the Vulgar: The Hallé Concerts and the Constitution of "High Culture" in Manchester *c.*1850–1880', *Journal of Victorian Culture*, 2 (1997), 208–28; Richard Sennett, *The Fall of Public Man* (Cambridge: Cambridge University Press, 1977); Barbara Maria Stafford, *Artful Science: Enlightenment, Entertainment, and the Eclipse of Visual Education* (Cambridge, Mass.: MIT Press, 1994).

[53] [Frederick Knight Hunt], 'The Hunterian Museum', *Household Words*, 14 December 1850, 279; Sophie Forgan, 'Building the Museum: Knowledge, Conflict, and the Power of Place', *Isis*, 96 (2005), 572–85.

[54] [Ham], 'Guide to the Pathological Museum', 69; Keir Waddington, 'Mayhem and Medical Students: Image, Conduct, and Control in the Victorian and Edwardian London Teaching Hospital', *Social History of Medicine*, 15 (2002), 45–64.

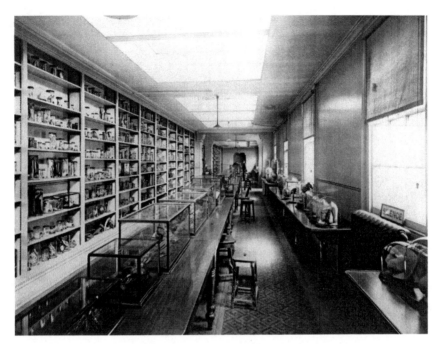

Fig. 6.3. The Guy's Hospital Museum in the late nineteenth century; note the sign on the right. London Metropolitan Archives, courtesy of the Gordon Museum, King's College London.

deep historical precedents; visitors have touched museum objects—or wanted to—for as long as there have been museums.[55] Handling specimens is perhaps the most intimate sensory encounter, and this had (and has) particular resonance with human remains—touch becomes a material connection between living and dead, person and once-person. Thomas de Quincey, faced with a skeleton in Charles White's collection, mused 'Who was he? It is not every day that one makes the acquaintance of a skeleton; and with regard to such a thing—thing, shall one say, or person?'[56] When the poet and civil servant Arthur Munby visited an anatomy exhibition in 1859, he gazed, fascinated, at the female of the two human skins on

[55] Fiona Candlin, *Art, Museums and Touch* (Manchester: Manchester University Press, 2010); Classen, 'Museum Manners'; Elizabeth Pye (ed.), *The Power of Touch: Handling Objects in Museum and Heritage Context* (London: UCL Institute of Archaeology, 2008); Mark M. Smith, *Sensing the Past: Seeing, Hearing, Smelling, Tasting, and Touching in History* (Berkeley: University of California Press, 2008); Stewart, 'From the Museum of Touch'.
[56] De Quincey, *Autobiographic Sketches*, 434.

display. Finally, he 'lifted the stiff hand, & touched the dusty hair'.[57] Touch verified sight, as reflected in William Hunter's emphasis on the pedagogic value of handling specimens, but was also a risky business for the integrity of the specimens:

> most of the preparations, must be sent round the company; that every student may examine them in his own hand. To prevent confusion, you will please observe, that, in the first seat, the preparations are to go round from right to left; in the second bench, from left to right; and so alternately, to the farthest seat of all. To prevent loss of time, when you give a preparation to your neighbour, be so good as to point out the part, or circumstance which is to be examined; as I shall do, when it is first handed round: and every student will recollect, that he is to confine his examination to that part only; for, were he to speculate upon other things in the preparation, he would not only wander form the subject at hand, which would reflect upon his understanding, but he would detain the preparation too long from the rest of the company. We expect that the preparations will not be injured, or destroyed, by your examination of them; and therefore, that they will only be looked at: no experiment is to be made, by pressing to bending, to try their strength or texture. With all possible care they are constantly wearing out, or growing the worse for use; any of them are the result of patient labour, and not easily restored; many of them are such rarities, as are not recoverable, when lost, by any great pains that can be taken.[58]

One of the principal roles of the museum, as we have seen, was to provide lecture courses with specimens to handle. Preservative techniques such as quicksilver injections, detailed in chapter 3, were intended to render specimens sufficiently robust to handle. Museums supplied objects for the dreaded medical viva voce (see figure 3.2) throughout the nineteenth century and beyond. Students fretted of the specimens that 'any one of them may suddenly be hurled at him (like a bolt out of the pathological blue) by a merciless examiner in a place where catalogues are not and labels are unknown'.[59] Central to the activities of the pathological societies that proliferated in Britain in the mid century was the tactile engagement with case study specimens at their meetings.

---

[57] Barry Reay, *Watching Hannah: Sexuality, Horror and Bodily De-Formation in Victorian England* (London: Reaktion, 2002), 36; Natalie Loveless, 'Affecting Bodies', in T. Christine Jespersen, Alicita Rodriguez, and Joseph Starr (eds.), *The Anatomy of Body Worlds: Critical Essays on the Plastinated Cadavers of Gunther Von Hagens* (Jefferson, NC: McFarland, 2009), 106–20.

[58] William Hunter, *Two Introductory Lectures, Delivered by Dr. William Hunter, to His Last Course of Anatomical Lectures* (London: Johnson, 1784), 112; Druin Burch, *Digging up the Dead: Uncovering the Life and Times of an Extraordinary Surgeon* (London: Chatto and Windus, 2007).

[59] [Ham], 'Guide to the Pathological Museum', 69.

While students and other visitors with privileged access continued to be allowed to handle collections, specimens had to be protected from the masses of untrained visitors, as touching came to be considered harmful in museums generally.[60] At La Specola in Florence, where the anatomical collection was opened to the Tuscan public as early as 1789, visitors soon set about stroking the specimens (especially the wax genitalia), a common way of engaging with statuary in the eighteenth century.[61] The integrity of specimens was already perceived to be under threat, and anatomists felt it was 'expedient to defend them as much as possible from injuries'.[62] With the expansion of museum access generally in the mid nineteenth century came a policing of touch that became the hallmark of museums until recently. At the Royal College of Surgeons of Edinburgh, 'the only visitors who ever touch the preparations are the medical students, who, in their desire to inspect an object, sometimes forget that it is prohibited to handle it'; as conservator, Frederick Knox disapproved even of students getting immediate access to his painstakingly preserved specimens.[63] Similarly in Glasgow,

> preparations are handed about in the Class-rooms among the Students, who are not likely to be very considerate in their mode of examining them, or of passing them to one another. Every one who is acquainted with anatomical preparations must be aware how unfavourable for their preservation in good condition such treatment must necessarily be.... Ten or twenty preparations, in progress of circulation through a class, must, it is obvious, form just as many sources of distraction to the Students from the discourse of their preceptor. [Rather,] It is from examining the preparations in their places on the shelves, with the aid of a printed catalogue, that Students are most likely to derive from them the greatest amount of benefit.

Accordingly, they kept their specimens in presses 'enclosed with doors of wire trellis in wooden frames, or a construction calculated (when not thrown open) in a considerable degree to impede the inspection of the

---

[60] Candlin, *Art, Museums and Touch.*

[61] Monika von Düring, Georges Didi-Huberman, and Marta Poggesi, *Encyclopaedia Anatomica: A Complete Collection of Anatomical Waxes* (Köln: Taschen, 1999); Francis Haskell and Nicholas Penny, *Taste and the Antique: The Lure of Classical Sculpture, 1500–1900* (New Haven: Yale University Press, 1981); Maerker, *Model Experts.*

[62] Thomas Pole, *The Anatomical Instructor; or, an Illustration of the Modern and Most Approved Methods of Preparing and Preserving the Different Parts of the Human Body* (2nd edn, London: Callow, 1813), 85.

[63] William MacGillivray, unidentified journal clipping, 21 November 1837, Royal College of Surgeons of Edinburgh Archive; Matthew H. Kaufman, 'Frederick Knox, Younger Brother and Assistant of Dr Robert Knox: His Contribution To "Knox's Catalogues"', *Journal of the Royal College of Surgeons of Edinburgh*, 46 (2001), 44–56; Knox, *Anatomist's Instructor.*

preparations', and only advanced students and faculty were granted access.[64] Likewise at Joseph Woodward's commercial gallery, 'visitors are particularly requested not to touch any of the illustrations'.[65]

And so just as the exhibits at La Specola had to be locked in display cases, Victorian collections were gradually removed from tactile range. The use of formal vitrines increased, standardizing museum displays and distancing the observer and specimen. In Dublin, the surgeons began to purchase glass cases for their museum from the mid 1830s, as well as erecting railings around the table cases in the centre of the gallery: a new edict was displayed:

> That no visitor shall handle or touch any of the preparations in the Museum. That visitors on entering the Museum shall leave their umbrellas or sticks at the door, or deliver them in charge to the Porter. That any visitor who shall Break Glass, or otherwise injure any of the preparations be required to pay for the damages so done, and that the Porter be authorized to insist on such reparation: in default of which, that he must repair the injury at his own expense.[66]

The objects were reified, rendered sacrosanct. In Manchester, the epidiascope was used instead of handing objects around the class,

> so as to be visible to all in the theatre at once, and the point of interest then engaging attention demonstrated. The advantage of this method of showing specimens to a class over that of handing them round for individual inspection is obvious. With the epidiascope the lecturer can demonstrate on the screen first a museum specimen preserved to show the naked eye and natural colour appearances of, say a tuberculous lung, then a lantern slide of the microscopic anatomy, then for contrast any plates from books which may further illustrate the point engaging the attention of the class.[67]

One reason why the intermediality discussed in the previous chapter was so important was to compensate for the removal of the haptic aspects of the encounter with the object.

Denial of touch and removal of sources of noise from the museum had some success. But still the museum experience could not be restricted to the visual: for objects that had once been alive tended to smell. Students in Rudolf Virchow's pathology museum in Berlin, for example, were positively encouraged to learn from specimens not only by handling, but also

---

[64] Commissioners for Visiting the University of Glasgow, *Report*, 89, 87.

[65] [Woodhead], *Descriptive Catalogue*, 23.

[66] Museum Committee Minutes, 9 February 1835 to 4 April 1835, Royal College of Surgeons in Ireland Archive RCSI/MUC/1.

[67] Victoria University, *Victoria University of Manchester Medical School*, 19–20.

by smelling them.[68] But for the most part, the olfactory associations were unintentional and unpleasant. Collections of wet anatomical specimens tended to be the most pungent and their aroma became associated with death and decay even though, ironically, it was the fluids involved in the very process of preservation that generated their distinctive smell. The close association of smell and disease in the presence of so much visual evidence of the morbid was overwhelming. The miasmatic notion of aroma as pathogenic—Chadwick's insistence that 'all smell is disease'—endured long after the advent of germ theory.[69] And death was never far way: pathological collections as we saw in chapter 2 were commonly stored adjacent to the post-mortem facilities. Even Thomas Hodgkin acknowledged 'the emphysematous state of the subject' and 'the odour exhaled by the bodies of the dead'.[70] His successor Samuel Wilks described a specimen as a 'Horny excrescence, from the head of a woman . . . When recent these were soft, waxy, and had a cheesy odour'.[71] It was common practice to smoke in the dissecting room to cover such noxious odours (if not in the museum, as indicated in the discussion of fire hazards in chapter 4).[72]

That such complaints endured, despite flues and ventilation in late-century custom-built premises, may be illustrative of the changing role of smell in modern society. During the Enlightenment, Alain Corbin has argued, the 'olfactory revolution' relegated smell from the sacred to the profane, from the realm of the religious to that of the sensual, sentimental.[73] As cities became more fragrant thanks to sanitary reforms, and the revolution in civic cleanliness was accompanied by similar changes in the personal realm, so the middle classes became less tolerant of stench. That

---

[68] Angela Matyssek, *Rudolf Virchow. Das Pathologische Museum: Geschichte Einer Wissenschaftlichen Sammlung Um 1900* (Darmstadt: Steinkopff, 2003). For a museum *of* smell (as opposed to the smell of museums), see Avery Gilbert, 'The Smell Museum: Preserving Odors from the Past', *What the Nose Knows: The Science of Scent in Everyday Life* (New York: Crown, 2008), 205–24.

[69] Peter Stallybrass and Allon White, *The Politics and Poetics of Transgression* (London: Methuen, 1986), 139.

[70] Thomas Hodgkin, 'On the Object of Post Mortem Examinations', *London Medical Gazette*, 2 (1828), 423–31 at 424.

[71] Samuel Wilks, *Pathological Catalogue of the Museum of Guy's Hospital. Diseases of the Nervous System, Integument, and Organs of the Senses* (London: MacKenzie, 1861), 53.

[72] John Harley Warner and James M. Edmonson, *Dissection: Photographs of a Rite of Passage in American Medicine 1880–1930* (New York: Blast, 2009).

[73] Constance Classen, David Howes, and Anthony Synnott, *Aroma: The Cultural History of Smell* (London: Routledge, 1994); Alain Corbin, *The Foul and the Fragrant: Odor and the French Social Imagination*, trans. Miriam L. Kochan, Roy Porter, and Christopher Prendegast (1982; Cambridge, Mass.: Harvard University Press, 1986).

any smell remained in the museum was unsatisfactory as the ideal public space became free from odour.

The medical museum remained, however, as one student tastefully put it, a store-house for 'dead meat'.[74] The association of dead specimens and food had been a common theme early in the century. At the Hunterian Museum in Glasgow, the preparations in the 'Hall of Anatomy' were displayed on 'presses'—that is, 'A large (usually shelved) cupboard...in Scotland, also for provisions, victuals, plates, dishes and other table requisites'.[75] The preservative techniques discussed in chapter 4 were detailed as recipes, and often involved isinglass, a pure form of gelatine, also used in cookery.[76] The bookselling firm Wheatley and Adlard, during the depression in the book trade in the 1820s, diversified into wine and medical specimens at the same time.[77] As they advertised at one sale, 'On the table is a superb assortment of various organs corroded: and almost unexampled injections of the hand and foot, inimitably dissected, with numerous other anatomical *chef-d'œuvres*'—a common culinary allusion. The sale in question was that of the collection of Joshua Brookes, whose classroom was said to have smelt like a ham shop; even Edward Osler (grandfather of William), who visited in 1816, 'recoiled in terror from the stench. He thought the odours themselves might poison him. The experience seemed to him like a descent into Hades.'[78]

Nevertheless, by the close of the Victorian era, odour-free museums were intended to be about sight: the sense of reason, rationality, education, and the chosen sensory mode of late nineteenth-century scientific enterprise (see figure 6.4).[79] Smell—emotive, savage, intuitive—was to be avoided, as were other sensory pollutants: destructive touch and unruly, chaotic sound. Sight was the sense of science.[80] We have seen that the sensescape of pathological collections had some elements in common with other museums, scientific or otherwise, and some particularities. The ways

[74] [Nathaniel Burnett Ham], 'Our Special Pathologist', *The Guyoscope*, 2/18 (1898), 42. On the gustatory experience of museum collections, see Classen, 'Museum Manners'.

[75] Oxford English Dictionary, s.v. 'Press'; James C. Laskey, *A General Account of the Hunterian Museum, Glasgow* (Glasgow: Smith, 1813).

[76] John James Edwards and M. J. Edwards, *Medical Museum Technology* (London: Oxford University Press, 1959).

[77] Benjamin Wheatley and George Adlard, *Museum Brookesianum. A Descriptive and Historical Catalogue of the Remainder of the Anatomical and Zootomical Museum, of Joshua Brookes, Esq.* (London: Taylor, 1830), viii.

[78] Michael Bliss, *William Osler: A Life in Medicine* (Oxford: Oxford University Press, 1999), 4; Hubert Cole, *Things for the Surgeon: A History of the Resurrection Men* (London: Heinemann, 1964), 39; Adrian Desmond, *The Politics of Evolution: Morphology, Medicine and Reform in Radical London* (Chicago: University of Chicago Press, 1989), 160.

[79] Candlin, *Art, Museums and Touch*.

[80] Lorraine Daston and Peter Galison, *Objectivity* (Boston: Zone, 2007).

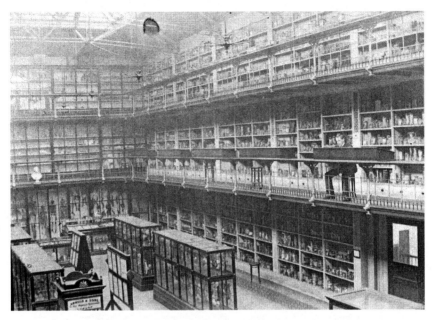

Fig. 6.4. Anatomy and Pathology Museum, St Bartholomew's Hospital, *c.* 1900, showing a student (apparently) quietly at work. Copyright St Bartholomew's Hospital Archive, Barts and the London Hospital Trust Archives and Museums.

that visitors responded to this experience—the subject of the remainder of this chapter—was more specific to their contents: deviant human remains.

THE GOOD, THE BAD, AND THE UGLY

As conditioned as the sensory experience of museum visiting was intended to be, not all reactions to morbid specimens matched curators' expectations. Traces of these diverse responses—from happiness to horror—have already emerged in the preceding discussion and this final section focuses in more detail on particular kinds of reactions to pathology displays. The topic at hand is therefore the relationship between object and observer; an engagement that was historically and culturally contingent, but never one-way.[81] However didactic and interpreted the exhibition, responses

[81] David Freedberg, *The Power of Images: Studies in the History and Theory of Response* (Chicago: University of Chicago Press, 1989). On visitor accounts to eighteenth-century

were a combination of that which was elicited by the display and that which came from within the visitor—things remembered and felt. Both memory and emotion therefore have powerful roles to play in the visiting experience.[82] Reactions are and were unpredictable and ungovernable, and to explore the history of different responses from a different era is necessarily to present a rather messy picture that defies an over-arching narrative. Rather, responses are here grouped according to their distance from that which was intended by the museums. By these criteria—which are admittedly from the perspective of the producers rather than the consumers—some responses were *good*: awe, wonder, and enlightenment. Prevalent among *bad* responses were horror, disgust, and titillation. Finally, some visitors responded in downright *ugly* ways—with anger and violence. This apparently trivial classification may not have great analytical value, but does have the virtue of allowing a brief illustration of a cross-section of the traces of responses to pathological displays.

We have seen that pathologists and anatomists intended their collections to be edifying. Like other curators of natural objects, they laid out the makings of the human body to illuminate the glory of nature and its workings. If the visit could be pleasurable, all the better—one St Thomas's student recorded 'I have been very much pleased in looking over the Museum'—but this should not trivialize the experience, as Frederick Knox argued: 'my leading object has been to make the student *really* fond of visiting museums; and, with this view, I have done every thing in my power to make him practically acquainted with the mechanism of anatomical and pathological museums'.[83] Whether within a secular framework or as a powerful element of natural theology (praising the work of the creator), they encouraged the powerful sense of wonder invoked by their

anatomical collections, see Chaplin, 'John Hunter', especially chapter 10. For a modern study of visitor responses to a medical museum, see Nora Jones, 'The Mütter Museum: The Body as Spectacle, Specimen, and Art' (Ph.D. thesis, Temple University, 2002).

[82] On the historical contingency of affect, and its significance in medical and cultural history, see Fay Bound Alberti, *Matters of the Heart: History, Medicine, and Emotion* (Oxford: Oxford University Press, 2010). On memory and/in museums, see Gaynor Kavanagh, *Dream Spaces: Memory and the Museum* (Leicester: Leicester University Press, 2000); Nick Merriman, 'Museum Collections and Sustainability', *Cultural Trends*, (2008), 3–21. On the affective impact of human bones in particular, see Jeanne Cannizzo, John Harries, and Joost Fontein (eds.), 'What Lies Beneath: Exploring the Affective Presence and Emotive Materiality of Human Bones', special issue of *Journal of Material Culture*, 15/4 (2010), especially Elizabeth Hallam, 'Articulating Bones', *Journal of Material Culture* 15 (2010), 465–92.

[83] Hampton Weekes to Richard Weekes 24 September 1801, in Ford, *A Medical Student*, 43; Knox, *Anatomist's Instructor*, vi, original emphasis.

displays.[84] 'No one who ever visited the Hunterian Museum', proclaimed David Murray, 'can forget the surprise and wonder he felt when he entered the building and saw the striking objects which presented themselves to view.'[85] True to form, the American neurosurgeon Harvey Cushing visited at the turn of the century and found it 'wonderful'—a visit that historians have since argued was fundamental in his later brain arching work.[86]

As one visitor commented of Kahn's museum, however, 'you come away with mingled humiliation and awe'.[87] Museums were perceived as morgues, as mausolea. One traveller to the Hunterian in Glasgow felt that 'these rare specimens excite various emotions, more allied, I fear, to sadness than to joy—to melancholy than to pleasure!'[88] The prevalence of death in medical museums tempered feelings of wonder for many visitors: that the expansion of museums in Britain coincided with the emergence of the Victorian cult of death may not have been accidental.[89] The medical museum, for many, was horrific—the servants of the anatomy teacher Joseph Jordan, for example, considered his museum to be haunted.[90] Cultural historians have made convincing connections between such imagined re-animation and Gothic narratives: certainly by the late century, medico-scientific discourses contributed to the somatic emphasis of Gothic fiction, which privileged racial degeneration, atavism,

[84] On wonder and/at museums, see Lorraine J. Daston and Katharine Park, *Wonders and the Order of Nature, 1150–1750* (New York: Zone, 1998); Stephen Greenblatt, 'Resonance and Wonder', in Ivan Karp and Steven D. Lavine (eds.), *Exhibiting Cultures: The Poetics and Politics of Museum Display* (Washington, DC: Smithsonian Institution Press, 1991), 42–56; Susan Stewart, *On Longing: Narratives of the Miniature, the Gigantic, the Souvenir, the Collection* (Durham, NC: Duke University Press, 1993).

[85] David Murray, *The Hunterian Museum in the Old College of Glasgow* (Glasgow: Jackson, Wylie and Co., 1925), 4.

[86] John F. Fulton, *Harvey Cushing: A Biography* (Springfield, Illinois: Thomas, 1946); Cathy Gere, 'A Brief History of Brain Archiving', *Journal of the History of the Neurosciences*, 12 (2003), 396–410.

[87] *London Era*, 30 March 1851, 11, also cited in Stephen Johnson, 'The Persistence of Tradition in Anatomical Museums', in Jespersen, Rodriguez, and Starr, *The Anatomy of Body Worlds*, 68–85 at 75.

[88] James Johnson, *The Recess, or Autumnal Relaxation in the Highlands and Lowlands* (London: Longman, Rees, Orme, Brown, & Co., 1834), 187.

[89] On the culture and history of death ways, see Elizabeth Hallam, Jenny Hockey, and Glennys Howarth, *Beyond the Body Death and Social Identity* (London: Routledge, 1999); Elizabeth Hallam and Jenny Hockey, *Death, Memory, and Material Culture* (Oxford: Berg, 2001); Christine Quigley, *The Corpse: A History* (Jefferson, NC: MacFarland, 1996); Julie-Marie Strange, *Death, Grief and Poverty in Britain, 1870–1914* (Cambridge: Cambridge University Press, 2005).

[90] G. A. G. Mitchell, 'Joseph Jordan 1787–1873 FRCS', in Willis J. Elwood and A. Félicité Tuxford (eds.), *Some Manchester Doctors: A Biographical Collection to Mark the 150th Anniversary of the Manchester Medical Society 1834–1984* (Manchester: Manchester University Press for the Manchester Medical Society, 1984), 65–74.

deviant sexualities, and monstrosity—examples of which could all be found in pathological museums.[91]

Perhaps more commonly than horror, the abundant evidence of disease in the medical museum prompted visitors across the century and the social spectrum to respond with that 'most embodied and visceral of emotions', disgust.[92] Arthur Munby was particularly detailed in his account of a life-like specimen at an anatomy show, recording that 'The woman's skin was quite perfect from head to foot: it was slit down the back, and hung loosely on a wooden cross, in hideous mockery of the living figure.' He continued, 'It was horrible to look at in the face—it was like a leather mask, every feature perfect, yet hanging helpless & collapsed—the nose awry, the lips drooping, the eyes wide and empty.'[93] Even a physician acknowledged that the Hunterian's display of morbid stomachs was 'not very pleasant to contemplate'.[94] Kahn's museum in particular was variously considered 'horrible' or 'revolting, filthy and disgusting'.[95] One medical student recorded in his diary in 1860:

DECEMBER 7TH: Went to Dr. Kahn's Museum in the afternoon. A decidedly indecent pseudo-scientific affair, founded by quack doctor... Lecture on Deleterious Influences was of course disgusting.

DECEMBER 8TH: Had a rather serious attack of diarrhœa, a malady to which I am seldom subject. Can it have been bestowed on me by an all-wise Providence as a just punishment for my having visited that sink of iniquity, Dr. Kahn's Museum yesterday? Who knows?[96]

Squeamishness such as this was testament to the widespread expansion of disgust since the eighteenth century, and the prevalence of disgust as a response to medical museums warrants a moment of reflection on its

---

[91] R. Hoberman, 'In Quest of a Museal Aura: Turn of the Century Narratives About Museum-Displayed Objects', *Victorian Literature and Culture*, 31 (2003), 467–82; Kelly Hurley, *The Gothic Body: Sexuality, Materialism, and Degeneration at the Fin De Siècle* (Cambridge: Cambridge: Cambridge University Press, 1996); Robert Mighall, *A Geography of Victorian Gothic Fiction: Mapping History's Nightmares* (Oxford: Oxford University Press, 1999).

[92] William Ian Miller, *The Anatomy of Disgust* (Cambridge, Mass.; London: Harvard University Press, 1997), xii; Winfried Menninghaus, *Disgust: The Theory and History of a Strong Sensation*, trans. Howard Eiland and Joel Golb (Albany: State University of New York Press, 2003).

[93] Reay, *Watching Hannah*, 35.

[94] Andrew Wynter, *Peeps into the Human Hive*, 2 vols. (London: Chapman and Hall, 1874), i. 268.

[95] H. G. Hibbert, *Fifty Years of a Londoner's Life* (London: Grant Richards, 1916), 41; *The Lancet*, 5 April 1856, 376–7.

[96] Shephard T. Taylor, *The Diary of a Medical Student During the Mid-Victorian Period, 1860–1864* (Norwich: Jarrold, 1927), 16.

wider social contexts. 'Disgust', writes one of its historians, 'has a key role to play in the civilizing process, working as it does to internalise norms of cleanliness, reserve and restraint.'[97] Over the last three centuries the sight of the corpse and the internal workings of the human body have increasingly been deemed disgusting, and in the Victorian period the anatomy museum was one of the few remaining legitimate sites for its display. While disgusting things were removed from the public sphere, that which constituted 'disgusting' expanded. Disgust was in part a reaction against the ugly, the abnormal (themselves categories in the process of redefinition)—an emotion working to police the norms of modern society, elevating the moral, the middle-class, the clean, from the squalors of poverty, filth, and diseased deformity. Further, revulsion also situated other forms of ugliness on display within the moral realm—monsters and even exotic ethnographic specimens, perpetuating the association in visitors' minds between the medical museum and the freak show, which endures today, as a study of recent visitor responses has demonstrated.[98]

Over the course of the nineteenth century, however, we can see evidence of efforts to eradicate disgust as a response. The wax models discussed in chapter 5 were widely employed as a means to eliminate distasteful elements of dissection. One anatomical gallery claimed that its model Venus could illuminate anatomy 'without in the slightest degree wounding delicacy', and another 'can be looked upon without any of those repulsive feelings that would strike many on inspecting a human subject dissected'; the *Athenaeum* advised its readers 'to avail themselves of a few general ideas on the subject of anatomy' from Signor Sarti's wax museum, 'which they may do so without labour or disgust'.[99] As such they were even suitable for a female audience.

The more general resistance to female visitors, however, was bound up with another reaction that the museum orthodoxy sought to eradicate (without much success): titillation. 'Most public museums now contain

---

[97] Miller, *Anatomy of Disgust*, 20; Norbert Elias, *The Civilizing Process: The History of Manners and State Formation and Civilization*, trans. Edmund Jephcott (new edn, Oxford: Blackwell, 1994).

[98] Jones, 'The Mütter Museum'. On the rich cultural history of freakery, see Mark S. Blumberg, *Freaks of Nature: What Anomalies Tell Us About Development and Evolution* (New York: Oxford University Press, 2008); Michael Mitchell, *Monsters: Human Freaks in America's Gilded Age* (2nd edn, Toronto: ECW, 2002); Rosemarie Garland Thomson (ed.), *Freakery: Cultural Spectacles of the Extraordinary Body* (New York; London: New York University Press, 1996).

[99] Burmeister, 'Popular Anatomical Museums', 46; *Athenaeum* 13 April 1839, 279; W. Mawhinney, *Anatomical & Physiological Description of the Late Signor Sarti's New Florentine Venus, Together with the Causes, Symptoms, and Treatment of the Diseases of the Principal Organs* (7th edn, London: Mallett, 1854).

fine views of the parts of generation', announced one curator in the 1830s, and these were not always viewed for educational purposes.[100] Joseph Kahn, whose museum displayed more generative parts than most, railed against 'false delicacy' that prevented the display of the complete human anatomy, and instead protested, 'my wish is not to gratify a prurient curiosity, but to present to the scientific observer with a general and correct view of the perfect and wonderful structure of the body'.[101] The morbid preparations, by contrast, played on their horrific aspect, shocking visitors into modifying their behaviour (and buying the remedies he sold). Rene Burmeister and Alan Bates have deftly demonstrated how the *volte-face* towards professional censure of Kahn's and other commercial anatomy museums in the 1860s centred around accusations of indecency.[102] 'Anatomical museums', raged the same *Lancet* that had once applauded them, 'offer to the sensual cravings of the more degraded members of the community genial recreation.'[103]

The hostile response to the possibility of titillation was part of a larger campaign to police the responses to anatomical displays. The medical museum audiences were to react soberly, without arousal or revulsion. *The Times* approved of Brookes's museum: 'what on a first view is not only displeasing to the sight, but even disgusting, becomes a matter of interest and examination, when considered as the means of improving science and assisting the cause of humanity'.[104] One pathologist later added sternly, 'Pathological specimens are frequently examined by students too much as though they were mere curios, concerning which an inquisitive examiner might some day desire enlightenment. An intelligent inspection of pathological material should be something very different from this.'[105] Curators set out to eradicate pleasure, any hint of the fairground. 'So long as mere amusement forms the inducement for visiting a museum, not the slightest benefit can accrue from such visits;—there can be nothing in an anatomical museum calculated to amuse any one', thundered Frederick Knox. 'All specific aberrations in Nature's productions unexamined and undissected, are mere objects of curiosity; and *amusement* should never form a feature in an *anatomical* museum.'[106]

---

[100] Knox, *Anatomist's Instructor*, 124.
[101] Kahn, *Catalogue of Dr. Kahn's Anatomical Museum*, iii; Kahn, *Catalogue of Dr. Kahn's Anatomical and Pathological Museum*.
[102] Bates, ' "Indecent and Demoralising Representations" '; Burmeister, 'Popular Anatomical Museums'; Johnson, 'The Persistence of Tradition'.
[103] *The Lancet*, 3 June 1865, 600.
[104] *The Times*, 26 February 1830, 3.
[105] T. N. Kelynack, 'Practical Pathology', *Manchester Royal Infirmary Students' Gazette*, 1/1 (1898), 13–14 at 14.
[106] Knox, *Anatomist's Instructor*, vi, 131, original emphasis.

Such policing of responses was intended to eradicate not only amusement but also sympathy. The fragmentation of the corpse and the distancing of object from subject in the museum discussed in chapter 3 was in part intended to imbue medical students with dispassion. As William Hunter famously claimed, dissection would introduce his students 'to a kind of necessary inhumanity'.[107] Sure enough, when Benjamin Silliman visited Hunter's collection he declined to detail what he saw: 'I could be particular, but the minds of those who have not been drilled into apathy, by a familiarity with the disgusting lacerated fragments of a dissecting room, cannot bear the exhibition of particular images of these things.'[108] As one US anatomy professor warned his students in the mid nineteenth century, 'anatomy, however indispensable it may be, tends certainly to freeze up the springs of human feeling, and destroy our sympathy for human suffering'.[109] Like dissection, exposure to human remains in the museum engendered what sociologists later dubbed the 'detached concern' of the medical practitioner.[110]

Even if medical practitioners trained in museums came away imbued with this 'necessary inhumanity', many other visitors reacted in ways that could not have been further removed from 'detached concern'. Visceral responses at times spilled over into violence, and there are many accounts of threats to the specimens themselves, from the trivial to the substantial. Minor vandalism in medical museums was often associated with the plentiful alcohol stored there, as for example the report of students in Edinburgh piercing the lids of jars to evaporate the alcohol (presumably out of mischief rather than for consumption) and elsewhere preservative

[107] Hunter, *Two Introductory Lectures*; Byron J. Good and Mary-Jo DelVecchio Good, 'Learning Medicine: The Constructing of Medical Knowledge at Harvard Medical School', in Shirley Lindenbaum and Margaret M. Lock (eds.), *Knowledge, Power, and Practice: The Anthropology of Medicine and Everyday Life* (Berkeley: University of California Press, 1993), 81–107; Lynda Payne, *With Words and Knives: Learning Medical Dispassion in Early Modern England* (Aldershot: Ashgate, 2007); Ruth Richardson, 'A Necessary Inhumanity?' *Journal of Medical Ethics*, 26 (2000), 104–6; Ruth Richardson, *Death, Dissection and the Destitute* (2nd edn, London: Phoenix, 2001); Roger Smith, *Being Human: Historical Knowledge and the Creation of Human Nature* (New York: Columbia University Press, 2007); John Harley Warner and James M. Edmonson, *Dissection: Photographs of a Right of Passage in American Medicine 1880–1930* (New York: Blast, 2009); John Harley Warner and Lawrence J. Rizzolo, 'Anatomical Instruction and Training for Professionalism from the 19th to the 21st Centuries', *Clinical Anatomy*, 19 (2006), 403–14.
[108] Silliman, *Journal of Travels*, ii. 75; Keppie, *William Hunter*.
[109] H. V. M. Miller writing in 1847, cited in Warner and Rizzolo, 'Anatomical Instruction', 404.
[110] Harold I. Lief and Renée C. Fox, 'Training for "Detached Concern" in Medical Students', in Harold I. Lief, Victor F. Lief, and Nina R. Lief (eds.), *The Psychological Basis of Medical Practice* (New York: Harper and Row, 1963), 12–35.

stocks were purloined or never arrived, as discussed in chapter 4.[111] Medical students, with a reputation for rowdiness, were generally perceived as a threat to collections ('Our preparations are liable to accidents', complained one anatomist, 'from the giddiness and wantonness of young men').[112]

Greater danger to the integrity of the collection came not from students but from other quarters, especially arising from the connection between institutions for anatomical education and body-snatching. Although pathology collections were rarely stocked from 'resurrected' corpses (see chapter 3), they were often caught in the cross-fire. A proposal to incorporate Glasgow University's anatomy facilities into the proposed Hunterian Museum was ruled out after a riot in which soldiers were called out.[113] When Joseph Jordan's cargo of preserved cadavers was held up en route to Scotland from Manchester the stench aroused suspicion, and when the contents of the barrels were revealed, a crowd besieged his anatomy school, breaking windows.[114] The Anatomy School in Sheffield was demolished entirely by one angry crowd, and in Cambridge attempts to commandeer a pauper's body under the auspices of the Anatomy Act so incensed a public meeting that a mob stormed the anatomical school, intent on liberating the body but turning instead on the Florentine waxes.[115] This violent end was also shared by at least one commercial anatomy museum's waxes, smashed with a hammer by the prosecuting solicitor after the proprietors were found guilty of obscenity in 1873.[116] It seems that curators themselves escaped such debacles unharmed, but others were not so lucky:

[111] Knox, *Anatomist's Instructor*; Michael G. Rhode and James Connor, 'Curating America's Army Medical Museum', in Amy Levin (ed.), *Defining Memory: Local Museums and the Construction of History in America's Changing Communities* (Lanham, Md.: Alta-Mira, 2007), 177–96.

[112] James Cleghorn to unknown correspondent, 29 January 1791, Trinity College Dublin Manuscript Room MUN/P/1/1972. See also Bates, '"Indecent and Demoralising Representations"'; Waddington, 'Mayhem and Medical Students'; Katherine A. Webb, 'The Development of the Medical Profession in Manchester 1750–1860' (Ph.D. thesis, University of Manchester, 1988).

[113] James Coutts, *A History of the University of Glasgow* (Glasgow: Maclehose, 1909).

[114] Mitchell, 'Joseph Jordan'; John V. Pickstone, *Medicine and Industrial Society: A History of Hospital Development in Manchester and Its Region, 1752–1946* (Manchester: Manchester University Press, 1985); Webb, 'Development of the Medical Profession'. See also Sean Burrell and Geoffrey Gill, 'The Liverpool Cholera Epidemic of 1832 and Anatomical Dissection—Medical Mistrust and Civil Unrest', *Journal of the History of Medicine and Allied Sciences*, 60 (2005), 478–98.

[115] F. K. Donnelly, 'The Destruction of the Sheffield School of Anatomy in 1835: A Popular Response to Class Legislation', *Transactions of the Hunter Archaeological Society*, 10/3 (1975), 167–72; Richardson, *Death, Dissection and the Destitute*; Weatherall, *Gentlemen, Scientists, and Doctors*.

[116] Bates, '"Indecent and Demoralising Representations"'.

a French tailor who decapitated his wife with a saw was alleged to have previously visited Kahn's exhibition to study the anatomy of the throat.[117]

Extreme a reaction as homicide may have been, we have seen that such violent sensory and affective behaviours were one end of a range of responses, some of which accorded with the intentions of the collectors and anatomists, but many of which did not. Characteristic of all these behaviours was a particular kind of human–object relationship that stemmed not so much from the materiality of the things themselves— which were after all physically very similar to the comparative anatomy specimens they sat beside—but rather the affective meanings applied to them by visitors. Passionate or dispassionate, these responses contributed to nineteenth-century constructions of the deviant body. We shall see in the following chapter how this relationship then changed over the course of the following century.

THE MUSEUM AFFECT

The 'museum effect' is that phenomenon observed by museologists whereby an object is radically dislocated from its point of origin, wrenched from its context and rendered a frozen work of art in the surrounds of the museum. The poor pun of this chapter's conclusion is an expression of my wish to present a complete account of this process, including not only the institution's role in the museum effect, but also the emotional and sensory experiences of the visitors—the museum *affect*.[118]

From this preliminary exploration of a variety of experiences, we can see a pattern not so much of changing reactions to human remains, but attempts by those displaying them to limit the range of acceptable responses. Just as art gallery audiences were trained in the appropriate tastes and behaviours, so too responses to anatomy displays were conditioned, both sensually and emotionally.[119] Distinctions were reinforced between street shows and worthy

---

[117] Kate Summerscale, *The Suspicions of Mr Whicher, or the Murder at Road Hill House* (London: Bloomsbury, 2008), 106.

[118] Alberti, 'Museum Affect'. On the museum effect, see Svetlana Alpers, 'The Museum as a Way of Seeing', in Ivan Karp and Steven D. Lavine (eds.), *Exhibiting Cultures: The Poetics and Politics of Museum Display* (Washington: Smithsonian Institution Press, 1991), 25–32; Susan Vogel, 'Always True to the Object, in Our Fashion', in Karp and Lavine, *Exhibiting Cultures*, 191–204.

[119] Freedberg, *The Power of Images*; Andrew Hemingway, 'Art Exhibitions as Leisure-Class Rituals in Early Nineteenth-Century London', in Brian Allen (ed.), *Towards a Modern Art World* (New Haven, Conn.; London: Yale University Press, 1995), 95–108; C. S. Matheson, '"A Shilling Well Laid out": The Royal Academy's Early Public', in David H. Solkin (ed.), *Art on the Line: The Royal Academy Exhibitions at Somerset House 1780– 1836* (New Haven, Conn.: Yale University Press, 2001), 38–54.

museums, between low and high medicine, between unruly crowd and well-behaved visitors. Curators sought to replace the perceptual promiscuity of the cabinet of curiosities with a regulated gaze, presenting the museum as a site for remote, reasoned observation of the morbid body rather than a gawking spectacle of deviance.[120] Sites for the display of anatomy and pathology were segregated, accessible only to those who knew how to react properly. By the end of the century, there were far fewer places where the uninitiated could experience dead bodies and their representations, as the medical profession asserted its dominion over the corpse more generally.[121] Gruesome specimens that were likely to provoke disgust were removed from the public view, especially that of women. Those who did gain access were subject to a new, strictly scopic regime, and the opportunity to experience the unruly sensations of the oral, tactile, and olfactory realms was restricted. In doing so the range of emotional responses available to them was ostensibly narrowed. Mere curiosity was discouraged; disgust controlled; titillation condemned. Those with access knew that the appropriate external reaction was sober contemplation, rather than revulsion or arousal. In terms of the institutions introduced at the very beginning of *Morbid Curiosities*, St Bartholomew's Hospital was to be as culturally and emotionally distant as possible from Bartholomew Fair.

But visitors were not passive dupes. Throughout this account there has been evident the tension between museum authorities controlling the visit and museum audiences constructing their experience and affective responses. Historians struggle to recover 'corporeal practices', one scholar of the senses has observed, because 'walking, eating, smelling and touching, while laden with social significance, are often so taken for granted that they are little commented on by their practitioners'.[122] We know that visitors chatted, touched things, and complained about the smell. That the objects had once been people, however, made reactions very difficult to standardize, to regulate, or even to gauge. Visitors trembled with fear or winced in empathy; they were aroused by models and repulsed by corpses. So far, so familiar—we may behave the same way ourselves. But even though the precious few traces of responses that remain may thus offer few surprises, nevertheless these reactions, and visitors' memories and imagination, were historically specific. Response theorists posit that reception is locally embedded within particular interpretive formations and social

[120] Tony Bennett, *The Birth of the Museum: History, Theory, Politics* (London: Routledge, 1995); Tony Bennett, *Pasts Beyond Memory: Evolution, Museums, Colonialism* (London: Routledge, 2004).

[121] Quigley, *Corpse*; Jonathan Simon, 'The Theatre of Anatomy: The Anatomical Preparations of Honoré Fragonard', *Eighteenth-Century Studies*, 36 (2002), 63–79.

[122] Classen, 'Museum Manners', 895.

conditions.[123] The wonder or disgust felt by visitors in 1800 were different from those experienced by their counterparts a century later, and again removed from nowadays, working for different reasons, in a different climate.

By studying curatorial intention alongside audience response it has become clear that as didactic as displays may have become, even in the revised sensory regime of the Edwardian museum, the museum–visitor encounter was dialogic. The increased conditioning of the museum visit that gave rise to the sanctity of the modern museum object—the museum *effect*—developed in response to the museum *affect*.

[123] Tony Bennett, 'Figuring Audiences and Readers', in James Hay, Lawrence Grossberg, and Ellen Wartella (eds.), *The Audience and Its Landscape* (Boulder: Westview, 1996), 145–59; James L. Machor and Philip Goldstein (eds.), *Reception Study: From Literary Theory to Cultural Studies* (New York: Routledge, 2000).

7

Conclusion

A Catalogue of Errors

Over the preceding chapters we have seen that medical museums were a prevalent aspect of nineteenth-century cultures of display and of medical education. Building on the Enlightenment 'museum oeconomy', collections owned by hospitals, colleges, entrepreneurs, and other individuals played key roles in the construction of the body, the material basis of medicine, and the exhibitionary complex more generally. Crucially, we have observed, most of the specimens within them were diseased body parts. These deviant fragments circulated through the medical marketplace, acquiring meanings as they were exchanged and objectified, rendered material culture. Preservation techniques then stabilized them physically and conceptually. Thus frozen, human remains were assembled into a series of bodies in medical museum galleries, each supported by models in wax and images on paper. Intended to be sober and edifying, visitors nevertheless responded with awe and horror.

Whereas these audiences may have been restricted by the turn of the nineteenth century, the collections themselves were huge. In 1905, for example, Guy's Hospital Museum, whose story has featured repeatedly in these pages, was re-housed in new premises as the 'Gordon Museum' (thanks to £5,000 from Robert Gordon, lawyer, businessman, governor and benefactor of the hospital).[1] The collection that Thomas Hodgkin began with 500 specimens had grown to over 12,000; and it was still just one of over one hundred medical museums, and was by no means the largest.

And yet only a handful of these collections are evident today, mostly in the royal colleges. What happened to the others in the intervening century? What was the fate of so many thousands of carefully extracted, prepared, and exchanged human remains?

---

[1] See the correspondence between Robert Gordon and the then treasurer, Cosmo Bonsor, London Metropolitan Archives H09/GY/1/155–156.

EVOLUTION OR EXTINCTION?

The absence of twentieth-century synthetic histories of museums generally, and of medical museums in particular, tempt the historian to write
them off after the First World War. And yet pathology collections
continued to grow, split, merge, and circulate. Until surprisingly late in
the century, museums were important sites for medical education; but in
different ways and with different media than their Victorian predecessors.
There can be no doubt, however, that the value and meaning of gross
pathology shifted significantly in the later century; and that the use and
display of human remains has very different meanings in recent years, as
evidenced by new legislation in the UK and the rigorous debates around
the *Body Worlds* exhibition.

Certainly as the Great War loomed, medical museums and the specimens therein held as significant a place in medical and museological
culture as ever they had. Although the foundation of the International
Association of Medical Museums in 1906 was in part promoted by the
perception of threats to the use and survival of the collections, its activities
indicate the energy and commitment of medical curators at the time. The
Association was in no small part maintained by Maude Abbott, long-
serving curator of the McGill University Pathology Museum, but also had
strong links with the United States Army Medical Museum.[2] A British
section was founded in 1911 by a group that included such luminaries
as the Canadian physician Sir William Osler (by then Regius Chair of
Medicine at Oxford) and Arthur Keith of the Hunterian in London.

The collections championed by the International Association and its
branches were, however, beginning to occupy different conceptual and
physical spaces than those outlined above, as the status and role of pathology
changed within medical practice and education. As chapter 2 revealed, many
of the new pathological, bacteriological, and public health laboratories
established in the early twentieth century housed collections, inherited or
new. For the most part, morbid and healthy anatomy collections parted

---

[2] Robin A. Cooke (ed.), *Scientific Medicine in the Twentieth Century: A Commemoration
of 100 Years of the International Association of Medical Museums and the International
Academy of Pathology* (Augusta, Ga.: United States and Canadian Academy of Pathology,
2006); Erin Hunter McLeary, 'Science in a Bottle: The Medical Museum in North
America, 1860–1940' (Ph.D. thesis, University of Pennsylvania, 2001). On the Army
Medical Museum, see Michael G. Rhode and James Connor, 'Curating America's Army
Medical Museum', in Amy Levin (ed.), *Defining Memory: Local Museums and the Construction of History in America's Changing Communities* (Lanham, Md.: AltaMira, 2007),
177–96.

company—in Manchester, for example, the former moving with pathology and the latter to what would eventually become the School of Biological Sciences; similar schisms are evident in Dublin and elsewhere.[3] Edinburgh University's collection spawned no fewer than four specialist offspring. As pathology diversified into chemical, physiological, clinical, and experimental sub-disciplines, museum collections also diversified and specialized.[4] Dedicated condition-specific institutions established in the twentieth century such as the National Heart Hospital and the institutes for Laryngology and even Psychiatry housed collections. Histo-pathological archives, often dedicated to a single disease entity, became an important clinical and research tool.

One new specialist collection of particular note was Henry Wellcome's Museum of Tropical Medicine and Hygiene in London. Founded in 1914, it became the Wellcome Museum of Medical Science in 1924 (although it retained its tropical focus).[5] Later situated on the upper ground floor of the impressive 1932 Wellcome Building at Euston, it operated within the research division of the foundation, displaying cutting-edge material. It offered specialists training in tropical diseases, building up a substantive collection of morbid specimens as well as pioneering use of intermedial visuals (see figures 7.1 and 7.2). And the Wellcome Museum was not the only medical collection dedicated to the study and promotion of hygiene and public health: the Parkes Museum of Hygiene had been founded at University College London in 1876 (in honour of Alexander Parkes, Professor of Military Hygiene at the Army Medical School), and by the twentieth century it was a core part of the Sanitary

[3] Duncan Wilson, *Reconfiguring Biological Sciences in the Late Twentieth Century: A Study of the University of Manchester* (Manchester: University of Manchester, 2008); Museum Committee Minutes, 2 February 1904, Royal College of Surgeons in Ireland Archive RCSI/MUC/2; Dugald L. Gardner, 'A Tale of Two Old and Historical Museums', in Cooke, *Scientific Medicine*, 92–8.

[4] Cathy Gere, 'A Brief History of Brain Archiving', *Journal of the History of the Neurosciences*, 12 (2003), 396–410; C. J. Hackett, 'A List of Medical Museums of Great Britain (1949–50)', *British Medical Journal*, 16 June 1951 (1951), 1380–3; Cay-Rüdiger Prüll, 'Pathology and Politics in the Metropolis, 1900–1945: London, Berlin and the Third Reich', in Margit Szöllösi-Janze (ed.), *Science in the Third Reich* (Oxford: Berg, 2001), 139–83.

[5] Wellcome Museum of Medical Science records, 1923–1983, Wellcome Library, London, GB 0120 WA/MMS; Antony J. Duggan, *How to Use the Wellcome Museum of Medical Science: A Guide for Teachers and Students* (London: Wellcome Foundation, 1973); Frances Larson, *An Infinity of Things: How Sir Henry Wellcome Collected the World* (Oxford: Oxford University Press, 2009); Wellcome Museum of Medical Science, *The Wellcome Museum of Medical Science, 1914–1964: An Account of Its Development, Content and Techniques* (London: Wellcome Foundation, 1964).

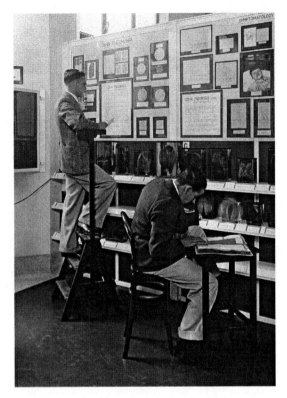

Fig. 7.1. The Wellcome Building, Euston Road, London: visitors at a lobar pneumonia display on the upper ground floor. Mid twentieth century. Wellcome Library, London.

Institute.[6] Elsewhere, public health exhibitions were especially prevalent during the First World War not only in and with medical collections but also across the museum sector. They reflected concerns about the poor physical state of conscripts during the Boer conflict a decade earlier, the challenges of food economy and the dangers of infant mortality. 'The war

[6] Ken Arnold, *Cabinets for the Curious: Looking Back at Early English Museums* (Aldershot: Ashgate, 2006); Beverly P. Bergman and Simon A. StJ. Miller, 'Historical Perspectives on Health: The Parkes Museum of Hygiene and the Sanitary Institute', *Journal of the Royal Society for the Promotion of Health,* 123 (2003), 55–61; Sophie Forgan, 'From Modern Babylon to the White City: Science, Technology and Urban Change in London, 1870–1914', in Miriam Levin, et al., *Urban Modernity: Cultural Innovation in the Second Industrial Revolution* (Cambridge, Mass.: MIT Press, 2010), 75–132; Jonathan Reinarz, 'The Age of Museum Medicine: The Rise and Fall of the Medical Museum of Birmingham's School of Medicine', *Social History of Medicine,* 18 (2005), 419–37.

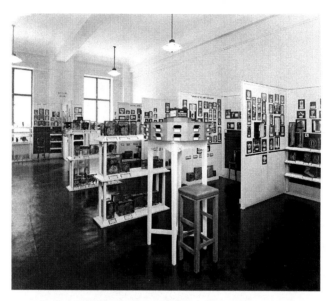

Fig. 7.2. Section 13 (neoplasms) in the Wellcome Museum of Medical Science, London, including a device for viewing photomicrographs, 1962. Wellcome Library, London.

is devouring the best of our manhood', warned the *Museums Journal* 'let museums help to save our babies.'[7] When Birmingham University established a new Department of Industrial Hygiene, plans involved a new collection.

Those collections that were not given over entirely to health and hygiene nevertheless often contributed to this field by loaning pathological specimens to any one of the numerous international, colonial, or health expositions, which were vast enterprises with huge attendance.[8] For example, anatomical preparations from medical school museums and Wellcome's collection were displayed as part of the sizeable medical section of the Hall of Science at the 1933 Chicago World's Fair that formed the basis of the Chicago Museum of Science and Industry. The fair attracted nearly 40 million visitors. Pathological collections thereby gained a very different and for the most part much larger audience than within their host institutions. On a smaller scale, but perhaps just as

[7] *Museums Journal*, 16 (1916), 56.
[8] Julie K. Brown, *Health and Medicine on Display: International Expositions in the United States, 1876–1904* (Cambridge, Mass.: MIT Press, 2009); Eben J. Carey, *Medical Science Exhibits: A Century of Progress* (Chicago: Cuneo, 1936).

significantly, medical congresses often gathered temporary museums from the local museums, especially the annual exhibition of the British Medical Association.[9]

Like other museums, medical collections were thereby in a healthy state in the inter-war period, as new institutions were founded and extant collections grew. The number of auto-bequests to medical science increased; acquisition routes stretched to the furthest reaches of the colonies; the preparation and preservation of new specimens was sufficiently widespread to support a sub-industry of equipment suppliers; and gross pathology remained part medical curricula.[10] We would expect advocacy of medical collections from Arthur Keith at the Hunterian, who considered the museum to be central to research, and from Sidney H. Daukes, Director of the Wellcome Museum of Medical Science (who proclaimed that 'the medical museum is regarded as a necessary adjunct to any well-equipped school of medicine'); but it seemed that their medical colleagues also agreed with them.[11] Although the Great War had put a stop to international meetings, the International Association of Medical Museums thrived, establishing a specimen exchange network in 1922. According to a survey undertaken under its aegis in 1951—albeit with a haphazard approach to historical data—over half of the 80 medical collections in the UK were founded in the 1900s, spread evenly over the first and second quarter of the century.[12]

Nevertheless, medical collections were not insulated from broader developments in medicine and the museum sector after the Second World War. The changing status of material culture within biomedicine, as in other disciplines such as anthropology, impacted negatively on the

---

[9] British Medical Association, *Catalogue of the Pathological Museum Held in the Histological Laboratory of the Department of Anatomy, Victoria University of Manchester* (Manchester: Morris and Yeaman, 1929); British Medical Association, *Catalogue of the Museum Held in the School of Anatomy, Trinity College, Dublin* (Dublin: Sackville, 1933).

[10] On body donation, see Elizabeth Hallam, 'Anatomical Bodies and Materials of Memory', in Belinda Brooks-Gordon, et al. (eds.), *Death Rites and Rights* (Oxford: Hart Publications, 2007), 279–98; Ruth Richardson, *Death, Dissection and the Destitute* (2nd edn, London: Phoenix, 2001); on acquisition routes, see Cressida Fforde, *Collecting the Dead: Archaeology and the Reburial Issue* (London: Duckworth, 2004); Larson, *Infinity of Things*; on techniques and suppliers, see John James Edwards and M. J. Edwards, *Medical Museum Technology* (London: Oxford University Press, 1959); McLeary, 'Science in a Bottle'; on gross pathology, see Cooke, *Scientific Medicine*.

[11] S. H. Daukes, *The Medical Museum: Modern Developments, Organisation and Technical Methods Based on a New System of Visual Teaching* (London: Wellcome Institute, 1929), 11; see also Arthur Keith, 'The museum as an engine of research', Royal College of Surgeons report, 16 June 1925, cited in Daukes, *Medical Museum*, 18–19; Elizabeth Hallam, *Anatomy Museum. Death and the Body Displayed* (London: Reaktion, 2011).

[12] Four established before 1800; twenty-nine in the period 1800–1900; twenty-four in 1900–25; twenty-four in 1925–1950. Hackett, 'List of Medical Museums'.

status of museums, and the use of objects within them.[13] More specifically, pathology increasingly drew from chemistry and was practised at the microscopic level, so that pathologists were less interested in morbid anatomy and more concerned with analytical and clinical work—from the pathology of death to disease in the living. 'Pots' were therefore no longer so central to medical training, and new pathologists were more likely to be immunologists and biochemists rather than anatomists. Although it should not be overstated, the reframing of the International Association of Medical Museums as the International Academy of Pathology in 1955 reflected this change.[14] Wider institutional changes were also afoot in the UK. The foundation of the National Health Service and the post-war expansion of universities increased resources for research, but they were not invested in museums. The renowned collection at St Thomas's, for example, was mostly destroyed in 1957.[15]

The function of museums more generally also continued to change. After the investment by the Carnegie United Kingdom Trust in the 1930s, the interruption of the War and its austere aftermath slashed museum funding.[16] Many curators turned their attention to educational activities and work with the public—something that medical curators were less inclined to do. For although specimens were lent out to expositions, access to the museums themselves had been carefully demarcated over the previous decades. The Wellcome Museum of Medical Science may have boasted prominent frontage on the Euston Road, but 'Access to the Museum [was] limited to certain categories of teachers and students... *The general public* [were] *not admitted*.'[17] Medical collections thereby became increasingly distanced from the rest of the heritage sector, and records of their use and even their existence become sparse.

A few collections did survive, however, staffed by a small new generation of post-war curators. Principal among them was Jessie Dobson, who guided the (London) Hunterian through its reconstruction after considerable Blitz damage.[18] Dobson had previously worked briefly for J. B. S.

---

[13] For a comparative study in natural history, archaeology, and anthropology, see Samuel J. M. M. Alberti, *Nature and Culture: Objects, Disciplines and the Manchester Museum* (Manchester: Manchester University Press, 2009).

[14] Cooke, *Scientific Medicine*.

[15] John M. T. Ford, *A Medical Student at St Thomas's Hospital, 1801–1802: The Weekes Family Letters*, *Medical History* Supplement 7 (London: Wellcome Institute for the History of Medicine, 1987).

[16] Cathy Pearson, 'Curators, Culture and Conflict: The Effects of the Second World War on Museums in Britain, 1926–1965' (Ph.D. thesis, University College London, 2008).

[17] Duggan, *How to Use the Wellcome Museum*, 6, original emphasis.

[18] William LeFanu, 'Jessie Dobson, MSc', *Medical History*, 29 (1985), 98.

Stopford, the Dean of Medicine at Manchester, where Tom Lawley curated the pathology museum for most of the second half of the century, including moving it into the massive faculty building named for Stopford.[19] The importance of individuals in shaping institutional collections, especially those with apparently never-ending energy and tenures, has always been a factor in the role and continued existence of museums, but this was especially important in the post-war decades.

The museums that survived were often those that continued to incorporate different media. Chapter 5 demonstrated that medical collections have always included textual, two- and three-dimensional representations of morbidity alongside specimens, and this principle continued as the form of the images evolved.[20] The Gordon Museum was substantially refreshed in the decades after the war, including a photographic unit and a new forensic medicine section. Increasingly sophisticated microphotographs were gathered and stored in extant collections, for example at the bustling Edinburgh University Pathology Museum; nearby, the Royal College established a radiology collection in 1971. Sidney Daukes had set out to make the Wellcome Museum of Medical Science a 'photographic storehouse' for such media, and by the 1960s, ten thousand clinicians, researchers, and students from all over the world visited per annum. Across town, six thousand members of the public each year visited the 'Health Exhibition Centre', that developed from the Parkes Museum under the auspices of the Royal Society for the Promotion of Health (as the Sanitary Institute had become).[21] New information and communication technologies for medical education in the late twentieth century (including the 'visible human') have often been considered the death knell for medical museums, and yet this need not have been the case. Indeed, in some places the converse was observable, as new imaging techniques worked in concert with material culture in the late twentieth century as their predecessors had in the nineteenth. Guy's was not the only museum to include a computer cluster among its objects, thus ensuring high footfall and protecting the space from encroachment. And so some collections were significant enough to be afforded space in new buildings in the higher

---

[19] University of Manchester Collection Curators' Forum records, pathology file, 1998, Manchester Museum Archive.

[20] See for example Rene L. Nerenberg and Nancy R. Swan, 'Pathology Museum in a Hallway', *Medical Teacher*, 3/1 (1981), 25–8. On the emergence of plastic and other new kinds of models, see Hallam, *Anatomy Museum*.

[21] Gardner, 'Tale of Two Old and Historical Museums'; Dawn Kemp with Sara Barnes, *Surgeon's Hall: A Museum Anthology* (Edinburgh: The Royal College of Surgeons of Edinburgh, 2009); Daukes, *Medical Museum*; Duggan, *How to Use the Wellcome Museum*; Wellcome Museum, *Wellcome Museum*; Bergman and Miller, 'Historical Perspectives'.

education expansion in the 1960s and 1970s, including for example the Stopford Building in Manchester and the new Edinburgh University Medical School buildings on George Square.[22]

REGULATION AND RE-INVENTION

Although the decline of medical collections over the twentieth century was not universal, then, there is no denying that many were closed or destroyed. As had always been the case, those without senior staff to champion them, or indeed those without any staff at all, were likely to fall prey to re-organisations and lose their space for offices, laboratories and (collection-free) computer clusters. Changes in the medical curriculum away from 'pots' undermined their value and resourcing, and the drastic reduction in the number of post-mortems stymied acquisitions.[23] The Health Exhibition Centre closed when the Royal Society for the Promotion of Health moved to new premises in 1971. The Edinburgh University Pathology Museum was consigned to storage later in the decade. The Manchester collection survived, but only after two severe 'thinning out' sessions; the bulk of it was transferred to the Manchester Royal Infirmary as space in the Stopford Building became limited. Even the Wellcome Museum of Medical Science was absorbed into the Wellcome Tropical Institute in 1985. That there were twenty-nine histopathology collections in London alone at the end of the decade is therefore perhaps surprising, but few were associated any longer with their gross counterparts, and thirteen of them were considered 'at risk'.[24]

A rear-guard action against these closures is evident in the formation of the Pathology Museums Group in 1991.[25] Curators including John Turk

[22] Gardner, 'Tale of Two Old and Historical Museums'; Manchester Museum Archive, University of Manchester Collection Curators' Forum records, pathology file. On the visible human, see Catherine Waldby, *The Visible Human Project: Informatic Bodies and Posthuman Medicine* (London: Routledge, 2000).

[23] For a survey of the changing function of the dead body and the 'disappearance of the corpse' in medical education' over the century, see Roger Cooter, 'The Dead Body', in Roger Cooter and John Pickstone (eds.), *Companion to Medicine in the Twentieth Century* (Amsterdam: Harwood, 2000), 469–85.

[24] Stephen Baycroft, et al., *Histopathology Collections in London* (London: London Museums Service, *c.* 1990); Bergman and Miller, 'Historical Perspectives'; Gardner, 'Tale of Two Old and Historical Museums'; Neil Handley (ed.), *Continuing in Trust: The Future of the Departmental Collections in the University of Manchester* (Manchester: University of Manchester, 1998); Wellcome Museum of Medical Science records, 1923–1983, Wellcome Library, London, GB 0120 WA/MMS.

[25] Papers of the Pathology Museums Group 1991–2002, Royal London Hospital Archives and Museum SO/PM/1–8; John L. Turk, 'The Future of Pathology Collections

at the English Royal College pointed to the value of specimens as the material record of rare or eliminated diseases, in military medicine in particular, and as important three-dimensional counterparts to medical images. The group 'rescued' several abandoned collections, including those of the Milford Hospital, the Royal Army Medical College at Milbank, and the Queen Elizabeth Hospital at Hackney, and in the course of their lobbying it transpired that a significant number of medical schools retained a pathology collection on some scale. The group's arguments and concerns, however, were not unique to the UK, to medical museums, nor to the late twentieth century.[26] All sorts of curators have often felt their collections to be under threat, and lobbied for greater resources; pathologists' peers in natural history and geology museums, for example, also felt they faced extinction in the late twentieth century. The challenges of space and the changing value of material culture had always been in flux; and although no single causal factor is evident, their particular configuration in the late twentieth century left medical collections more vulnerable than they had been when a significant change in legislation would alter their management and standing once again.

The practice of keeping body parts from post-mortems has a long history, as we have seen throughout this book. Relatives of the dead were rarely appraised of this, and if they found out, their concerns were given little heed. So neither the practice itself nor the (understandable) reaction were new in the well-publicized cases of retaining paediatric organs post-mortem at the Royal Liverpool Children's Hospital (Alder Hey) and the Bristol Royal Infirmary at the turn of the century; but their effects were unprecedented. 'My baby's body was on a dirty table in 36 jars', quoted *The Sun* furiously, 'I put them in a carrier bag'.[27] Both institutions had been removing and storing children's internal parts without consent, as was customary, but doing so in what was for the UK an unusually large-scale, misleading, and even incompetent manner—stockpiled organs in Liverpool were used neither for teaching nor research. Two major enquiries ensued and published in 2001, which gave rise to the

in the United Kingdom', *Museum Management and Curatorship*, 13 (1994), 295–9; Turk, 'The Medical Museum and Its Relevance to Modern Medicine', *Journal of the Royal Society of Medicine*, 87 (1994), 40–2.

[26] Denis Wakefield, 'The Future of Medical Museums: Threatened but Not Extinct', *Medical Journal of Australia*, 187 (2007), 379–80.

[27] Cited in Hugh Pennington, 'Myrtle Street', *London Review of Books*, 8 March 2001, 21–3 at 23. For a brief but expert outline of the scandals and their impact see Bronwyn Parry, 'The Afterlife of the Slide: Exploring Emotional Attachment to Artefactualised Bodily Traces', in Ilana Loewy and Nick Hopwood (eds.), *Microscope Slides: Investigating a Neglected Scientific Resource* (conference preprint: Institut Pasteur, Paris; Max Planck Institute for the History of Science, 2009).

Retained Organs Commission. Chaired by Professor Margot Brazier from the University of Manchester School of Law, the commission undertook widespread consultation over three years, and mooted 'a regulatory framework for museums and archives of material obtained from post mortem examinations'. Although acknowledging that 'specimens in pathology museums are a largely irreplaceable resource for medical education', given that there was no specific training and insufficient guidance for medical curators, the commission concluded with a call for statutory regulation.[28] This would be under the auspices of the Human Tissue Authority (HTA) thanks to a new Human Tissue Act (2004), which came into force in 2006, quickly followed by the Human Tissue (Scotland) Act (2006).[29] The Act's principal function is to license cadaver supply for medical education, but it also had a significant effect on museums, which now had to obtain expensive licenses to keep body parts with a British provenance from the previous 100 years and to demonstrate *consent* for them—as defined in the twenty-first century.

Three elements of the discussions of the commission and their manifestation in the HTA chime with particular historical resonance in light of the historical analysis of the retention of human remains in previous chapters. First is the framing of organ retention as transgressing a gift relationship. We saw in chapter 3 that many body parts arrived at museums as gift exchanges, but between practitioners rather than from patients; this practice, when revealed in the twenty-first century, met with disapproval. Secondly, the post-mortem fragmentation of the human body remained a key issue in the debate. While whole body donation has in general increased over the twentieth century, the removal and dispersal of particular organs has remained an emotive issue. Finally, many of those who spoke to the commission demanded respect for both the living and the dead, and insisted on informed consent for retention, thus emphasizing the personhood of the body parts and resisting their

---

[28] Retained Organs Commission, *A Consultation Document on Unclaimed and Unidentifiable Organs and Tissue: A Possible Regulatory Framework* (London: Department of Health, 2002), 4, 26; Retained Organs Commission, *Remembering the Past, Looking to the Future: The Final Report of the Retained Organs Commission* (London: Department of Health, 2004); Bristol Royal Infirmary Inquiry, *Learning from Bristol: The Report of the Public Inquiry into Children's Heart Surgery at the Bristol Royal Infirmary 1984–1995* (Norwich: The Stationery Office, 2001); Royal Liverpool Children's Inquiry, *Report* (London: House of Commons, 2001).

[29] M. D. Dominic Bell, 'The UK Human Tissue Act and Consent: Surrendering a Fundamental Principle to Transplantation Needs?' *Journal of Medical Ethics*, 32 (2006), 283–86; Gareth Jones and Maja I. Whitaker, *Speaking for the Dead: Cadavers in Biology and Medicine* (2nd edn, Aldershot: Ashgate, 2009); J. C. E. Underwood, 'The Impact on Histopathology Practice of New Human Tissue Legislation in the UK', *Histopathology*, 49 (2006), 221–8.

objectification and the associated 'necessary inhumanity'. The passage of the Human Tissue Act was therefore not an abrupt event horizon, but rather the latest manifestation of ongoing shifts in post-mortem meanings and practices. Legislation since the Second World War—including the 1961 and 1984 Human Tissue Acts, the 1984 Coroner's Rules and the 1988 Anatomy regulations—had moved gradually towards regulation and consent. The Royal College of Pathologists had issued guidelines shortly after the scandals came to light, encouraging greater sensitivity and communication (but unsurprisingly the college was not in favour of statutory regulation).[30] The HTA was also a manifestation of a more general phenomenon within healthcare and the UK public sector generally, giving users more involvement, voice, and choice in service provision. Hospital patients and museum visitors alike became 'clients' in a Thatcherite market economy and 'users' under New Labour, and therefore deserved consultation and 'informed consent'.[31] But as this volume was going to press, the political context shifted again, and it seems the HTA will be disbanded by the Conservative–Liberal Democrat coalition government elected in 2010.[32]

However short-lived it may turn out to have been there is no way of knowing how many poorly documented and staffed collections quietly disappeared or were disbanded at the prospect of HTA scrutiny or in the wake of the Act. The pathology collection at Edinburgh University, to cite only one prominent example, was dispersed in 2004. In Manchester the remains of the pathology collection are currently under threat as the space they occupy is ripe for re-allocation. But such developments stand in stark contrast to the other end of the exhibitionary complex, where informed consent was at the core of the debates around a phenomenon that by contrast brought human remains back into the public experience like nothing in the previous century. Across the country, as one senior pathologist noted in 2009,

> The use of preserved anatomical specimens stopped—a lot of research stopped—while we worked out what would be socially and legally acceptable in due course. Paradoxically, we now have the controversial situation of Gunther von Hagens and his *Body Worlds* exhibition drawing the crowds,

---

[30] Royal College of Pathologists, *Guidelines for the Retention of Tissues and Organs at Post-Mortem Examination* (London: Royal College of Pathologists, 2000).

[31] For patient-centred healthcare see Nicola Mead and Peter Bower, 'Patient-Centredness: A Conceptual Framework and Review of the Empirical Literature', *Social Science and Medicine*, 51 (2000), 1087–110; Andrew G.H. Thompson, 'The Meaning of Patient Involvement and Participation in Health Care Consultations: A Taxonomy', *Social Science and Medicine*, 64 (2007), 1297–310.

[32] Department of Health, *Liberating the NHS: Report of the Arm's-Length Bodies Review* (London: Department of Health, 2010).

and having been to one of his exhibitions (I was looking at the people, not the exhibits, because I've seen the exhibits before), what the people were interested in, they were glued to his disease process examples, which are actually the modern equivalents of the museum pots. So we have been obliged to stop using the very sort of material that the public was saying, 'this is fascinating'.[33]

In recent decades, artists have used—or rather, continued to use—human remains and fluids to provoke reflection and debate, as for example in the work of Anthony Noel Kelly or Marc Quinn. But no exhibition (the Chicago Worlds' Fair notwithstanding) has attracted the sheer numbers as German anatomist Gunther von Hagens's *Body Worlds*.

In 1977, von Hagens had patented a method of preservation using silicone-impregnation that he dubbed 'plastination'. He set up the Institute for Plastination in Heidelberg in 1994, and launched the first manifestation of *Body Worlds*, an exhibition of these 'plastinates', in Japan in 1995. Now in its fourth manifestation, the exhibitions have been staged over 50 times, attracting some 25 million paying visitors. Although it included a large number of healthy and diseased body parts, the attention of visitors and commentators alike has been focussed on whole bodies arranged in sporting or imaginative poses. Von Hagens provoked an ongoing debate about the artistic or education merit of the exhibition, and the ethics of his acquisition methods, that would be futile to seek to resolve here.[34] More pertinent is the extent to which *Body Worlds* is simply the latest manifestation of the ongoing culture of displaying human remains, earlier manifestations of which have been detailed in previous chapters.

Certainly von Hagens explicitly positions *Body Worlds* as the heir to Renaissance anatomical art and display. But others have compared the exhibition to freak shows and popular anatomy museums, and von Hagens

---

[33] Peter Furness, interviewed on 'The High Price of Alder Hey', radio programme, presented by Sue Armstrong, 13 August 2009, BBC Radio 4.

[34] Gunther von Hagens and Angelina Whalley (eds.), *Body Worlds—the Anatomical Exhibition of Real Human Bodies* (Heidelberg: Institut für Plastination, 2002). The large body of literature devoted to *Body Worlds* includes Lawrence Burns, 'Gunther Von Hagens' Body Worlds: Selling Beautiful Education', *The American Journal of Bioethics*, 7 (2007), 12–23; J. T. H Connor, '"Faux Reality" Show? The Body Worlds Phenomenon and Its Reinvention of Anatomical Spectacle', *Bulletin for the History of Medicine*, 81 (2007), 848–65; Jane Desmond, 'Postmortem Exhibitions: Taxidermied Animals and Plastinated Corpses in the Theaters of the Dead', *Configurations*, 16 (2008), 347–77; José F. T. M. van Dijck, 'Bodyworlds: The Art of Plastinated Cadavers', *Configurations*, 9 (2001), 99–126; Peter M. McIsaac, 'Gunther Von Hagens' Body Worlds: Exhibitionary Practice, German History, and Difference', in Daniel J. Sherman (ed.), *Museums and Difference* (Bloomington: Indiana University Press, 2007), 155–202; Elizabeth Stephens, 'Inventing the Bodily Interior: *Écorché* Figures in Early Modern Anatomy and Von Hagens' *Body Worlds*', *Social Semiotics*, 17 (2007), 313–26.

is the inheritor, wittingly or not, of many of the practices of eighteenth- and nineteenth-century anatomy and pathology museums more generally.[35] Plastination may not be such an innovative technique, but rather is redolent, for example, of the methods deployed by Honoré Fragonard in eighteenth-century France. The specimens are intermedially supported by text, image, and word (the audioguide replacing the museum lecture) and the quantitative majority of the specimens on display are fragmented body parts rather than the iconic whole-body mounts. Female remains are in the minority, largely concerned with reproduction, and are pathologized; the displays draw moral conclusions from deviant behaviour, as Joseph Kahn and his peers did; and the identity of the patients is ostensibly erased. How, then, to explain the different responses to *Body Worlds*? Similar as the content may be, its visitor constituency is very different to its nineteenth-century forbears—not only in sheer quantity but also qualitatively—a different range of individuals with different education, operating within a very different topography of affect and museum sensescape. Death and the body have very different places in society in the early twenty-first century than they had in the nineteenth.

Besides which, the cultures of collecting and display in twenty-first-century Britain may include similar institutions and objects to the Victorian exhibitionary complex, but they are now configured very differently; and as we have seen already in this chapter, anatomical preparations have different values in both biomedicine and (elsewhere) in society. This is vividly demonstrated by those pathology collections that continue to thrive in *Body Worlds'* shadow and under the watchful eye of the Human Tissue Authority. Staff of several of the larger museums whose histories featured in this volume have reframed them as vital aspects of medical and social heritage, those closing a century-long gap between medical collections and other kinds of museums. The royal college collections in both London and Edinburgh appointed directors from the museum sector rather than the medical ranks to oversee successful high-profile renovations (see figure 7.2). The Wellcome Trust opened a new museum, Wellcome Collection, in the same building that once housed its Museum of Medical Science. Like the royal colleges, they invite a general public, who have attended in increasing numbers. Further afield, the US

---

[35] T. Christine Jespersen, Alicita Rodriguez, and Joseph Starr (eds.), *The Anatomy of Body Worlds: Critical Essays on the Plastinated Cadavers of Gunther Von Hagens* (Jefferson, NC: McFarland, 2009); Uli Linke, 'Touching the Corpse: The Unmaking of Memory in the Body Museum', *Anthropology Today*, 21/5 (2005), 13–19; Jonathan Simon, 'The Theatre of Anatomy: The Anatomical Preparations of Honoré Fragonard', *Eighteenth-Century Studies*, 36 (2002), 63–79; Jonathan Simon, 'Honoré Fragonard, Anatomical Virtuoso', in Bernadette Bensaude-Vincent and Christine Blondel (eds.), *Science and Spectacle in the European Enlightenment* (Aldershot: Ashgate 2008), 141–58.

Army Medical Museum has been reinvented as the National Museum of Health and Medicine, the Virchow Museum in Berlin and Museion in Copenhagen are prominent and active.[36] All seek to provide a resource in 'medical humanities', 'that promising space between the hard science and technology of medicine and the softer lives of those involved in its practice', giving them a 'a refashioned vitality'.[37]

MATERIAL MORBIDITY

If you were to visit the renovated Hunterian Museum at the Royal College of Surgeons shown in figure 7.3 (and I hope that you will), and were to turn your attention to case 11 bay 3, you would find there specimen RCSHC/P998, the normal-abnormal specimen which began this study (chapter 1, figure 1.3). Readers of *Morbid Curiosities* and the interpretation provided in the Hunterian will view it not only as an important pathological specimen, but also a unique historical artefact. Taken from the body of a woman, it was rendered partible and re-fashioned into a dividual morbid body. It has survived generations of curators, pathologists, medical students, and other visitors. It has meant different things to different people, as subject and object, person and thing; it has been elucidated by images, texts, and models. These conceptual changes have been closely associated with physical trans-formation, involving not only the labour of John Hunter, but also of those who curated his collection over the following two centuries. It has endured numerous physical and conceptual re-organizations, several moves, and terrible bomb damage. It is the physical embodiment of the processes of material culture. It is pathological knowledge materialized.

The central thesis of *Morbid Curiosities* has been that this and other diseased corpses were fragmented, circulated, preserved, and displayed in order to construct the abnormal in the medical collection. If, as Canguil-hem bleakly observed, 'life gambles against growing entropy', then the medical museum displayed those who lost.[38] Curators regulated the dead body materially as other professionals regulated the living body's sexuality,

---

[36] Thomas Söderqvist, Adam Bencarda, and Camilla Mordhorst, 'Between Meaning Culture and Presence Effects: Contemporary Biomedical Objects as a Challenge to Museums', *Studies In History and Philosophy of Science*, 40 (2009), 431–8; see also Jane E. Dahlstrom and Gerlese S. kerlind, 'An Innovation in the Teaching of Pathology—The Surgical Specimen Museum of the Australian National University Medical School', in Cooke, *Scientific Medicine*, 99–101.

[37] Arnold, *Cabinets for the Curious*, 172.

[38] Georges Canguilhem, *The Normal and the Pathological*, trans. Carolyn R. Fawcett (1943; 2nd edn, New York: Zone, 1989), 236.

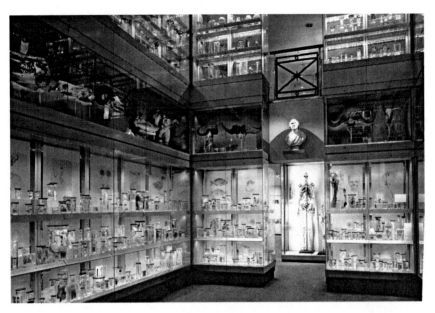

Fig. 7.3. The new 'Crystal Gallery' at the Royal College of Surgeons of England, 2005. Copyright the Hunterian Museum at the Royal College of Surgeons of England.

behaviour, politics, and race. Morbidity was embedded in the exhibitionary complex alongside other forms of the 'other', be they exotic animals, strange peoples, or ancient artefacts. By breaking up the body and locating disease, the medical establishment—and some beyond its ranks—at once produced corporeal norms and demarcated abnormality. Deviant bodies were classified and policed, no longer displayed as freaks, prodigies or curiosities, but rather as partible, reducible, explicable variations on the norm. 'How, then,' asked Foucault of the nineteenth century, 'could the species of great exceptional monstrosity end up being divided up into this host of little abnormalities, of both abnormal and familiar characters?'[39] The category of 'monster'—the unpredictable deviant—became narrower and narrower, teratology reduced to the uncontrollable afterword in the museum. Here was the transition from monstrosity to abnormality Foucault observed—in nuanced, located, *material* terms. It was a transformation that came about thanks to the concerted efforts of a community of

[39] Michel Foucault, *Abnormal: Lectures at the Collège De France 1974–1975*, ed. Valerio Marchetti, Antonella Salomoni, and Arnold I. Davidson, trans. Graham Burchell (1975; London: Verso, 2003), 110.

practice that emerged, slowly, around these most gruesome of objects. Morbid anatomists commandeered the dead body and used it to build pathological anatomy; and so to understand pathology as a discipline we must understand the museum as an institution, and vice versa.

Which is not to say that this was the only function of the medical museum, nor that pathologists enjoyed a monopoly over preparations' meanings. Curatorial intention and visitor experience do not precisely correspond in any museum display, especially when the objects in question have such potentially affective connections with death, disease, and self. Furthermore, when we assesses not only display but also the many other significant episodes in the trajectory of a museum object, all the individuals and institutions that engaged with the body part re-emerge, together with the meanings they afforded it. Both before and after the post-mortem corporeal fragmentation, the identity of the originating patient—the source of this raw material—was obscured by those of surgeons and physicians, anatomists and pathologists, collectors and curators. It was not only a piece of a person but also a piece of work, a virtuoso performance of the preparator. Nineteenth-century medical thought broke the body into parts conceptually; anatomists did so physically.

Even the apparently simple act of referring to body parts as 'objects', then, is indicative of a radical meaning shift experiences by corporeal fragments on their way to and within the medical museum. Living bodies began to be objectified, pathologized, as soon as they were diagnosed, and both technical and conceptual practices continued this process after death. We have seen in particular how significant fragmentation was in objectifying the body, dislocating and isolating morbidity before re-assembly. Crucially, once they were objects, things, then body parts were property, and could be *owned* (whether in law or in practice). The notion of (patients') consent so central to contemporary debates around human remains held little sway in the nineteenth-century medical marketplace. On the contrary, as we saw in chapter 3, dying persons or their families had no right to deprive surgeons and physicians of the raw material from which museum specimens would be manufactured. In this context of 'necessary inhumanity', objects derived from living people occupied a liminal space between person and thing, self and other. The diseased dead held up a mirror to the healthy living, emphasizing both the fallibility and the materiality of the self. But these changes were neither one-way nor permanent. The flexibility of these specimens, whose person-ness and thing-ness could vary in different contexts, demonstrates the permeability of the barrier between people and things.

The object that this human fragment became had very different meanings in the museum. It was now intended to be related not to other body parts of the patient, but rather to other examples of the disease, to other media, and to other things collected by that collector. By framing the human remains in medical museums as 'dividual bodies', I have argued in these chapters that these collections are composed of multi-authored, partible systems, each of them representing a set of relations. They are more than composites, they are unique re-arrangements of unique pieces. But even this framing, as a conglomerate, intermedial dividual, could not impede the polysemic character of human remains. Their 'human-ness' stubbornly endured, eliciting wonder, horror, fear, and sympathy. Objects that were once alive have very particular biographies, and the social life—afterlife—of these things is revealing of the place of death and disease in Western society. They are embedded in a complex configuration of flesh and bone, wax and paper, with changing meanings over time and between groups, with complex layered meanings drawing from their varied contexts.

Medical museums were characterized not only by these qualities, but also by the sheer quantity of material they held. Like other collections, they were dynamic beasts, at first formed or acquired, subsequently exchanged and sometimes dispersed. But for the most part they simply grew, incrementally acquiring new meanings with their manifold new acquisitions. Like natural history collections, they reached their peak in quantity and prestige in the decades around 1900. And yet, as we have seen in this final chapter, this was not to last, in part due to the sheer inertia of so many thousands of preparations. As fascinating as it may be for the historian, such relentless accrual condemned to obsolescence too many of institutions that housed them, as medical research, social mores, and even the value afforded to things changed over the twentieth century. The meaning of individual specimens may be flexible, but the combined physicality of thousands of them is not. The bodies in the medical museum are both its blessing and its curse.

Selected Bibliography

Adams, Rachel, *Sideshow U.S.A.: Freaks and the American Cultural Imagination* (Chicago: University of Chicago Press, 2001).

Alberti, Samuel J. M. M., 'Objects and the Museum', *Isis*, 96 (2005), 559–71.

—— 'Owning and Collecting Natural Objects in Nineteenth-Century Britain', in Marco Berretta (ed.), *From Private to Public: Natural Collections and Museums* (New York: Science History Publications, 2005), 141–54.

—— 'The Museum Affect: Visiting Collections of Anatomy and Natural History', in Fyfe and Lightman, *Science in the Marketplace*, 371–403.

—— 'Wax Bodies: Art and Anatomy in Victorian Medical Museums', *Museum History Journal*, 2 (2009), 7–35.

Altick, Richard D., *The Shows of London: A Panoramic History of Exhibitions, 1600–1862* (Cambridge, Mass.: Belknap, 1978).

Andrews, Lori and Nelkin, Dorothy, *Body Bazaar: The Market for Human Tissue in the Biotechnology Age* (New York: Crown, 2001).

Appadurai, Arjun (ed.), *The Social Life of Things: Commodities in Cultural Perspective* (Cambridge: Cambridge University Press, 1986).

Arnold, Ken, 'Time Heals: Making History in Medical Museums', in Gaynor Kavanagh, (ed.), *Making Histories in Museums* (London: Leicester University Press, 1996), 15–29.

—— 'Museums and the Making of Medical History', in Robert Bud, Bernard Finn, and Helmuth Trischler (eds.), *Manifesting Medicine: Bodies and Machines* (Amsterdam: Harwood Academic, 1999), 145–74.

—— *Cabinets for the Curious: Looking Back at Early English Museums* (Aldershot: Ashgate, 2006).

—— and Olsen, Danielle (eds.), *Medicine Man: The Forgotten Museum of Henry Wellcome* (London: British Museum Press, 2003).

Baillie, Matthew, *The Morbid Anatomy of the Most Important Parts of the Human Body* (London: Johnson, 1793).

Bates, Alan W., ' "Indecent and Demoralising Representations": Public Anatomy Museums in Mid-Victorian England', *Medical History*, 52 (2008), 1–22.

Bell, Charles, *A System of Dissections, Explaining the Anatomy of the Human Body, the Manner of Displaying the Parts, and Their Varieties in Disease*, 2 vols. (Edinburgh: Mundell, 1798–1803).

—— (ed.), *Letters of Sir Charles Bell* (London: Murray, 1870).

Bell, John, *Engravings, Explaining the Anatomy of the Bones, Muscles and Joints* (Edinburgh: Paterson, 1794).

Bending, Lucy, *The Representation of Bodily Pain in Late Nineteenth-Century English Culture* (Oxford: Clarendon, 2000).

Bennett, Tony, 'The Exhibitionary Complex', *New Formations*, 4 (1988), 73–102.

—— *The Birth of the Museum: History, Theory, Politics* (London: Routledge, 1995).

—— *Pasts Beyond Memory: Evolution, Museums, Colonialism* (London: Routledge, 2004).

Bichat, Xavier, *Physiological Researches on Life and Death*, trans. F. Gold (1799; London: Longman, Hunt, Rees, Orme and Browne, 1815).

—— *Pathological Anatomy* (Philadelphia: John Grigg, 1827).

Black, Peter (ed.), '*My Highest Pleasure': William Hunter's Art Collection* (Glasgow: University of Glasgow in association with Paul Holberton, 2007).

Bliss, Michael, *William Osler: A Life in Medicine* (Oxford: Oxford University Press, 1999).

Blumberg, Mark S., *Freaks of Nature: What Anomalies Tell Us About Development and Evolution* (New York: Oxford University Press, 2008).

Bogdan, Robert, *Freak Show: Presenting Human Oddities for Amusement and Profit* (Chicago: University of Chicago Press, 1988).

Bonner, Thomas Neville, *Becoming a Physician: Medical Education in Great Britain, France, Germany and the United States 1750–1945* (New York: Oxford University Press, 1995).

Bound Alberti, Fay, *Matters of the Heart: History, Medicine, and Emotion* (Oxford: Oxford University Press, 2010).

Boyle, Robert, *Some Considerations Touching the Usefulnesse of Experimental Naturall Philosophy*, 2 vols. (Oxford: Hall, 1663).

Brennan, Teresa and Jay, Martin (eds.), *Vision in Context: Historical and Contemporary Perspectives on Sight* (London: Routledge, 1996).

Brock, C. Helen (ed.), *The Correspondence of Dr William Hunter*, 2 vols. (London: Pickering and Chatto, 2008).

Brown, Julie K., *Health and Medicine on Display: International Expositions in the United States, 1876–1904* (Cambridge, Mass.: MIT Press, 2009).

Burch, Druin, *Digging up the Dead: Uncovering the Life and Times of an Extraordinary Surgeon* (London: Chatto and Windus, 2007).

Burmeister, Maritha Rene, 'Popular Anatomical Museums in Nineteenth-Century England' (Ph.D. thesis, Rutgers University, 2000).

Burney, Ian A., *Bodies of Evidence: Medicine and the Politics of the Inquest 1830–1926* (Baltimore: Johns Hopkins University Press, 2000).

Bynum, Caroline Walker, *Fragmentation and Redemption: Essays on Gender and the Human Body in Medieval Religion* (New York: Zone, 1991).

Bynum, William F. and Porter, Roy (eds.), *William Hunter and the Eighteenth-Century Medical World* (Cambridge: Cambridge University Press, 1985).

Candlin, Fiona, *Art, Museums and Touch* (Manchester: Manchester University Press, 2010).

Canguilhem, Georges, *The Normal and the Pathological*, trans. Carolyn R. Fawcett (1943; 2nd edn, New York: Zone, 1989).

Carswell, Robert, *Pathological Anatomy. Illustrations of the Elementary Forms of Disease* (London: Longman, Orme, Brown, Green and Longman, 1838).

Chadarevian, Soraya de and Hopwood, Nick (eds.), *Models: The Third Dimension in Science* (Stanford, Calif.: Stanford University Press, 2004).

Chalmers-Hunt, J. M. (ed.), *Natural History Auctions 1700–1972: A Register of Sales in the British Isles* (London: Sotheby Parke Bernet, 1976).

Chaplin, Simon, 'John Hunter and The "Museum Oeconomy", 1750–1800' (Ph.D. thesis, King's College London, 2009).

——, 'Emotion and Identity in John Hunter's Museum', in Karen Ingham, *Narrative Remains* (London: Royal College of Surgeons of England, 2009), 8–15.

Classen, Constance, 'Museum Manners: The Sensory Life of the Early Museum', *Journal of Social History*, 40 (2007), 895–914.

——, Howes, David, and Synnott, Anthony, *Aroma: The Cultural History of Smell* (London: Routledge, 1994).

Cole, Francis Joseph, 'History of the Anatomical Museum', in Oliver Elton (ed.), *A Miscellany Presented to John Macdonald Mackay* (Liverpool: Liverpool University Press, 1914), 302–17.

——*A History of Comparative Anatomy: From Aristotle to the Eighteenth Century* (London: Macmillan, 1944).

Connor, J. T. H, '"Faux Reality" Show? The Body Worlds Phenomenon and Its Reinvention of Anatomical Spectacle', *Bulletin for the History of Medicine*, 81 (2007), 848–65.

Cooke, Robin A. (ed.), *Scientific Medicine in the Twentieth Century: A Commemoration of 100 Years of the International Association of Medical Museums and the International Academy of Pathology* (Augusta, Ga.: United States and Canadian Academy of Pathology, 2006).

Cooper, Bransby Blake, *The Life of Sir Astley Cooper, Bart.*, 2 vols. (London: Parker, 1843).

Corbin, Alain, *The Foul and the Fragrant: Odor and the French Social Imagination*, trans. Miriam L. Kochan, Roy Porter, and Christopher Prendegast (1982; Cambridge, Mass.: Harvard University Press, 1986).

Crary, Jonathan, *Techniques of the Observer: On Vision and Modernity in the Nineteenth Century* (Cambridge, Mass.: MIT Press, 1990).

Cross, Stephen J., 'John Hunter, the Animal Oeconomy, and Late Eighteenth-Century Physiological Discourse', *Studies in History of Biology*, 5 (1981), 1–110.

Cunningham, Andrew and Williams, Perry (eds.), *The Laboratory Revolution in Medicine* (Cambridge: Cambridge University Press, 1992).

Cunningham, George J., *The History of British Pathology*, ed. G. Kemp McGowan (Bristol: White Tree, 1992).

Dacome, Lucia, 'Resurrecting by Numbers in Eighteenth-Century England', *Past and Present*, 193 (2006), 73–110.

Daston, Lorraine (ed.), *Things That Talk: Object Lessons from Art and Science* (New York: Zone, 2004).

—— and Galison, Peter, *Objectivity* (Boston: Zone, 2007).

—— and Park, Katharine, *Wonders and the Order of Nature, 1150–1750* (New York: Zone, 1998).

Daukes, S. H., *The Medical Museum: Modern Developments, Organisation and Technical Methods Based on a New System of Visual Teaching* (London: Wellcome Institute, 1929).

Desmond, Adrian, *The Politics of Evolution: Morphology, Medicine and Reform in Radical London* (Chicago: University of Chicago Press, 1989).

Desmond, Jane, 'Postmortem Exhibitions: Taxidermied Animals and Plastinated Corpses in the Theaters of the Dead', *Configurations*, 16 (2008), 347–77.

Dickenson, Donna, *Body Shopping: The Economy Fuelled by Flesh and Blood* (Oxford: Oneworld, 2008).

Dijck, José F. T. M. van, 'Bodyworlds: The Art of Plastinated Cadavers', *Configurations*, 9 (2001), 99–126.

Dixon-Woods, Mary, et al., 'Human Tissue And "The Public": The Case of Childhood Cancer Tumour Banking', *BioSocieties*, 3 (2008), 57–80.

Dobson, Jessie, 'Some Eighteenth Century Experiments in Embalming', *Journal of the History of Medicine*, 8 (1953), 431–41.

—— 'The Architectural History of the Hunterian Museum', *Annals of The Royal College of Surgeons of England*, 21 (1961), 113–26.

—— 'The Place of John Hunter's Museum', *Annals of the Royal College of Surgeons of England*, 33 (1963), 32–40.

Durbach, Nadja, *The Spectacle of Deformity: Freak Shows and Modern British Culture* (Berkeley: University of California Press, 2010).

Durey, Michael J., 'Bodysnatchers and Benthamites: The Implications of the Dead Body Bill for the London Schools of Anatomy, 1820–42', *The London Journal*, 2 (1976), 200–25.

Düring, Monika von, Didi-Huberman, Georges, and Poggesi, Marta, *Encyclopaedia Anatomica: A Complete Collection of Anatomical Waxes* (Köln: Taschen, 1999).

Edwards, John James and Edwards, M. J., *Medical Museum Technology* (London: Oxford University Press, 1959).

Elwood, Willis J. and Tuxford, A. Félicité (eds.), *Some Manchester Doctors: A Biographical Collection to Mark the 150th Anniversary of the Manchester Medical Society 1834–1984* (Manchester: Manchester University Press for the Manchester Medical Society, 1984).

Fforde, Cressida, *Collecting the Dead: Archaeology and the Reburial Issue* (London: Duckworth, 2004).

Findlen, Paula, *Possessing Nature: Museums, Collecting, and Scientific Culture in Early Modern Italy* (Berkeley: University of California Press, 1994).

Finnegan, Diarmid, 'The Spatial Turn: Geographical Approaches in the History of Science', *Journal of the History of Biology*, 41 (2008), 369–88.

Fleetwood, John, *History of Medicine in Ireland* (2nd edn, Dublin: Skellig, 1983).

—— *The Irish Body Snatchers: A History of Body Snatching in Ireland* (Dublin: Tomar, 1988).

Flower, William Henry, *Essays on Museums and Other Subjects Connected with Natural History* (London: Macmillan, 1898).

Ford, John M. T., *A Medical Student at St Thomas's Hospital, 1801–1802: The Weekes Family Letters, Medical History* Supplement 7 (London: Wellcome Institute for the History of Medicine, 1987).

Forgan, Sophie, 'Bricks and Bones: Architecture and Science in Victorian Britain', in Galison and Thompson (eds.), *The Architecture of Science*, 181–208.

—— 'Building the Museum: Knowledge, Conflict, and the Power of Place', *Isis*, 96 (2005), 572–85.

Foster, W. D., *Pathology as a Profession in Great Britain and the Early History of the Royal College of Pathologists* (London: Royal College of Pathologists, 1983).

Foucault, Michel, *The Birth of the Clinic: An Archaeology of Medical Perception*, trans. Alan M. Sheridan (London: Tavistock, 1976).

—— *Discipline and Punish: The Birth of the Prison*, trans., Alan M. Sheridan (London: Allen Lane, 1977).

—— *Abnormal: Lectures at the Collège De France 1974–1975*, ed. Valerio Marchetti, Antonella Salomoni, and Arnold I. Davidson, trans. Graham Burchell (1975; London: Verso, 2003).

Fowler, Chris, *The Archaeology of Personhood: An Anthropological Approach* (London: Routledge, 2004).

Fox, Daniel M. and Lawrence, Christopher, *Photographing Medicine: Images and Power in Britain and America since 1840* (New York: Greenwood, 1988).

Fox, Renée C. and Swazey, Judith P., *Spare Parts: Organ Replacement in American Society* (Oxford: Oxford University Press, 1992).

Fraser, Andrew G., *The Building of Old College: Adam, Playfair and the University of Edinburgh* (Edinburgh: Edinburgh University Press, 1989).

Freedberg, David, *The Power of Images: Studies in the History and Theory of Response* (Chicago: University of Chicago Press, 1989).

Fyfe, Aileen and Lightman, Bernard (eds.), *Science in the Marketplace: Nineteenth-Century Sites and Experiences* (Chicago: University of Chicago Press, 2007).

Galison, Peter and Thompson, Emily (eds.), *The Architecture of Science* (Cambridge, Mass.: MIT Press, 1999).

Gannal, Jean Nicolas, *History of Embalming, and Preparations in Anatomy, Pathology and Natural History*, ed. and trans. Richard Harlan (1838; Philedelphia: Dobson, 1840).

Gefland, Toby, *Professionalising Modern Medicine: Paris Surgeons and Medical Science and Institutions in the Eighteenth Century* (Westport, Conn.: Greenwood, 1980).

Gere, Cathy, 'A Brief History of Brain Archiving', *Journal of the History of the Neurosciences*, 12 (2003), 396–410.

Geyer-Kordesch, Johanna, Macdonald, Fiona, and Hull, Andrew, *Physicians and Surgeons in Glasgow: The History of the Royal College of Physicians and Surgeons of Glasgow 1599–1858* (London: Hambledon, 1999).

Gieryn, Thomas F., *Cultural Boundaries of Science: Credibility on the Line* (Chicago: University of Chicago Press, 1999).

Gilman, Sander L., *Health and Illness: Images of Difference* (London: Reaktion, 1995).

Gosden, Chris and Larson, Frances, with Petch, Alison, *Knowing Things: Exploring the Collections at the Pitt Rivers Museum 1884–1945* (Oxford: Oxford University Press, 2007).

Guerrini, Anita, 'Duverney's Skeletons', *Isis*, 94 (2003), 577–603.

—— 'Anatomists and Entrepreneurs in Early Eighteenth-Century London', *Journal of the History of Medicine and Allied Sciences*, 59 (2004), 219–39.

Hackett, C. J., 'A List of Medical Museums of Great Britain (1949–50)', *British Medical Journal*, 16 June 1951 (1951), 1380–83.

Haigh, Elizabeth, *Xavier Bichat and the Medical Theory of the Eighteenth Century*, *Medical History* Supplement 4 (London: Wellcome Institute for the History of Medicine, 1984).

Hallam, Elizabeth, 'Anatomical Bodies and Materials of Memory', in Belinda Brooks-Gordon, et al. (eds.), *Death Rites and Rights* (Oxford: Hart Publishing, 2007), 279–98.

—— *Anatomy Museum: Death and the Body Displayed* (London: Reaktion, 2011).

—— 'Articulating Bones', *Journal of Material Culture*, 15 (2010) 465–92.

—— and Hockey, Jenny, *Death, Memory, and Material Culture* (Oxford: Berg, 2001).

—— —— and Howarth, Glennys, *Beyond the Body: Death and Social Identity* (London: Routledge, 1999).

Hamilton, David, *The Healers: A History of Medicine in Scotland* (2nd edn, Edinburgh: Mercat, 2003).

Hansen, Julie V., 'Resurrecting Death: Anatomical Art in the Cabinet of Dr. Frederik Ruysch', *Art Bulletin*, 78 (1996), 663–79.

Harries, Elizabeth Wanning, *The Unfinished Manner: Essays on the Fragment in the Later Eighteenth Century* (Charlottesville, VA: University of Virginia Press, 1994).

Harrison, Robert, *The Dublin Dissector: Or, Manual of Anatomy* (Dublin: Hodges and McArthur, 1827).

Heinrich, Larissa N., *The Afterlife of Images: Translating the Pathological Body between China and the West* (Durham, NC: Duke University Press, 2008).

Herle, Anita, Elliott, Mark, and Empson, Rebecca, *Assembling Bodies: Art, Science and Imagination* (Cambridge: University of Cambridge Museum of Archaeology and Anthropology, 2009).

Hillman, David A. and Mazzio, Carla (eds.), *The Body in Parts: Fantasies of Corporeality in Early Modern Europe* (New York: Routledge, 1997).

Hoeyer, Klaus, 'Person, Patent and Property: A Critique of the Commodification Hypothesis', *Biosocieties*, 2 (2007), 327–48.

Hogle, Linda F., *Recovering the Nation's Body: Cultural Memory, Medicine, and the Politics of Redemption* (New Brunswick, NJ: Rutgers University Press, 1999).

Hooper-Greenhill, Eilean, *Museums and the Shaping of Knowledge* (London: Routledge, 1992).

—— *Museums and the Interpretation of Visual Culture* (London: Routledge, 2000).

Hopwood, Nick, *Embryos in Wax: Models from the Ziegler Studio* (Cambridge: Whipple Museum of the History of Science, 2002).

—— 'Artist Versus Anatomist, Models against Dissection: Paul Zeiller of Munich and the Revolution of 1848', *Medical History*, 51 (2007), 279–308.

Hoskins, Janet, 'On Losing and Getting a Head: Warfare, Exchange, and Alliance in a Changing Sumba, 1888–1988', *American Ethnologist*, 16 (1989), 419–40.

Howes, David (ed.), *Empire of the Senses: The Sensual Culture Reader* (Oxford: Berg, 2004).

Hughes, Jessica, 'Fragmentation as Metaphor in the Classical Healing Sanctuary', *Social History of Medicine*, 21 (2008), 217–36.

Hunter, William, *Anatomia Uteri Humani Gravidi Tabulis Illustrata* (Birmingham: Baskerville, 1774).

—— *Two Introductory Lectures, Delivered by Dr. William Hunter, to His Last Course of Anatomical Lectures* (London: Johnson, 1784).

Hurley, Kelly, *The Gothic Body: Sexuality, Materialism, and Degeneration at the Fin de Siècle* (Cambridge: Cambridge University Press, 1996).

Hurren, Elizabeth T., 'A Pauper Dead-House: The Expansion of the Cambridge Anatomical Teaching School under the Late-Victorian Poor Law, 1870–1914', *Medical History*, 48 (2004), 69–94.

—— 'Whose Body Is It Anyway?: Trading the Dead Poor, Coroner's Disputes, and the Business of Anatomy at Oxford University, 1885–1929', *Bulletin of the History of Medicine*, 82 (2008), 775–818.

—— *Dying for Victorian Medicine: English Anatomy and Its Trade in the Dead Poor, 1870 to 1929* (London: Palgrave Macmillan, forthcoming).

Hyde, Ralph, *Panoramania! The Art and Entertainment of The 'All-Embracing' View* (London: Trefoil, 1988).

Jacyna, L. Stephen, 'The Laboratory and the Clinic: The Impact of Pathology on Surgical Diagnosis in the Glasgow Western Infirmary 1875–1910', *Bulletin for the History of Medicine*, 62 (1988), 384–406.

—— '"A Host of Experienced Microscopists": The Establishment of Histology in Nineteenth-Century Edinburgh', *Bulletin of the History of Medicine*, 75 (2001), 225–53.

Jenner, Mark S. R. and Wallis, Patrick (eds.), *Medicine and the Market in England and Its Colonies, c. 1450–c. 1850* (New York: Palgrave Macmillan, 2007).

Jespersen, T. Christine, Rodriguez, Alicita, and Starr, Joseph (eds.), *The Anatomy of Body Worlds: Critical Essays on the Plastinated Cadavers of Gunther Von Hagens* (Jefferson, NC: McFarland, 2009).

Jones, Gareth and Whitaker, Maja I., *Speaking for the Dead: Cadavers in Biology and Medicine* (2nd edn, Aldershot: Ashgate, 2009).

Jones, Nora, 'The Mütter Museum: The Body as Spectacle, Specimen, and Art' (Ph.D. thesis, Temple University, 2002).

Jordanova, Ludmilla J., *Sexual Visions: Images of Gender in Science and Medicine between the Eighteenth and Twentieth Centuries* (Hemel Hempstead: Harvester Wheatsheaf, 1989).

Karp, Ivan and Lavine, Steven D. (eds.), *Exhibiting Cultures: The Poetics and Politics of Museum Display* (Washington: Smithsonian Institution Press, 1991).

Kass, Amalie M. and Kass, Edward H., *Perfecting the World: The Life and Times of Dr. Thomas Hodgkin 1798–1866* (Boston: Harcourt Brace Jovanovich, 1988).

Kaufman, Matthew H., *Medical Teaching in Edinburgh During the 18th and 19th Centuries* (Edinburgh: Royal College of Surgeons of Edinburgh, 2003).

Kemp, Dawn with Barnes, Sara, *Surgeon's Hall: A Museum Anthology* (Edinburgh: The Royal College of Surgeons of Edinburgh, 2009).

Kemp, Martin, *Dr William Hunter at the Royal Academy of Art* (Glasgow: University of Glasgow Press, 1975).

—— *Bodyscapes: Images of Human Anatomy from the Collections of St Andrews* (St Andrews: Crawford Arts Centre, 1995).

—— and Wallace, Marina, *Spectacular Bodies: The Art and Science of the Human Body from Leonardo to Now* (London; Berkeley: Hayward Gallery; University of California Press, 2000).

Keppie, Lawrence, *William Hunter and the Hunterian Museum in Glasgow, 1807–2007* (Edinburgh: Edinburgh University Press, 2007).

Knox, Frederick John, *The Anatomist's Instructor, and Museum Companion: Being Practical Directions for the Formation and Subsequent Management of Anatomical Museums* (Edinburgh: Black, 1836).

Larson, Frances, *An Infinity of Things: How Sir Henry Wellcome Collected the World* (Oxford: Oxford University Press, 2009).

Latour, Bruno and Weibel, Peter (eds.), *Making Things Public: Atmospheres of Democracy* (Cambridge, Mass.: MIT Press, 2005).

Lawrence, Susan C., *Charitable Knowledge: Hospital Pupils and Practitioners in Eighteenth-Century London* (Cambridge: Cambridge University Press, 1996).

—— 'Beyond the Grave—The Use and Meaning of Human Body Parts: A Historical Introduction', in Robert F. Weir (ed.), *Stored Tissue Samples: Ethical, Legal and Public Policy Implications* (Iowa City: University of Iowa Press, 1998), 111–42.

—— and Bendixen, Kae, 'His and Hers: Male and Female Anatomy Texts for U.S. Medical Students, 1890–1989', *Social Science and Medicine*, 7 (1992), 925–34.

Learmount, Brian, *A History of the Auction* (Iver: Barnard and Learmount, 1985).

Lederer, Susan E., *Flesh and Blood: Organ Transplantation and Blood Transfusion in Twentieth-Century America* (Oxford: Oxford University Press, 2008).

Levin, Miriam, Forgan, Sophie, Hessler, Martina, Kargon, Robert H., and Low, Morris, *Urban Modernity: Cultural Innovation in the Second Industrial Revolution* (Cambridge, Mass.: MIT Press, 2010).

Livingstone, David N., *Putting Science in Its Place: Geographies of Scientific Knowledge* (Chicago, Ill.: University of Chicago Press, 2003).

Lock, Margaret, *Twice Dead: Organ Transplants and the Reinvention of Death* (Berkeley: University of California Press, 2002).

Lohman, Jack and Goodnow, Katherine (eds.), *Human Remains and Museum Practice* (Paris and London: UNESCO and the Museum of London, 2006).

McCormack, Helen, 'A Collector of the Fine Arts in Eighteenth-Century Britain: Dr William Hunter 1718–1783' (Ph.D. thesis, University of Glasgow, 2010).

McCulloch, N. A., Russell, D., and McDonald, Stuart W., 'William Hunter's Casts of the Gravid Uterus at the University of Glasgow', *Clinical Anatomy*, 14 (2001), 210–17.

Macdonald, Sharon, 'Accessing Audiences: Visiting Visitor Books', *Museum and Society*, 3 (2006), 119–36.

MacDonald, Helen, *Human Remains: Dissection and Its Histories* (London: Yale University Press, 2006).

—— *Possessing the Dead: The Artful Science of Anatomy* (Melbourne: Melbourne University Publishing, 2010).

McGrath, Roberta, *Seeing Her Sex: Medical Archives and the Female Body* (Manchester: Manchester University Press, 2002).

MacGregor, Arthur, *Curiosity and Enlightenment: Collectors and Collections from the Sixteenth to the Nineteenth Century* (New Haven, Conn.: Yale University Press, 2007).

McLeary, Erin Hunter, 'Science in a Bottle: The Medical Museum in North America, 1860–1940' (Ph.D. thesis, University of Pennsylvania, 2001).

MacLeod, Suzanne (ed.), *Reshaping Museum Space: Architecture, Design, Exhibitions* (London: Routledge, 2005).

Maerker, Anna, *Model Experts: Wax Anatomies and Enlightenment in Florence and Vienna, 1775–1815* (Manchester: Manchester University Press, 2011).

Malcolm, Elizabeth and Jones, Greta (eds.), *Medicine, Disease and the State in Ireland, 1650–1940* (Cork: Cork University Press, 1999).

Maleuvre, Didier, *Museum Memories: History, Technology, Art* (Stanford, Calif.: Stanford University Press, 1999).

Markus, Thomas A., *Buildings and Power: Freedom and Control in the Origin of Modern Building Types* (London: Routledge, 1993).

Mason, Michael, *The Making of Victorian Sexuality* (Oxford: Oxford University Press, 1994).

Matthews, Paul, 'Whose Body? People as Property', *Current Legal Problems*, 36 (1983), 197–200.

Matyssek, Angela, *Rudolf Virchow. Das Pathologische Museum: Geschichte einer Wissenschaftlichen Sammlung um 1900* (Darmstadt: Steinkopff, 2003).

Maulitz, Russell C., *Morbid Appearances: The Anatomy of Pathology in the Early Nineteenth Century* (Cambridge: Cambridge University Press, 1987).

Mauss, Marcel, *The Gift* (1925; New York: Norton, 1976).

Mazumdar, Pauline M. H., 'Anatomical Physiology and the Reform of Medical Education: London 1825–1835', *Bulletin of the History of Medicine*, 57 (1983), 230–46.

Menninghaus, Winfried, *Disgust: The Theory and History of a Strong Sensation*, trans. Howard Eiland and Joel Golb (Albany: State University of New York Press, 2003).

Merriman, Nick, 'Museum Collections and Sustainability', *Cultural Trends* (2008), 3–21.

Mighall, Robert, *A Geography of Victorian Gothic Fiction: Mapping History's Nightmares* (Oxford: Oxford University Press, 1999).

Miller, William Ian, *The Anatomy of Disgust* (Cambridge, Mass.; London: Harvard University Press, 1997).

Mitchell, Michael, *Monsters: Human Freaks in America's Gilded Age* (2nd edn, Toronto: ECW, 2002).

Mohr, Peter and Jackson, Bill, 'The University of Manchester Medical School Museum: Collection of Old Instruments or Historical Archive?' *Bulletin of the John Rylands University Library of Manchester*, 87 (2005), 209–23.

Moscucci, Ornella, *The Science of Woman: British Gynaecology 1849–1890* (Cambridge: Cambridge University Press, 1990).

Moser, Stephanie, *Wondrous Curiosities: Ancient Egypt at the British Museum* (Chicago: University of Chicago Press, 2006).

Murray, David, *Museums: Their History and Their Use*, 3 vols. (Glasgow: MacLehose, 1904).

—— *The Hunterian Museum in the Old College of Glasgow* (Glasgow: Jackson, Wylie and Co., 1925).

Nochlin, Linda, *The Body in Pieces: The Fragment as a Metaphor of Modernity* (London: Thames and Hudson, 1994).

Nussbaum, Martha Craven, *Sex and Social Justice* (New York: Oxford University Press, 1999).

Nutton, Vivian and Porter, Roy (eds.), *The History of Medical Education in Britain* (Amsterdam: Rodopi, 1995).

Nys, Lisbet, 'The Public's Signatures: Visitors' Books in Nineteenth-Century Museums', *Museum History Journal*, 2 (2009), 163–80.

O'Connor, Erin, *Raw Material: Producing Pathology in Victorian Culture* (Durham, NC: Duke University Press, 2000).

Offer, Avner, 'Between the Gift and the Market: The Economy of Regard', *Economic History Review*, 50 (1997), 450–76.

Paget, James, *Memoirs and Letters of Sir James Paget*, ed. Stephen Paget (London: Longmans, Green, 1901).

Panzanelli, Roberta (ed.), *Ephemeral Bodies: Wax Sculpture and the Human Figure* (Los Angeles, Calif.: Getty Research Institute, 2008).

Park, Katharine, *Secrets of Women: Gender, Generation and the Origins of Human Dissection* (New York: Zone, 2006).

Parry, Bronwyn, *Trading the Genome: Investigating the Commodification of Bio-Information* (New York: Columbia University Press, 2004).

—— and Gere, Cathy, 'Contested Bodies: Property Models and the Commodification of Human Biological Artefacts', *Science as Culture*, 15 (2006), 139–58.

Payne, Lynda, *With Words and Knives: Learning Medical Dispassion in Early Modern England* (Aldershot: Ashgate, 2007).

Peachey, George C., *John Heaviside Surgeon* (London: St Martin's Press, 1931).

Pearce, Susan M., *On Collecting: An Investigation into Collecting in the European Tradition* (London: Routledge, 1995).

Pearson, Cathy, 'Curators, Culture and Conflict: The Effects of the Second World War on Museums in Britain, 1926–1965' (Ph.D. thesis, University College London, 2008).

Peck, Robert M., 'Alcohol and Arsenic, Pepper, and Pitch: Brief Histories of Preservation Techniques', in Sue Ann Prince (ed.), *Stuffing Birds, Pressing Plants, Shaping Knowledge: Natural History in North America, 1730–1860* (Philadelphia: American Philosophical Society, 2003), 27–53.

Petherbridge, Deanna and Jordanova, Ludmilla J. (eds.), *The Quick and the Dead: Artists and Anatomy* (London: Hayward Gallery, 1997).

Pickstone, John V., *Medicine and Industrial Society: A History of Hospital Development in Manchester and Its Region, 1752–1946* (Manchester: Manchester University Press, 1985).

—— 'Museological Science? The Place of the Analytical/Comparative in 19th-Century Science, Technology and Medicine', *History of Science*, 32 (1994), 111–38.

—— *Ways of Knowing: A New History of Science, Technology and Medicine* (Manchester: Manchester University Press, 2000).

—— 'Working Knowledges before and after *circa* 1800: Practices and Disciplines in the History of Science, Technology and Medicine', *Isis*, 98 (2007), 489–516.

Pole, Thomas, *The Anatomical Instructor; or, an Illustration of the Modern and Most Approved Methods of Preparing and Preserving the Different Parts of the Human Body* (London: Couchman and Fry, 1790).

Pomian, Krzysztof, *Collectors and Curiosities: Paris and Venice, 1500–1800*, trans. Elizabeth Wiles-Portier (Cambridge: Polity, 1990).

Prüll, Cay-Rüdiger (ed.), *Traditions of Pathology in Western Europe: Theories, Institutions and Their Cultural Setting* (Herbolzheim: Centaurus, 2003).

Pye, Elizabeth (ed.), *The Power of Touch: Handling Objects in Museum and Heritage Context* (London: UCL Institute of Archaeology, 2008).

Quigley, Christine, *The Corpse: A History* (Jefferson, NC: MacFarland, 1996).

Reay, Barry, *Watching Hannah: Sexuality, Horror and Bodily De-Formation in Victorian England* (London: Reaktion, 2002).

Reinarz, Jonathan, 'The Age of Museum Medicine: The Rise and Fall of the Medical Museum of Birmingham's School of Medicine', *Social History of Medicine*, 18 (2005), 419–37.

Rhode, Michael G. and Connor, James, 'Curating America's Army Medical Museum', in Amy Levin (ed.), *Defining Memory: Local Museums and the Construction of History in America's Changing Communities* (Lanham, Md.: AltaMira, 2007), 177–96.

Richardson, Ruth, 'A Necessary Inhumanity?' *Journal of Medical Ethics*, 26 (2000), 104–6.

—— 'A Potted History of Specimen-Taking', *The Lancet*, 11 March 2000, 935–36.

—— *Death, Dissection and the Destitute* (2nd edn, London: Phoenix, 2001).

—— *The Making of Mr. Gray's Anatomy* (Oxford: Oxford University Press, 2008).

Roach, Mary, *Stiff: The Curious Lives of Human Cadavers* (London: Viking, 2003).

Rodin, Alvin E. (ed.), *The Influence of Matthew Baillie's Morbid Anatomy: Biography, Evaluation and Reprint* (Springfied, Ill.: Charles C. Thomas, 1973).

Rosenman, Ellen Bayuk, 'Body Doubles: The Spermatorrhea Panic', *Journal of the History of Sexuality*, 12 (2003), 365–99.

Roth, Michael S., Lyons, Claire, and Merewether, Charles (eds.), *Irresistible Decay: Ruins Reclaimed* (Los Angeles: Getty Research Institute, 1997).

Rupke, Nicolaas A., *Richard Owen: Biology without Darwin* (2nd edn, Chicago: University of Chicago Press, 2009).

Sandell, Richard, Dodd, Jocelyn, and Garland-Thomson, Rosemarie (eds.), *Re-Presenting Disability: Activism and Agency in the Museum* (Abingdon: Routledge, 2010).

Sappol, Michael, *A Traffic of Dead Bodies: Anatomy and Embodied Social Identity in Nineteenth-Century America* (Princeton: Princeton University Press, 2002).

—— *Dream Anatomy* (Bethesda, Md.: National Library of Medicine, 2006).

Scheper-Hughes, Nancy, and Wacquant, Loïc J. D. (eds.), *Commodifying Bodies* (London: Sage, 2002).

Schiebinger, Londa, *The Mind Has No Sex? Women in the Origins of Modern Science* (Cambridge, Mass.: Harvard University Press, 1991) 42–82.

Schnalke, Thomas, *Diseases in Wax: The History of the Medical Moulage*, trans. Kathy Spatschek (Chicago: Quintessence, 1995).

Secord, Anne, 'Botany on a Plate: Pleasure and the Power of Pictures in Promoting Early Nineteenth-Century Scientific Knowledge', *Isis*, 93 (2002), 28–57.

Seigel, Jerrold, *The Idea of the Self: Thought and Experience in Western Europe since the Seventeenth Century* (New York: Cambridge University Press, 2005).

Sennett, Richard, *The Fall of Public Man* (Cambridge: Cambridge University Press, 1977).

Shapin, Steven, 'The Invisible Technician', *American Scientist*, 77 (1989), 554–63.

Sharp, Lesley A., 'The Commodification of the Body and Its Parts', *Annual Review of Anthropology*, 29 (2000), 287–328.

—— *Strange Harvest: Organ Transplants, Denatured Bodies, and the Transformed Self* (Berkeley: University of California Press, 2006).

—— *Bodies, Commodities, and Biotechnologies: Death, Mourning, and Scientific Desire in the Realm of Human Organ Transfer* (New York: Columbia University Press, 2007).

Sherman, Daniel J. (ed.), *Museums and Difference* (Bloomington: Indiana University Press, 2007).

Siegel, Jonah, *Desire and Excess: The Nineteenth-Century Culture of Art* (Princeton: Princeton University Press, 2000).

Simmons, Samuel Foart and Hunter, John, *William Hunter, 1718–1783: A Memoir*, ed. C. Helen Brock (1783; East Kilbride: University of Glasgow Press, 1983).

Simon, Jonathan, 'The Theatre of Anatomy: The Anatomical Preparations of Honoré Fragonard', *Eighteenth-Century Studies*, 36 (2002), 63–79.

—— 'Honoré Fragonard, Anatomical Virtuoso', in Bernadette Bensaude-Vincent and Christine Blondel (eds.), *Science and Spectacle in the European Enlightenment* (Aldershot: Ashgate, 2008), 141–58.

Smith, Charles W., *Auctions: The Social Construction of Value* (New York: Free Press, 1989).

Smith, Laurajane, 'The Repatriation of Human Remains—Problem or Opportunity?' *Antiquity*, 78 (2004), 404–13.

Smith, Mark M., *Sensing the Past: Seeing, Hearing, Smelling, Tasting, and Touching in History* (Berkeley: University of California Press, 2008).

Smith, Roger, *Being Human: Historical Knowledge and the Creation of Human Nature* (New York: Columbia University Press, 2007).

Söderqvist, Thomas, Bencarda, Adam, and Mordhorst, Camilla, 'Between Meaning Culture and Presence Effects: Contemporary Biomedical Objects as a Challenge to Museums', *Studies in History and Philosophy of Science*, 40 (2009), 431–8.

Sofaer, Joanna R., *The Body as Material Culture: A Theoretical Archaeology* (Cambridge: Cambridge University Press, 2006).

Stafford, Barbara Maria, *Artful Science: Enlightenment, Entertainment, and the Eclipse of Visual Education* (Cambridge, Mass.: MIT Press, 1994).

Stallybrass, Peter and White, Allon, *The Politics and Poetics of Transgression* (London: Methuen, 1986).

Star, Susan Leigh and Griesemer, James R., 'Institutional Ecology, "Translations" And Boundary Objects: Amateurs and Professionals in Berkeley's Museum of Vertebrate Zoology, 1907–39', *Social Studies of Science*, 19 (1989), 387–420.

Stephens, Elizabeth, 'Inventing the Bodily Interior: *Écorché* Figures in Early Modern Anatomy and Von Hagens' *Body Worlds*', *Social Semiotics*, 17 (2007), 313–26.

—— 'Venus in the Archive: Anatomical Waxworks of the Pregnant Body', *Australian Feminist Studies*, 25 (2010), 133–45.

Stewart, Susan, *On Longing: Narratives of the Miniature, the Gigantic, the Souvenir, the Collection* (Durham, NC: Duke University Press, 1993).

Strange, Julie-Marie, *Death, Grief and Poverty in Britain, 1870–1914* (Cambridge: Cambridge University Press, 2005).

Strathern, Marilyn, *The Gender of the Gift: Problems with Women and Problems with Society in Melanesia* (Berkeley: University of California Press, 1988).

Swan, Joseph, *An Account of a New Method of Making Dried Anatomical Preparations* (London: Cox, 1815).

Tansey, Violet and Mekie, D. E. C., *The Museum of the Royal College of Surgeons of Edinburgh* (Edinburgh: The Royal College of Surgeons of Edinburgh, 1982).

Taylor, Charles, *Sources of the Self: The Making of the Modern Identity* (Cambridge, Mass.: Harvard University Press, 1989).

Taylor, Shephard T., *The Diary of a Medical Student During the Mid-Victorian Period, 1860–1864* (Norwich: Jarrold, 1927).

Terry, Jennifer and Urla, Jacqueline (eds.), *Deviant Bodies: Critical Perspectives on Difference in Science and Popular Culture* (Bloomington: Indiana University Press, 1995).

Thomas, Julian, *Understanding the Neolithic* (2nd edn, London: Routledge, 1999).

Thomas, Sophie, 'Assembling History: Fragments and Ruins', *European Romantic Review*, 14 (2003), 177–86.

Thomson, Rosemarie Garland (ed.), *Freakery: Cultural Spectacles of the Extraordinary Body* (New York; London: New York University Press, 1996).

Thornton, John Leonard, 'A Diary of James Macartney (1770–1843) with Notes on His Writings', *Medical History*, 12 (1968), 164–75.

Tompsett, D. H., *Anatomical Techniques* (2nd edn, Edinburgh: Livingstone, 1970).

Tulk, Alfred and Henfrey, Arthur, *Anatomical Manipulation, or, the Methods of Pursuing Practical Investigations in Comparative Anatomy and Physiology* (London: Van Voorst, 1844).

Turk, John L., 'The Future of Pathology Collections in the United Kingdom', *Museum Management and Curatorship*, 13 (1994), 295–99.

Verdery, Katherine, *The Political Lives of Dead Bodies: Reburial and Postsocialist Change* (New York: Columbia University Press, 1999).

Vialles, Noélie, *Animal to Edible*, trans. J. A. Underwood (Cambridge: Cambridge University Press, 1994).

Waddington, Keir, 'Mayhem and Medical Students: Image, Conduct, and Control in the Victorian and Edwardian London Teaching Hospital', *Social History of Medicine*, 15 (2002), 45–64.

—— *Medical Education at St Bartholomew's Hospital, 1123–1995* (Woodbridge, Suffolk: Boydell, 2003).

Waldby, Catherine, *The Visible Human Project: Informatic Bodies and Posthuman Medicine* (London: Routledge, 2000).

—— and Mitchell, Robert, *Tissue Economies: Blood, Organs and Cell Lines in Late Capitalism* (Durham, NC: Duke University Press, 2006).

Wall, Cynthia, 'The English Auction: Narratives of Dismantlings', *Eighteenth-Century Studies*. 31 (1997), 1–25.

Warner, John Harley and Edmonson, James M., *Dissection: Photographs of a Rite of Passage in American Medicine 1880–1930* (New York: Blast, 2009).

—— and Rizzolo, Lawrence J., 'Anatomical Instruction and Training for Professionalism from the 19th to the 21st Centuries', *Clinical Anatomy*, 19 (2006), 403–14.

Weatherall, Mark, *Gentlemen, Scientists, and Doctors: Medicine at Cambridge, 1800–1940* (Woodbridge; Rochester, NY: Boydell, 2000).

Webb, Katherine A., 'The Development of the Medical Profession in Manchester 1750–1860' (Ph.D. thesis, University of Manchester, 1988).

Weiner, Annette B., *Inalienable Possessions: The Paradox of Keeping-While-Giving* (Berkeley: University of California Press, 1992).

Whitehead, Christopher, *Museums and the Construction of Disciplines: Art and Archaeology in Nineteenth-Century Britain* (London: Duckworth, 2009).

Wilkinson, Stephen, *Bodies for Sale: Ethics and Exploitation in the Human Body Trade* (London: Routledge, 2003).

Wilson, Duncan, 'Whose Body (of Opinion) Is It Anyway? Historicising Tissue Ownership and Problematising Public Opinion in Bioethics', in Barbara Katz Rothman, Elizabeth M. Armstrong, and Rebecca Tiger, (eds.) *Bioethical Issues, Sociological Perspectives* (*Advances in Medical Sociology* 9; Amsterdam: Elsevier, 2008), 9–32.

Woodward, Christopher, *In Ruins: A Journey through History, Art, and Literature* (London: Chatto and Windus, 2001).

Worboys, Michael, *Spreading Germs: Disease Theories and Medical Practice in Britain, 1865–1900* (Cambridge: Cambridge University Press, 2000).

Wordsworth, William, *The Prelude; or, the Growth of a Poet's Mind. An Autobiographical Poem* (1805; New York: Appleton, 1850).

Yanni, Carla, *Nature's Museums: Victorian Science and the Architecture of Display* (London: Athlone, 1999).

Youngquist, Paul, *Monstrosities: Bodies and British Romanticism* (Minneapolis: University of Minnesota Press, 2003).

Index